VITAMINS AND HORMONES

VOLUME 29

VITAMINS AND HORMONES

ADVANCES IN RESEARCH AND APPLICATIONS

Edited by

ROBERT S. HARRIS
University of Minnesota
Minneapolis, Minnesota

PAUL L. MUNSON
University of North Carolina
Chapel Hill, North Carolina

EGON DICZFALUSY
Karolinska Sjukhuset
Stockholm, Sweden

JOHN GLOVER
University of Liverpool
Liverpool, England

Consulting Editors

KENNETH V. THIMANN
University of California, Santa Cruz
Santa Cruz, California

IRA G. WOOL
University of Chicago
Chicago, Illinois

JOHN A. LORAINE
Medical Research Council
Edinburgh, Scotland

Volume 29
1971

ACADEMIC PRESS, New York and London

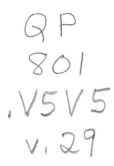

QP
801
.V5V5
v. 29

ACADEMIC PRESS, INC.
111 Fifth Avenue, New York, New York 10003

United Kingdom Edition published by
ACADEMIC PRESS, INC. (LONDON) LTD.
24/28 Oval Road, London NW1 7DD

LIBRARY OF CONGRESS CATALOG CARD NUMBER: 43-10535

PRINTED IN THE UNITED STATES OF AMERICA

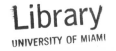

Contents

The Hypothalamic Hypophysiotropic Thyrotropin-Releasing Factor

ROGER GUILLEMIN, ROGER BURGUS, AND WYLIE VALE

The Chemistry of Parathyroid Hormone and the Calcitonins

JOHN T. POTTS, JR., HENRY T. KEUTMANN, HUGH D. NIALL, AND GEOFFREY W. TREGEAR

Protein-Polypeptide Hormones of the Human Placenta

BADRI N. SAXENA

The Biosynthesis of Vitamins E and K and Related Compounds

D. R. THRELFALL

The Excretion of Steroid Hormone Metabolites in Bile and Feces

W. TAYLOR

The Action of Thyrotropin on Thyroid Metabolism

J. E. DUMONT

Contributors to Volume 29

Numbers in parentheses indicate the pages on which the authors' contributions begin.

ROGER BURGUS, *The Salk Institute for Biological Studies, La Jolla, California* (1)

J. E. DUMONT, *Laboratory of Nuclear Medicine, School of Medicine, University of Brussels, Waterloo, Brussels, Belgium* (287)

ROGER GUILLEMIN, *The Salk Institute for Biological Studies, La Jolla, California* (1)

HENRY T. KEUTMANN, *Endocrine Unit, Massachusetts General Hospital, and Department of Medicine, Harvard Medical School, Boston, Massachusetts* (41)

HUGH D. NIALL, *Endocrine Unit, Massachusetts General Hospital, and Department of Medicine, Harvard Medical School, Boston, Massachusetts* (41)

JOHN T. POTTS, JR., *Endocrine Unit, Massachusetts General Hospital, and Department of Medicine, Harvard Medical School, Boston, Massachusetts* (41)

BADRI N. SAXENA, *Department of Medicine Firm II, Christian Medical College Hospital, Vellore-4 (Tamil Nadu), India* (95)

W. TAYLOR, *Department of Physiology, The Medical School, The University, Newcastle upon Tyne, England* (201)

D. R. THRELFALL, *Department of Biochemistry and Agricultural Biochemistry, University College of Wales, Aberystwyth, Wales* (153)

GEOFFREY W. TREGEAR, *Endocrine Unit, Massachusetts General Hospital, and Department of Medicine, Harvard Medical School, Boston, Massachusetts* (41)

WYLIE VALE, *The Salk Institute for Biological Studies, La Jolla, California* (1)

ix

Preface

The Editors take pardonable pride in presenting this, the twenty-ninth volume of *Vitamins and Hormones*.

This issue contains timely, critical reviews on the following: the hypothalamic hypophysiotropic thyrotropin-releasing factor (Guillemin, Burgus, and Vale); the chemistry of parathyroid hormone and the calcitonins (Potts, Keutmann, Niall, and Tregear); the protein-polypeptide hormones of the human placenta (Saxena); the biosynthesis of vitamins E and K (Threlfall); the excretion of steroid hormone metabolites in the bile and feces (Taylor); and the action of thyrotropin on thyroid metabolism (Dumont).

We are deeply indebted to these eleven authors in six universities and institutes located in five countries (Belgium, England, India, the United States, and Wales) for generously donating their time and sharing their wisdom in this cause.

As previously announced, Dr. John Glover, Professor of Biochemistry at the University of Liverpool, Liverpool, England, has become a co-editor of *Vitamins and Hormones* beginning with the present volume. The continuing editors heartily welcome him to the editorial board, for they realize that this competent and respected scientist will add new dimensions and strengths to their enterprise.

ROBERT S. HARRIS
PAUL L. MUNSON
EGON DICZFALUSY
JOHN GLOVER

The Hypothalamic Hypophysiotropic Thyrotropin-Releasing Factor*

ROGER GUILLEMIN, ROGER BURGUS, AND WYLIE VALE

The Salk Institute for Biological Studies, La Jolla, California

I. Introduction

To write a review on a subject that has occupied many years of one's life is almost an enjoyable proceeding if it can be done in some sort of a *post facto* manner, that is when the major questions that constituted that subject have been satisfactorily answered. Even though no question in science is ever fully answered, there are some times in the evolution of a research program when one can stop for a while and take stock of what has been accomplished. Such a point has recently been reached in the efforts of many investigators over the last 20 years at characterizing the "elusive hypothalamic hormones," with the isolation, determination of the molecular structure, and total synthesis of one of these, the thyrotropin releasing factor (TRF). This review will be essentially what its title implies. Thus there will be no attempt at framing the subject of this review with the much broader problem of the hypothalamic control of the secretion of the adenohypophysial hormones. This has been done in other reviews over the last few years (Meites and Nicoll, 1966;

*Our own studies quoted in this review have been supported over the years by research grants from the USPH, NIH AM 08290-01-06, HD 02577-01, and presently by contract No. AID/csd-2785 (AID), the Ford Foundation and the Rockefeller Foundation.

1

Guillemin, 1967; Martini and Ganong, 1967; McCann and Porter, 1969; Everett, 1969; Meites, 1970) to which the interested reader could refer.

II. Methods of Assay for TRF

At the moment there are no methods available, such as radioimmuno-assays or double isotope dilution methods, which would allow direct measurement of TRF in biological fluids; such methods will most likely become available within one to two years after the writing of this review (completed February 1971). All presently available methods for measuring TRF activity are based on bioassays *in vivo* or *in vitro* in which the end points are:

1. *In vivo:* (a) measurement of the amount of ^{125}I-labeled thyroid hormones released into peripheral blood in response to the amount of thyroid-stimulating hormone (TSH) released by the dose of TRF injected; (b) changes in plasma TSH levels in response to TRF (Ducommun *et al.*, 1965), as measured by bioassay (McKenzie, 1958) or specific radioimmunoassay (Martin and Reichlin, 1970) for rat or mouse TSH.

2. *In vitro:* measurement by subsequent bioassay or radioimmunoassay of the amount of TSH secreted by rat hemipituitaries surviving in short-term incubation.

A reference standard preparation for TRF was proposed by Guillemin and Sakiz (1965). One unit of biological TRF activity was defined as the biological activity present in 1 mg of that reference standard preparation. Pure natural TRF of ovine origin was shown later to have a specific activity of 50,000 TRF U/mg using that reference standard preparation; this figure was independent of the assay method used. Synthetic TRF (PCA-His-Pro-NH$_2$·monoacetate) has the same specific activity within the confidence limits of the assays. For reasons which do not appear to have real scientific grounds (see Schally *et al.*, 1968, p. 497), the only other group besides ours seriously engaged in the characterization of TRF never expressed its data as a function of the unit defined by us, or of any other biological unit for that matter; they used instead the concept of "minimal active dose." The concept and the use of the TRF unit with availability of highly quantitative assay methods was proved to be of major significance and interest during the isolation studies in our hands, since the results obtained were totally independent of the method of assay as long as the reference preparation was used concomitantly—a favorable set of circumstances which is never encountered when working within the concept of "minimal active dose." The use of the TRF unit and the concept of specific activity (TRF U/mg) are proving of considerable facility and use in current studies dealing with the biological activity of a large number of synthetic analogs of TRF (see Section V).

1. *In vivo* assay for TRF

a. A routine assay of moderate sensitivity but of great ease of preparation. Sensitivity of the assay, approximately 1.5 U TRF or 30 ng pure synthetic TRF.

Rats, males, 50–70 gm body weight, strain practically irrelevant, are received in the laboratory, kept on normal diet (Purina Laboratory Chow, Ralston Purina Co., St. Louis, Missouri) and tap water; the next morning they are given, by intraperitoneal injection, 4.0 μCi ^{125}I. Approximately 48 hours later they are anesthetized with ether, a sample of blood (0.2 ml) is taken from a jugular vein and the sample of TRF active material to be tested is immediately injected into the same jugular vein [0.2 ml or 0.3 ml—diluted in 1% bovine serum albumin (BSA) in physiological saline]. The rats are left to recover, and 2 hours later they are anesthetized again and another sample of blood (0.2 ml) is taken from the same or the opposite jugular vein. The two aliquots of blood are counted [γ radiation, counts per minute (cpm)] in a scintillation counter. After $\log_{10}$ transformation (of all cpm), counts of the second blood sample are adjusted by covariance to those of the first blood sample, and classical mathematics of 4- or 6-point assays are carried out with the covariance adjusted values (see Sakiz and Guillemin, 1964, for a complete description of the mathematical analysis involved—computer programs are available from several sources for carrying out these routine calculations).

This assay is highly specific for TRF. It shows no response to even large amounts of α-MSH or β-MSH (Yamazaki *et al.*, 1963b). One of its further advantages is that it is not very sensitive to TSH ($\leq$1.5 mU/rat administered as above is required to give a statistical response). One should use no fewer than five animals per point (dose) when precise statistical analysis of data are required; average $\lambda = 0.250$.

With no further treatment, the rats can usually be used once more 24 hours later for another assay; the precision of the second assay is usually not as good as that of the first.

b. A highly sensitive *in vivo* bioassay using mice.

This assay requires a longer preparation of the animals than the one above; however, it is much more sensitive (limit of sensitivity: 250 mU TRF or 5 ng synthetic TRF always gives a statistically significant response); it is not uncommon to have very sensitive animals respond in a statistically significant manner to 1 ng pure TRF or 50 mU TRF activity.

Mice, males, 15–20 gm at the time they are received in the laboratory, Swiss Albino (Taconic Farms)—probably any local strain should work just as well as long as one can rely on its consistency—are placed for 10 days on a low iodine diet (such as obtained from Nutritional Biochemicals Corp., Cleveland, Ohio), and are given distilled water to drink to increase the thyroid uptake of radioiodine. They are then injected i.p. with 4 μCi ^{125}I and simultaneously with a minimal dose of thyroxine (approximately 0.45 μg, the exact dose usually being adjusted to take account of seasonal variation in sensitivity). The animals are immediately placed in an elevated temperature environment (35°C $\pm$ 0.5°C); 48–50 hours after injection of ^{125}I and thyroxine, a sample of blood (0.2 ml) is taken from the jugular vein under ether anesthesia, the material to be tested for TRF activity is injected into the same jugular vein (0.3 ml in BSA/saline as above), and 2 hours later a second sample of blood is taken from the same or the contralateral jugular vein. The mice are preferably kept at 35°C during the entire 2-hour period. Both plasma samples are counted (γ radiation cpm); all cpm are transformed ($\log_{10}$); results are calculated as above in the assay using rats (see Sakiz and Guillemin, 1964).

All samples of TRF reference standard and unknowns are preferably diluted in 0.1% bovine serum albumin solution in physiological saline. One should use a minimum of 5 animals per point (dose) for good precision in statistical analysis; average λ for this assay = 0.18.

In all *in vivo* assays for TRF, the use of "Δ cpm", i.e., the simple arithmetic difference between γ counts in the two samples of blood obtained, as the metameter with which to perform mathematical analyses is definitely not recommended; this type of metameter is not amenable to classical parametric statistical analysis and, indeed, always yields considerable heteroscedasticity when employed. The method of choice, and the only one strictly valid even by simple statistical criteria, is that of transformation of the original data ($\log_{10}$ is the simplest and most efficient) and performance of a classical analysis of covariance between the two variables (the independent variable is first blood γ counts; and the dependent variable is second blood γ counts).

2. *In vitro* assay for TRF

The most sensitive method of assay for TRF (200 μU TRF or 40 pg pure synthetic TRF) is based on measurement of amounts of TSH released *in vitro* during short-term incubation of rat pituitary tissues.

The method is recommended only for use with highly purified preparations (adding ≤ 1 μg/ml incubation fluid); it is not recommended as a routine technique to follow a purification procedure as spurious results may be obtained with crude materials or plasma extracts (see Guillemin and Vale, 1970, for a complete description of the limitations of these *in vitro* methods). TSH secreted into the incubation fluid is then measured by a radioimmunoassay or by the bioassay for TSH (McKenzie, 1958; Sakiz and Guillemin, 1964).

For this method, the preferred routine protocol presently used in this laboratory (see Guillemin and Vale, 1970) is as follows: Use 3 paired hemipituitaries from 100 gm body weight male rats per beaker (Teflon, 10 ml capacity) in 2.0 ml TC 199 incubation fluid. "Preincubate" (37°C for 30 minutes) in a metabolic shaker in an atmosphere of 95% O_2-5% CO_2; remove and discard the preincubation fluids by suction. Add fresh medium as above with the material to be tested (for TRF activity) in less than 50 μl; incubate for 30 minutes; remove both incubation fluids; add to the control fluid the same quantity of the material to be tested that had been added to the experimental beaker at the beginning of the incubation (cross-treatment). Fluids can be frozen for subsequent assay for TSH as above.

Potency ratios are calculated by classical factorial analysis of 4-point assays between experimental/control fluids; 10^{-10} to $10^{-8} M$ synthetic or natural TRF give TSH-potency ratios ranging from 2.0 to as high as 7–10.

III. Purification, Isolation, Characterization of TRF

Despite earlier claims based on questionable methodology and which proved to be wrong regarding conclusions as to the chemical characterization of TRF but which turned out also to be (unwittingly) correct in much of their physiological conclusions (what we term in this laboratory "the prophetic literature"), the first incontrovertible evidence for the existence and early purification of a hypothalamic TSH-releasing factor (TRF) appeared in 1962 (Guillemin *et al.*, 1962). A 2 N acetic acid extract of several hundred sheep hypothalamic fragments was filtered on Sephadex G-25, and in the bioassay animals (Yamazaki *et al.*, 1963a) two zones of activity were found in the effluent. One corresponded to non-retarded materials and was active in hypophysectomized as well as intact animals, thus showing that these were substances with TSH-like activity present in the hypothalamic extract. The other zone, which was strongly retarded on the gel (elution volume similar to that of α-MSH, preceding that of arginine-vasopressin), was active in the assay animals with an intact pituitary, and its biological activity (release of TSH) was inhibited by pretreatment with thyroxine. Furthermore, it stimulated secretion of TSH *in vitro* when added directly to incubated fragments of rat pituitary tissues. The conclusion was drawn that the material so purified corresponded to the then hypothetical TRF of hypothalamic origin. The biological activity of this crude preparation was resistant to heating and to incubation with trypsin but was destroyed during incubation with pepsin (Jutisz *et al.*, 1963a) or by 6 *N* HCl hydrolysis (110°C, 24 hours). The material having TRF activity, obtained from gel filtration, considered to be polypeptide in nature, was rapidly further purified by ion exchange chromatography on carboxymethylcellulose (CMC) (Jutisz *et al.*, 1963b).

These early observations were amply confirmed by subsequent investigators using extracts of the hypothalamus of sheep, pig, beef, rats, guinea pigs, mice, rabbits, and fragments of human brain origin (reviews in Guillemin, 1964, 1967; Schally *et al.*, 1968; McCann and Porter, 1969).

Guillemin *et al.* later reported (1965) purification of ovine TRF from 2 *N* acetic acid extracts of acetone powder from 80,000 sheep hypothalamic fragments by gel filtration, countercurrent distribution (CCD), ion-exchange chromatography on IRC-50, and finally thin-layer chromatography (TLC), obtaining 400 μg of material active at approximately 100 ng/dose *in vivo*. TRF activity was found in a ninhydrin-positive, Pauly-positive zone on TLC; amino acid composition after 6 *N* HCl hydrolysis was Lys, His 4, Thr, Ser, Glu 3, Pro 3, Gly, Ala, Met, Leu, Tyr. However, a final quantitative analysis was not claimed because of the small quantities of peptide available, and it was noted that a much larger quantity of brain fragments would be needed in order to approach the amino acid sequence.

Partial purification of bovine TRF was described by Schally *et al.* (1966a, 1968) and by Tsuji *et al.* (1968); bovine TRF showed properties similar to those of ovine TRF on gel-filtration and CMC chromatography (Schally *et al.*, 1966a, 1968) and was reported to be retarded by Sephadex G-50 and DEAE-cellulose (Tsuji *et al.*, 1968).

In a sequence of purification reported by Schally *et al.* (1966b), which included gel-filtration of 2 *N* acetic acid-glacial acetic acid extracts of 20,000 lyophilized hypothalami, phenol extraction, CMC chromatography and CCD, porcine TRF showed properties similar or identical to those obtained for bovine and ovine TRF. Free-flow electrophoresis of this material yielded 900 μg of a TRF reported to be active at 10 ng *in vivo* and 0.1 ng *in vitro*, which on hydrolysis gave the amino acid analysis: Gly 1, His 5, Pro 5, Thr 6, Leu 0.5, Ser 0.6, and Lys 0.4. After a private communication from our laboratory, Schally later revised this amino acid analysis to Glu 6 instead of Thr 6.

By that time (1966) it had become obvious (Guillemin, 1964) that huge quantities of hypothalamic tissue would have to be procured and processed in order to obtain sufficient amounts of any of the releasing factors before meaningful chemical studies could be performed. There was rather slow progress in the elucidation of the structure of TRF during the next 3 to 4 years; during this time two independent laboratories organized the logistics of collecting and extracting large quantities of hypothalamic fragments—Schally and co-workers working primarily with porcine TRF and Guillemin and co-workers working with ovine TRF. During this period, a number of preliminary reports appeared from both laboratories reporting progress and tribulations in the development of purification schemes and observations on the chemical nature of TRF (Schally *et al.*, 1966a, 1968, 1969; Guillemin *et al.*, 1964, 1968, 1970; Burgus *et al.*, 1966a,b; Burgus and Guillemin, 1967; Guillemin, 1968), describing the processing of about ¾ million ovine hypothalamic fragments and approximately ¼ million porcine hypothalamic fragments. Schally *et al.* (1968) summarized at the 1967 Laurentian Hormone Conference, and more recently with some additional data (1969), their latest purification scheme for porcine TRF, and Burgus and Guillemin (1970) presented their most recent purification sequence for ovine TRF in early 1969. Although there were some differences in the final versions of extraction methods and the order of application of certain purification steps, the final schemes utilized by the two laboratories were essentially identical in several purification steps and very similar in others.

Schally *et al.* (1966c, 1968) described the purification of TRF from 100,000 porcine hypothalami according to the sequence that they had previously published (1966b), with an additional partition chromatography stage, recording a yield of 2.8 mg TRF, reported to be active at doses <1 ng *in vivo*. This material, which was judged to be homogeneous by TLC and thin-layer electrophoresis (TLE) contained the amino acids Glu, His, Pro in essentially equimolar ratio, accounting for 30% of the weight of the preparation. It was later subjected to additional stages of partition chromatography, adsorption chromatography on charcoal, analytical gel-filtration, and finally paper chromatography (Schally *et al.*, 1969). No change in the amino acid content or specific biological activity was reported. Another batch of 165,000 porcine hypothalamic fragments was purified by the same scheme, producing essentially an identical material with a slightly higher amino acid content (33.6%), with a reported total yield from 265,000 hypothalami of 7.2 mg "pure TRF."

The final scheme for purification of ovine TRF described by Burgus and Guillemin (1970) utilized an organic solvent extraction; the extract was then further purified by ultrafiltration through an ion-exchange membrane, gel-filtration, partition chromatography, adsorption chromatography on charcoal, and finally partition chromatography in a second system. Each of the chromatographic steps was repeated before proceeding to the next step.

The alcohol-chloroform extraction procedure, including a glacial acetic acid-ether precipitation step as in the Kamm procedure (Kamm et al., 1928), had the advantage over procedures used previously in that a considerable weight reduction was achieved in a batch process; together with the ultrafiltration step it yielded a material of a sufficiently high specific activity so that the extract from over a quarter of a million hypothalamic fragments could be applied to a single preparative column (15 by 150 cm) for gel filtration, whereas 20–25 columns of this size would have been required otherwise (Guillemin et al., 1965, 1968; Schally et al., 1966c). However, these two steps introduced some difficulties, which arose from some rather interesting properties of the crude materials. The solvent extraction procedure yielded a TRF-active material which was not as firmly bound to CM-Sephadex as material derived from 2 N acetic acid extraction and gel filtration (Guillemin, 1968; Guillemin et al., 1968; Burgus et al., 1966b; Burgus and Guillemin, 1967). It was also observed that the TRF activity which passed through the ultrafiltration membrane was not retarded to the same extent as the original extract on refiltration; the same observation appeared to hold true for material which had passed unadsorbed through the CM-Sephadex columns. These were the first observations that indicated that the molecular weight of TRF could be much below 1000. Second, it is tempting to speculate that the apparent changes in behavior observed in the early stages of purification of the hypothalamic factor may have resulted from binding of the low molecular weight materials to a larger molecule whose size and/or charge governed the behavior of the complex—an observation that may have significance for the purification of other hypothalamic-releasing factors. Such a hypothesis would also explain the retention of TRF on anion exchange columns observed by Tsuji et al. (1968), an observation that is not consistent with the structure of isolated TRF (see below) since the molecule has no free anionic groups.

The yield from 270,000 sheep hypothalamic fragments was 1 mg of TRF having a biological activity of 57,000 ± 9900 TRF U/mg (see Guillemin and Sakiz, 1965, for a definition of the TRF unit) and which was active at ≤15 ng in vivo in the mouse assay described by Redding et al. (1966) and less than 0.1 ng in vitro (see Guillemin and Vale, 1970). Although the last steps of purification of ovine TRF indicated a constant specific biological activity by statistical criteria and the material appeared to be homogeneous as assessed by TLC in 4 different systems at 5-μg loads using a variety of visualization tests, we did not claim "isolation" or homogeneity of the material at that time because of the difficulties of proving this point without wasting precious supplies; we pointed out that, as proof of homogeneity, such simple methods as multiple TLC should be considered with caution—a view that we were happy to see shared later by others working in the field (Folkers et al., 1969; Bøler et al., 1969).

Total recovery of ovine TRF in terms of units of biological activity based on 4-point bioassays was about 20% for nine steps of purification (about 85% average recovery per step). Schally et al. (1969) claimed a recovery of porcine TRF of over 90% during each purification step for eleven steps of purification (theoretical overall recovery at 90% per step is calculated to be about 30% for 11 steps); however, it is unclear upon what these figures were based: if we calculate total number of minimal effective doses in vivo based on the weights, and the minimal effective dose reported for porcine TRF at each step, there appears to be a fluctuation between two million to 18 million total doses throughout the purification scheme with an overall recovery of 115%.

For some time it had been open to question whether ovine TRF was a simple (homomeric) polypeptide; the low content of amino acids (5–8%) in HCl hydrolyzates of ovine TRF preparations which had been carried through several purification steps and were apparently homogeneous in TLC and TLE with a variety of visualization tests, together with the observation that amino acids did not appear to concentrate during the last few stages of purification (Guillemin et al., 1968) had led us to question the long-held hypothesis that TRF was a simple polypeptide. Subsequent observations that pepsin, trypsin, pronase, carboxypeptidase A and B, and leucineaminopeptidase failed to inactivate TRF (Burgus et al., 1966a), that the biological activity always accompanied a Pauly-positive, but ninhydrin-negative zone on TLC or TLE, that dansylation followed by two dimensional chromatoelectrophoresis gave no evidence of free amino groups, and finally that an apparently constant specific biological activity was maintained in the last stages of purification (Burgus et al., 1966b; Burgus and Guillemin, 1967) did nothing to shake this hypothesis. However, IR and high resolution NMR spectra suggested an alicyclic or heterocyclic structure and were still compatible with a polypeptide (Guillemin, 1967; Burgus et al., 1966b; Burgus and Guillemin, 1967).

Schally et al. made similar observations regarding the nature of porcine TRF (Schally et al., 1968, 1966c), finding that all the enzymes that had been tested for ovine TRF (Burgus et al., 1966a), plus papain, subtilisin, and Nagarse, failed to inactivate porcine TRF (Schally et al., 1969). Porcine TRF activity was also associated with a ninhydrin-negative, Pauly-positive zone in all chromatographic and electrophoretic systems tested (Schally *et al.*, 1966c, 1968, 1969). Schally *et al.* thus concluded that their results were consistent with the hypothesis that TRF was not a simple polypeptide; however, the material which they considered to be homogeneous consistently yielded approximately 30% total amino acid content as Glu, His, and Pro in equimolar ratio. They reasoned that these three amino acids were part of the TRF molecule since on TLC or TLE, TRF activity was always associated with a Pauly-positive zone which yielded the three amino acids on hydrolysis; moreover, they observed that treatment of porcine TRF with Pauly reagent (Schally *et al.*, 1966c, 1968, 1969) or *N*-bromosuccinimide (Schally *et al.*, 1968, 1969) resulted in loss of biological activity. [The loss of biological activity of ovine TRF after treatment with Pauly reagent in solution (Guillemin, 1968; Burgus and Guillemin, 1970) had also been observed.] Schally *et al.* (1968, 1969) further observed that 8 synthetic tripeptides containing Glu, His, Pro or Gln in equimolar ratios were inactive in doses up to 10,000 times greater than those of natural porcine TRF and thus concluded that the "nonpeptide moiety which formed up to 70% of the TRF molecule was necessary for biological activity."

In January 1969, with the new supply of highly purified ovine TRF available (Burgus and Guillemin, 1970), amino acid analysis of 6 N HCl hydrolyzates of this preparation revealed only the amino acids Glu, His, and Pro, which occurred in exactly equimolar ratios and accounted for 81% of the preparation (theoretical contribution of His, Pro, and Glu for a tripeptide monoacetate calculates to 86%). Furthermore the ultraviolet (UV), infrared (IR), and nuclear magnetic resonance (NMR) spectra obtained with that preparation of TRF were consistent with those of a polypeptide and upon close examination most of the characteristics of those spectra could be accounted for by the structural features of the amino acids found in the hydrolyzates of TRF. Moreover, the solubility properties and the lack of volatility observed in attempts to obtain mass spectra or to perform gas chromatography (Burgus *et al.* 1966b; Burgus and Guillemin, 1967; Guillemin, 1968), as well as other analytical data, were consistent with those of a polypeptide; also, the lack of effect of proteolytic enzymes could be related to the particular amino acids observed. With the analyses of the more highly purified material unmistakably showing a significant contribution of amino acids to the total weight of the preparation, the hypothesis that TRF could not be a simple polypeptide was therefore abandoned in favor of the possibility that TRF might be a cyclic or a protected peptide, a view compatible with the failure to detect an N-terminus (Schally *et al.*, 1966c, 1968, 1969; Burgus *et al.*, 1966b; Burgus and Guillemin,

1967, 1970; Guillemin, 1968) or a C-terminus (Schally *et al.*, 1969; Burgus and Guillemin, 1970) as well as the resistance of the biological activity to proteases.

The knowledge that the amino acids His, Pro, and Glu not only occurred in equimolar ratio in porcine and ovine TRF but indeed accounted for almost the theoretical total weight of the molecule in the case of ovine TRF, along with the previous knowledge of a lack of an N-terminal amino acid, led us to reexamine derivatives of polypeptides containing equimolar ratios of these amino acids to serve at least as possible models for the methodology to be used in the characterization of ovine TRF. Burgus *et al.* (1969c) tested for TRF activity 6 tripeptide isomers containing L-His, L-Pro, and L-Glu synthesized by Gillessen *et al.* (1970) (containing only the peptides involving the α-carboxyl group of glutamic acid). The tripeptides proved to be devoid of TRF activity, confirming the earlier results of Schally *et al.* (1968, 1969). However, following treatment of each of the six tripeptides by acetic anhydride in an effort to protect the N-terminus as in natural TRF, the acetylation mixture from one, and only one of the peptides, namely H-Glu-His-Pro-OH, showed biological activity qualitatively indistinguishable from that of natural TRF. It was active in *in vivo* and in *in vitro* assays specific for TRF and its action *in vivo* was blocked by prior injection of the animals with thyroxine. The same preparation had no luteinizing hormone-releasing factor (LRF) activity (Burgus *et al.*, 1969c). The specific activity of the material obtained (15 TRF U/mg) was lower than that of purified natural TRF, and preliminary experiments with TLC of the acetylation mixture of Glu-His-Pro demonstrated several zones, Pauly-positive or negative, having TRF activity. The nature of several possible reaction products was considered: mono- or diacetyl- derivatives, polymers of Glu-His-Pro, and cyclic peptide derivatives or derivatives containing pyroglutamic acid (PCA) as the N-terminus. Subsequently we reported (Burgus *et al.*, 1969a) that the major product, by weight, of this procedure was indeed PCA-His-Pro-OH. The material was isolated from the reaction mixture and its structure was confirmed by mass spectrometry of the methyl ester and by its identity to authentic PCA-His-Pro-OH (Gillessen *et al.*, 1970) on TLC, the IR spectrum as well as similarity of specific biological activity *in vivo* (7–15 TRF U/mg). This represented the first demonstration of a fully characterized synthetic molecule, based on the known composition of natural TRF, to reproduce the biological activity of a releasing factor.

Several other products present in the acetylation mixture, some possibly having higher specific activity than PCA-His-Pro-OH, were not characterized. It is of interest that acetyl-Glu-His-Pro-OH obtained by total synthesis (Gillessen *et al.*, 1970) was devoid of TRF activity in the *in vivo* assay at doses up to 250 μg (Burgus *et al.*, 1969a).

Because of the differences between the specific biological activities of PCA-His-Pro-OH and natural ovine TRF and the different behavior of these two compounds in various chromatographic systems, it was evident that TRF was not PCA-His-Pro-OH as such. It was thought that a likely candidate for the structure of the natural material would be PCA-His-Pro-NH₂ and its synthesis was approached through the simple procedure of methanolysis of the methyl ester, PCA-His-Pro-OMe (Burgus *et al.*, 1969a, 1970a,b). The ester, prepared by treatment of the pure synthetic PCA-His-Pro-OH with methanolic HCl, was purified by partition chromatography and identified as PCA-His-Pro-OMe, on the basis of its behavior on TLC, its IR spectrum, and by mass spectrometry (Burgus *et al.*, 1970a,b). It had biological activity *in vivo* (28,600 ± 6700 TRF U/mg) approaching half of the specific activity of isolated ovine TRF (57,000 ± 9900 TRF U/mg); the compound was active *in vivo* at ≥10 ng (Burgus *et al.*, 1970a,b) and *in vitro* at 1.0 ng. Ammonolysis of the methyl ester in methanol produced a material which upon partition chromatography gave a small yield of a substance presumably PCA-His-Pro-NH₂, occurring in a Pauly-positive zone separated from the starting material, which had a higher specific activity *in vivo* (44,000 ± 1000 TRF U/mg) with a minimal active dose *in vivo* at ≤5 ng/animal, and *in vitro* at ≤1.0 ng. The properties of PCA-His-Pro-OMe and PCA-His-Pro-NH₂ were compared to the totally synthetic compounds (see also Gillessen *et al.*, 1970), PCA-His-Pro-OH and PCA-His-Pro-NH₂. Among the derivatives tested, the properties of ovine TRF most closely matched that of the amide, failing to separate from the synthetic compound in four different systems of TLC when run in mixtures. The IR spectra of several of the more highly purified preparations of the amide, including PCA-His-Pro-NH₂ prepared by total synthesis, were almost identical to that of ovine TRF, showing only minor differences in two regions of the spectra. The nitrogen analysis as obtained earlier by Dohrmann's method (Burgus and Guillemin, 1970) on the highly purified ovine TRF was judged to be open to question, since errors in handling of small samples in this method would not allow a clear distinction between a tripeptide and its amide. These new observations, together with the demonstration that the specific activity of the PCA-His-Pro-NH₂ was not statistically different from that of natural ovine TRF, led us to reconsider (Burgus *et al.*, 1970a) our earlier hypothesis (Burgus *et al.*, 1969a) that ovine TRF may have a secondary or tertiary amide on the C-terminal proline, rather than correspond to the primary amide of the tripeptide PCA-His-Pro.

Subsequently, Folkers *et al.* (1969) and Bowers *et al.* (1969a) reported that they had demonstrated biological activity in a mixture of derivatives of a synthetic peptide H-Glu-His-Pro-OH. The synthetic preparation, judged to be not over 80% pure, was treated in a manner very similar to that previously described by Burgus *et al.* (1969a), i.e., ammonolysis of the methyl ester, with the exception that the ammonolysis was carried out at a lower temperature. These conditions would be expected to produce both PCA- and the amide derivative; the material obtained, called "preparation A" was ninhydrin-negative and Pauly-positive, indicating that closure of Glu to PCA had indeed occurred. Samples of "preparation A" were subjected directly to biological tests without purification; doses of 6–54 ng were claimed to be active *in vivo*, 2–18 ng of porcine TRF giving similar responses (Folkers *et al.*, 1969; Bowers *et al.*, 1969b). The activity of the synthetic reaction mixture appeared to be inhibited by triiodothyronine and by incubation with human plasma in agreement with the results obtained by Burgus *et al.* (1969a). The reported lack of response by oral administration (Folkers *et al.*, 1969; Bowers *et al.*, 1969a) was in disagreement with the results of Vale *et al.* (1970) using pure tripeptide-OMe or amide, which showed activity at <1 μg/dose. Probably, the doses administered by Folkers *et al.* (1969) and Bowers *et al.* (1969a) of the crude material were too low to give a response; indeed Bowers *et al.* later (1970b) reported oral activity of PCA-His-Pro-NH$_2$ at doses essentially similar to those used by us. Similar reactions carried out by Folkers *et al.* (1969) on the derivatives Glu-Pro-His, Pro-His-Gln, Pro-His-Glu, gave no TRF activity, confirming the results obtained with acetylation mixtures of the various tripeptides (Burgus, 1969c) and in accord with the sequence "Glu-His-Pro" for porcine TRF, reported by Schally *et al.* (1969, see addendum). "Preparation A" was not subjected to any form of purification, which is unfortunate since the yield of amide prepared according to this procedure might be expected to be low and the methyl ester, PCA-His-Pro-OMe, may have been the major component of the mixture (Burgus *et al.*, 1969a, 1970). Moreover, the specific biological activity of the methyl ester being about half that of PCA-His-Pro-NH$_2$ (Burgus *et al.*, 1970a), the bioassay used by Bowers *et al.* may not have allowed Folkers *et al.* to distinguish between the methyl ester or the amide in their "preparation A" on the basis of biological activity.

Shortly after the publication of these preliminary communications, evidence was presented (Burgus *et al.*, 1969b), based primarily on low and high resolution mass spectrometry, that the ovine TRF preparation originally obtained (Burgus and Guillemin, 1970) was essentially homogeneous and had the structure PCA-His-Pro-NH$_2$. Both synthetic PCA-

His-Pro-NH$_2$ (Burgus et al., 1969a, 1970a) and highly purified ovine
TRF (Burgus and Guillemin, 1970) were introduced by direct probe into
a low resolution mass spectrometer after treatment with diazomethane
or trifluoroacetic anhydride-trifluoroacetic acid to give the methyl or
trifluoroacetyl (TFA) derivatives, respectively. All preparations gave
volatile materials in the temperature range of 150–200°C ($\leq 10^{-6}$ torr).
Several mass spectra taken throughout the range of the thermal gradient
(7 in the case of ovine TRF derivatives) showed fragmentation patterns
corresponding to a single component. Although none of the spectra revealed a molecular ion, fragments arising from the structures PCA,
methyl-PCA, His, methyl-His, Pro, Pro-NH$_2$, CONH$_2$, PCA-His, and
His-Pro-NH$_2$ were observed. The low-resolution mass spectra of the corresponding derivatives of synthetic PCA-His-Pro-NH$_2$ and TRF were
essentially identical. Fragments arising from unsubstituted PCA or His
were observed in the spectra of both types of derivatives.

The elemental composition of all the fragments, except m/e 221, the
intensity of which was too weak for it to be observed on the photoplate
used, were confirmed by high resolution mass spectroscopy of the methyl
derivatives. The methyl derivatives of natural TRF, as well as of PCA-
His-Pro-NH$_2$, presented a rather interesting problem in the interpretation
of the mass spectra. Since no molecular ion was present, the proof of the
sequence of the tripeptides required presence of ions unique to the
PCA-His and the His-Pro-NH$_2$ sequences. However, as an examination of
the structure will show, a form of symmetry about the α-carbon atom of
His exists such that the combinations of methylated or unmethylated
fragments of either dipeptide would produce fragments of the same
nominal masses and in some cases the same elemental compositions. Thus
the fragments m/e 234, 235, 248, and 249 could arise from PCA-His-Pro-
NH$_2$, or as another combination, as Schally et al. had previously reported
for porcine TRF (1968, 1969), the diketopiperazine of His,Pro. The
strength of high resolution mass spectroscopy as a tool is illustrated by
the fact that the nominal mass m/e 248 was shown by exact mass measurement to have the elemental composition $C_{11}H_{14}N_5O_2$, which distin-
guishes it as arising from His-Pro-NH$_2$ (-2H) resulting from a cleavage
between the α-carboxyl carbon of PCA and the α-amino group of His.
This fragment, together with others, such as PCA-His, m/e 221, considered with the qualitative identity of the mass spectra of the two types
of derivatives of ovine TRF with those of the synthetic material, establishes the structure of ovine TRF as PCA-His-Pro-NH$_2$.

More evidence confirms this structure. We have now repeatedly observed the molecular ions of ovine TRF ($m/e = 361$) in mass spectrometry by the use of chemical ionization probes or modified electron
impact probes. Chromatographic analysis of the hydrolyzate of ovine

TRF showed no basis constituents other than His separating from the ammonia peak (Burgus *et al.*, 1969b). The amino acid analysis of 6 N HCl hydroiyzates of ovine TRF corrected for contamination by ammonia in the reagents and atmospheric sources gave essentially a 1:1 ratio of ammonia to His; in the same series of experiments, methylamine, ethylamine, and dimethylamine could be distinguished from the ammonia peak on the basis of their retention values. The presence of both methylated and unsubstituted PCA and His in the diazomethane-treated materials provides strong evidence that the α-amino group in PCA and the imidazole nitrogen of His are unsubstituted in the isolated TRF. The positive Pauly reaction had already essentially ruled out substitution of the imidazole group (see also Bøler *et al.*, 1969). Furthermore, the NMR spectrum of ovine TRF (obtained by time averaging in D_2O) is essentially identical to that of synthetic PCA-His-Pro-NH$_2$.

In addition, a pyroglutamyl peptidase isolated by Fellows *et al.* (1971) destroys the biological activity of ovine TRF. The enzyme appears to be specific for the cleavage of PCA from PCA-terminal peptides and releases a similar fragment, presumably His-Pro-NH$_2$, from both TRF and synthetic PCA-His-Pro-NH$_2$, as determined by TLC (Pauly reagent) and by the dansyl method (Burgus *et al.*, 1970a).

Therefore, the structure of ovine TRF as *isolated* from the hypothalamus has been established as PCA-His-Pro-NH$_2$. However, we did point out (Burgus *et al.*, 1969b) that the possibility was not excluded that, as opposed to the isolated material, the *native* molecule of TRF may occur as Gln-His-Pro-NH$_2$ either free or conjugated to another structure such as a protein, which would not be necessary for biological activity *in vivo* or *in vitro;* there are such precedents in the chemistry of the eledoisins (Schröder and Lubke, 1966).

Bøler *et al.* (1969) compared the properties of porcine TRF with those of a synthetic preparation which they claimed to be characterized as PCA-His-Pro-NH$_2$ by "its hydrolysis to the 3 amino acids," its NMR spectrum, and by paper and thin-layer chromatography employing 17 different systems of solvent and adsorbents using Pauly reagent for visualization. The authors refer only to their "preparation A" as in Folkers *et al.* (1969) and no details of purification of that mixture were given; it would appear that the data presented were inadequate to distinguish PCA-His-Pro-NH$_2$ from other constituents in the mixture such as Glu-His-Pro, PCA-His-Pro-OH, PCA-His-Pro-OMe, and up to 20% impurities in the starting material.

In several subsequent reports, porcine TRF, prepared as described by Schally *et al.* (1969), was acknowledged to contain 50–70% impurities by weight including what appeared to be myristoleic acid and dioctylphthalate, and therefore was judged to have been 30–50% pure. Mass spectra were obtained and reported although neither the natural nor the synthetic product showed a molecular ion in mass spectrometry. The synthetic "preparation A" as well as a sample of PCA-His-Pro-NH$_2$ synthesized by Flouret (Abbott Laboratories) and the natural product were reported to have essentially identical R_f values (Pauly color) in the 17 chromatographic systems; data were presented representing graded responses of biological activity *in vivo* over a dose range of 1–18 ng/dose with no significant difference between responses of the natural or synthetic products. Possibilities of structures other than PCA-His-Pro-NH$_2$ for TRF were considered, including substitution of the PCA or a Gln residue by hydrolyzable groups on the nitrogen atom, or modification of the Pro-NH$_2$ groups, in other words as in a secondary or tertiary amide group. The possibility of substitution of the imidazole ring of His was ruled out because of the positive Pauly reaction. It was further reasoned (Bøler *et al.*, 1969) that "any structural modification of (Pyro)Glu-His-Pro-(NH$_2$) would necessitate another compound having identical R_f

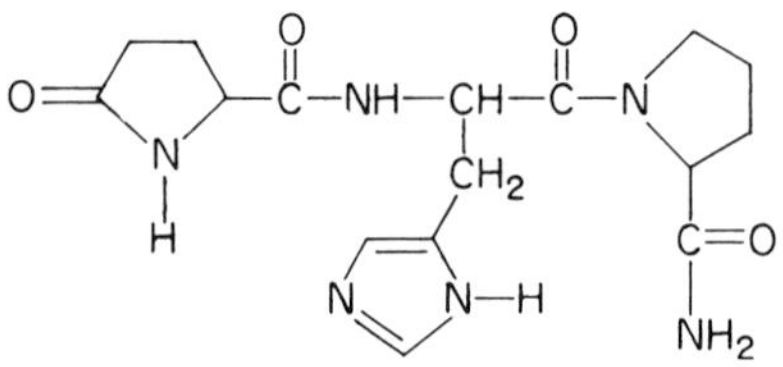

Fig. 1. Structure of the hypothalamic thyrotropin-releasing factor (PCA-His-Pro-NH$_2$) of ovine or porcine origin.

values to those of (Pyro)Glu-His-Pro-(NH$_2$) in all seventeen [chromatographic] systems" and that a "certain lack of structural specificity and potency [would have to exist] for the hormonal activity of TRH." On the basis of the mass spectrometric data, IR, NMR spectroscopy and all the above observations, Nair *et al.* (1970) finally concluded that porcine TRF had indeed the structure PCA-His-Pro-NH$_2$.

It is most interesting that TRF from two widely different species of mammals should have the same structure (Fig. 1) and apparently the same specific (biological) activity in similar assays; as we shall see below, TRF shows no evidence of species specificity for its biological actions, PCA-His-Pro-NH$_2$ being readily active in humans.

IV. METHODS OF CHEMICAL SYNTHESIS OF TRF

We have reported in some detail above (Section III) how our laboratory originally synthesized the first TRF-active molecules of known chemical composition by treatment with acetic anhydride of a series of tripeptide isomers containing equimolar ratios of the amino acids Glu, His, Pro; also how we synthesized what turned out to be the actual structure of TRF by first making the methyl ester of the tripeptide PCA-His-Pro-OH, producing PCA-His-Pro-NH$_2$ by ammonolysis of the tripeptide methyl ester (Burgus et al., 1969a,b). An essentially similar methodology was later used by (Folkers et al., 1969). The first complete de novo synthesis of the structure PCA-His-Pro-NH$_2$ was accomplished and reported by Gillessen et al. (1970). The method of Gillessen et al. has essentially been duplicated in our own laboratory on a relatively large scale, replacing the last stage of purification of the synthetic product by ion exchange on diethylaminoethyl-cellulose instead of the countercurrent distribution system used by Gillessen et al. We have thus synthesized TRF in quantities of more than 5 gm of the final pure product. In the method of Gillessen et al., the synthesis of TRF is effected by the successive coupling of carbobenzoxy-PCA to His-OCH$_3$ by dicyclohexyl-carbodiimide and the resulting deprotected dipeptide, by the azide method to Pro-NH$_2$.

Flouret (1970) has recently reported a method of synthesis of TRF based on the coupling of pentachlorophenylpyroglutamate with histidyl-proline amide. The dipeptide in this case was made by condensation of t-butyloxycarbonylhistidine with prolineamide mediated by dicyclo-hexylcarbodiimide, removal of the t-butyloxycarbonyl group by HCl and treatment of the peptide hydrochloride with a basic ion-exchange resin.

In the same report, Flouret also presented a method of solid phase synthesis using the BOC-amino acid derivatives, the final tripeptide being released from the resin as the amide by treatment with NH$_3$/MeOH-dimethylformamide (DMF) at 0°C for 24 hours. Two other methods of solid phase synthesis of TRF have recently been reported by Baugh et al. (1970) and Rivaille and Milhaud (1971). In our own laboratory, several methods of solid-phase synthesis of TRF have been devised and successfully utilized. The most convenient of these for the synthesis of TRF as well as TRF analogs is carried out on a benzhydrylamine-resin support as developed by Pietta and Marshall (1970). N^α-t-butyloxycarbonyl amino acids have been used exclusively here except for pyroglutamic acid. In the latter case, both the unprotected and the N^α-benzyloxy-carbonyl derivative were used. In the case of histidine, the N^α-butyloxy-carbonyl im-p-toluenesulfonyl derivative was utilized. Usually one or two couplings with dicyclohexylcarbodiimide (DCC) are sufficient to bring about complete coupling. The final product is removed from the resin by treatment with double-distilled anhydrous hydrogen fluoride

(Monahan, 1971). In most cases, the resulting peptides have been found to be homogeneous on several TLC systems.

Dunn (1971) synthesized TRF by a variation of an active ester synthesis. Dicarbobenzoxyhistidine was coupled by DCC to proline p-nitrophenyl ester. The α-Z group was removed with HBr in dioxane and the resulting dipeptide, after neutralization *in situ* with N-methyl-morpholine, was coupled with DCC to Z-PCA. Removal of the N-terminal Z group with HBr in dioxane followed by reaction with ammonia in methanol yielded TRF. However, poor yields during the neutralization and second coupling step, make it not a synthesis of choice.

It is our experience that the "classical" method of synthesis is the method of choice for obtaining large to very large quantities of TRF (5 gm or more); the Merrifield method can yield very rapidly, in a matter of hours, or at most a couple of days, up to a few hundred milligrams of biologically active product; in some cases, more time is spent on the purification of the final product to obtain it in homogeneous form than on its actual synthesis by the solid phase method. Use of the benzhydryl-amine-resin, which allows the direct cleavage of the peptide as the amide, is a considerable improvement on the early methods of solid phase synthesis used by us or others to synthesize TRF.

V. Synthetic Analogs of TRF and Their Biological Activity

A molecule as relatively simple as that of TRF with such high specific activity as well as such high specificity of action is obviously a model of choice for the synthesis of a series of analogs that would allow the study of relationships between specific changes in the molecular structure and modifications of biological activity, including the possibility of obtaining antagonists to TRF. Indeed, at the time of writing this review, only a few months after the elucidation of the structure of TRF, nearly 50 analogs of TRF have already been prepared by total synthesis and studied for their biological activity. For the sake of simplicity, developed structures of these various peptides will not be shown here. For the same reason, they will be grouped into simple categories corresponding to substitutions on or of each of the three amino acids of the molecule of TRF. It should be borne in mind that the overall biological activity of any given analog is affected by several different factors, such as excretion and degradation rates, and transport to the "molecular site of action" as well as the performance of the analog at that site. Therefore, conclusions to be drawn in comparing the various analogs are subject to limitations until all these factors can be identified and controlled (see·also section on mechanisms of action) (see Table I).

Most of these analogs show little or no biological activity, indicating that the changes in the molecule have been too drastic. TRF can be considered a neutral or weakly basic compound since its N-terminus is blocked by internal cyclization into PCA and its C-terminus is an amide. Formal charged entities on either end of the molecule reduce considerably the biological activity. In all cases so far observed, replacement of either PCA or His led to a drastic decrease in activity whereas replacement of Pro-NH_2 by closely related substituents still permitted retention of some significant activity. One dipeptide, PCA-His-(N^{3im}-Me)-OMe, which does not have a bulky C-terminal group similar to proline, shows some biological activity. This could mean that the Pro-NH_2 residue is of relatively less importance in comparison with PCA-His. Obviously many more derivatives need to be studied to sustain this statement.

The imidazole ring, however, may be suspected *a priori* to be of some importance (pK^* of $-N^{2-}$ in histidine $= 6.00$–6.10) (Edsall, 1943). PCA-Pyr(3)Ala-Pro-NH_2 (Hofmann and Bowers, 1970) was synthesized for that precise reason and showed little activity, from which the authors suggested that the acid-base properties [pK^* of $-N^{2-}$ in pyrazolyl-(3) alanine·HCl $=$ ca. 2.1] (Schneider and Schaeg, 1962) of the imidazole ring are not essential for thyrotropin-releasing activity. Two interesting derivatives, PCA-His(N^{1im}-Me)-Pro-NH_2 and PCA-His(N^{3im}-Me)-Pro-NH_2 were synthesized and showed very different biological activities: (1-Me)-TRF has a very low specific activity whereas (3-Me)-TRF is 10 times as active as the natural hormone. Substitution by a methyl group does increase the pK values on either position because of a positive inductive effect [pK^* of $-N^{2-}$ in 3-methylhistidine $= 6.56$ (Schneider and Schaeg, 1962), pK^* of $-N^{2-}$ in 1-methylhistidine $= 6.48$ (Edsall, 1943)].

More than one explanation can fit these data. One is that the increase in biological activity results from the increased basicity of the (1-*im*) position. In this instance the basicity of the imidazole ring will indeed be of great importance. An alternative explanation is that the 3-methyl group exerts a positive steric effect on biological action. In the case of (1-Me)-TRF, decrease of the biological activity could be explained either by a steric hindrance or by a negative influence of increased electron density on the 3 position.

Similarly, it is of interest that secondary amides on the C-terminus have activities intermediate between those of the corresponding primary and tertiary amides. This might be explained on the basis of a compromise between (1) positive inductive effect and (2) negative steric effect.

* It should be kept in mind that these pK values refer to those of the free amino acids. Variations of these values have been observed when the amino acids were part of a sequence (Schneider, 1963, among others).

TABLE I

ACTIVITY OF ANALOGS OF THYROTROPIN-RELEASING FACTOR (TRF) GROUPED
ACCORDING TO SUBSTITUTIONS ON OR OF THE AMINO ACIDS
OF THE TRF MOLECULE

	Specific activity (TRF U/mg)[a]	Relative activity (×% of TRF)	References[b]
1. Proline modifications[c]			
PCA-His-Hyp-NH₂	100	ca. 0.2	N
PCA-His-Ala-NH₂	—	ca. 0.1–1	F[d]
PCA-His-Gly-NH₂	—	No activity	F
PCA-His-Leu-NH₂	100	ca. 0.2	N
PCA-His-Val-NH₂	—	ca. 0.1–1	F
PCA-His-aminocyclopentane methylcarboxylate	11	ca. 0.1–1	N
PCA-His-sarcosineamide	160	0.3	N
PCA-DL-His-pipicolineamide	1300	2.5	N
PCA-His-OMe	No activity	No activity	B
PCA-His-(N³ⁱᵐ-Me)-OMe	10	0.02	R
PCA-His-azetidine carboxamide	800	1.5	N
PCA-His-pyrrolidineamide	100	0.2	N
PCA-His-piperidineamide	300	0.5	N
PCA-His-morpholineamide	80	0.2	N
PCA-His-hexamethyleneimineamide	20	0.2	N
PCA-His-Pro-OH	10	0.02	B
PCA-His-Pro-OMe	20000	40	B
PCA-His-Pro-OMe	—	ca. 2	F
PCA-His-Pro-OEt	200	0.4	N
PCA-His-Pro-NHMe	—	ca. 2–5	F
PCA-His-Pro-NH-Et	7000	14	N
PCA-His-Pro-NH-CH₂CH₂OH	8000	15	N
PCA-His-N-cyclopentylamide	<2	<0.004	N
PCA-His-Pro-NH-CH₂-(C₆H₆)	8000	15	N
PCA-His-Pro-N(Me)₂	—	ca. 2–5	F
PCA-His-Pro-N(Et)₂	20	0.04	N
PCA-His-Pro-Tyr-NH₂	No activity	No activity	N
2. Histidine modifications[c]			
PCA-His(N³ⁱᵐ-Me)-Pro-NH₂	400,000	1000	R
PCA-His(N¹ⁱᵐ-Me)-Pro-NH₂	20	0.04	R
PCA-Arg-Pro-NH₂	10	0.02	R
PCA-Pyr(3) Ala-Pro-NH₂		ca. 0.5	H[d]
3. Histidine and proline modifications combined[c]			
PCA-His(Bzl)-Pro-NH₂	—	ca. 0.2	F
PCA-His(Bzl)-Pro-NHMe	—	No activity	F
PCA-His(Bzl)-Val-NH₂	—	No activity	F
PCA-His(Bzl)-Leu-NH₂	—	No activity	F

TABLE I (Continued)

	Specific activity (TRF U/mg)[a]	Relative activity (×% of TRF)	References[b]
PCA-His(Bzl)-Ala-NH₂	—	No activity	F
PCA-His(Bzl)-Gly-NH₂	—	No activity	F
PCA-His(Bzl)-Phe-NH₂	—	No activity	F
4. *PCA modifications*[c]			
Cyclobutoyl-His-Pro-NH₂	<4	0.01	N
Cyclopentoyl-His-Pro-NH₂	8	0.02	N
Pro-His-Pro-NH₂	10	0.02	N
Gln-His-Pro-NH₂		ca. 0.01	F[e]
Glu-His-Pro-NH₂	20	0.04	M,D[e]
Glu-His-Pro-OH	No activity	No activity	G
Acetyl-Glu-His-Pro-OH	No activity	No activity	G

[a] TRF, PCA-His-Pro-NH₂ = 50,000 U/mg.

[b] Key to references: N: Nicolaides et al., 1971; F: Bowers et al., 1970a; B: Burgus et al., 1970a; R: Rivier et al., 1971; M: Monahan et al., 1971; H: Hofmann and Bowers, 1970; G: Gillessen et al., 1970; D: Dunn et al., 1971.

[c] All amino acids, L-configuration, unless shown otherwise.

[d] Data from references H and F cannot be expressed in specific activity (U/mg) as no true classical 4-point assays were performed; results reported are in "changes of cpm" (see p. 4 for comments on this procedure).

[e] Derivatives having a Glu or Gln may contain some contaminant of cyclized N-terminal (TRF).

In the case of tertiary amides, steric hindrance would be the prevailing phenomenon, thus diminishing the response by almost the same factor as going from the primary amide to the secondary amide. In this case a positive steric effect clearly does not exist. Other synthetic compounds where the N-terminus would be different (of the type R-CO-Gly-His-Pro-NH₂: R being electron withdrawing such as CF_3, or electron donating such as CH_3), might give some insight on the inductive effect in this N-terminal position.

None of these synthetic analogs has been reported, as yet, to have antagonistic properties against the biological activity of TRF.*

VI. BIOSYNTHESIS OF TRF

There is evidence that TRF can be synthesized by fragments of hypothalamic tissues or stalk median eminence surviving *in vitro* in short-term incubations in various media added with labeled amino acids (Mitnik and

* Discussion in this chapter was prepared by J. Rivier, whose contribution we gratefully acknowledge.

Reichlin, 1971; Guillemin, 1971b). The statement is based on evidence of incorporation of one or several of the (labeled) amino acid components of the TRF molecule, the newly synthesized TRF showing chromatography or electrophoresis behavior similar to that of cold TRF or ^{125}I-labeled synthetic TRF. In these preliminary experiments it would appear that this biosynthesis of TRF *in vitro* is not affected by pretreatment of the tissues with cycloheximide, suggesting that the biosynthesis of the small tripeptide amide may be nonribosomal in its mechanism. Studies now in progress should lead to definite answers on this important question in the near future.

VII. PHYSIOLOGY OF TRF

Availability over the last few years of highly purified TRF and more recently of synthetic TRF in unlimited quantities has helped to clarify many questions concerning the physiology of the secretion of TSH; on the other hand, if much new knowledge has recently been obtained on the physiology of secretion of TRF, there are still several questions which remain unanswered at the time of writing this review (see below). These should not remain unanswered for too long since apparently methodology is now becoming available, particularly the use of labeled TRF of high specific activity, to approach the subject in a meaningful manner.

Even the fairly crude early preparations of TRF contributed to the investigation and eventual clarification of one of the most classical problems of physiology since the early 1920's, i.e., the nature of the feedback between the secretion of the thyroid gland and that of the adenohypophysis with respect to TSH. Whereas the question for years had been whether thyroid hormones exerted their feedback inhibition of the secretion of TSH at the level of the pituitary or at the level of the hypothalamus, the first preparation of partially purified TRF made it possible to demonstrate that the feedback by the thyroid hormones was at the level of the adenohypophysial tissues since thyroxine added to pituitary tissues surviving *in vitro* or injected *in vivo* prior to removal of the pituitary for *in vitro* incubation could prevent the release of TSH induced *in vitro* by this crude preparation of TRF (Guillemin *et al.*, 1962, 1963). Later studies showed that there was an inverse relationship between the amount of thyroid hormones necessary to prevent the release of TSH due to variable amounts of TRF, so that in a classical physiological demonstration of the cybernetic concept of a feedback system with resetting point, there would always be a dose of TRF that could overcome the blockade due to a certain dose of thyroxine and there would always be a dose of thyroxine that would inhibit the release of TSH due to any dose of TRF (Vale *et al.*, 1967c). This relation between the antagonistic amounts of thyroid hormones and TRF had led investigators in the field, for awhile, to consider the possibility that the antagonistic effects of thyroid hormones and TRF involved competition for common binding sites at the level of the pituitary tissues. This hypothesis was never considered too seriously, as it was soon realized that TRF acts very rapidly (in a matter of seconds) to stimulate the release of TSH (Ducommun *et al.*, 1965), whereas it takes several hours for thyroid hormones to produce *in vivo* their inhibition of the activity of a subsequently administered dose of TRF and no less than 15 minutes in the case of *in vitro* incubations of the pituitary. The mechanism of this physiological antagonism between TRF and thyroid hormone regarding the secretion of TSH is now well understood and is discussed in detail in Section VIII, on the mode of action of TRF, and will not be further elaborated here.

TRF activity has been reported in blood collected from severed capillaries descending from median eminence along the pituitary stalk (Averill, 1970). Increased secretion of TRF as collected in blood from hypothalamopituitary portal vessels has been reported following acute electrical stimulation of the preoptic anterior hypothalamic area (Porter *et al.*, 1970; Averill *et al.*, 1966). It should be pointed out that, in all these experiments, the assays for TRF demonstrated only marginal effects; this question should be reinvestigated when radioimmunoassays for TRF become available. Nothing is known at the moment about the secretion rate of TRF under various physiological conditions. Studies aimed at this question by assessing hypothalamic TRF content by bioassay during various experimental conditions obviously cannot provide the correct answer to this difficult question: A multivariate function, such as the secretory rate of any hormone, simply cannot be defined by observing only one value of that function. Since TRF activity (or TRF-like activity) has been reportedly recovered from the blood of the hypothalamohypophysial portal system draining the hypothalamic area, when collected in animals under maximal stress of the surgical procedure (see below), it may be hypothesized that TRF is constantly secreted by the pertinent elements of the hypothalamic hypophysiotropic area and released into the primary plexus of the hypothalamohypophysial portal vessels, through which it is carried to the adenohypophysial tissue. There it will stimulate the secretion of TSH in such amount as determined by the levels of circulating free thyroxine or free triiodothyronine as in the mechanism discussed above. This basal (or resting) secretion of TRF by the hypothalamus can be modulated in its amplitude, i.e., rapidly increased as a function of time, by specific exteroceptive stimuli such as exposure to cold. An acutely increased secretion of TRF at times $t + dt$

would be able to override the level of inhibition of TSH secretion determined at time t by the then available levels of thyroid hormones, thus stimulating the secretion of TSH and in turn of thyroid hormones. The new elevated level of thyroid hormones would reset the level at which TRF could continue to stimulate secretion of TSH according to the mechanism described and discussed above. The secretion rate of TSH would then be altered anew according to the further secretion of TRF that could increase, remain constant or decrease from what it was at $t + dt$ depending on the then prevalent condition of the (TRF-stimulating) exteroceptive stimulus.

An interesting and not fully understood aspect of the physiology of TRF is probably related to the now well-known effect of "nonspecific stress" in somehow inhibiting the secretion of TSH, while at the same time it stimulates the secretion of ACTH (Ducommun et al., 1966). The results reported so far by several laboratories are compatible with the hypothesis that nonspecific stress, while stimulating the secretion of ACTH, inhibits the secretion of TSH by inhibiting the hypothalamic secretion of TRF (Sakiz and Guillemin, 1965). Methods are becoming available with which to test this working hypothesis; a primary role of TRF in these acute changes in the secretion of TSH in response to stress remains to be demonstrated.

There is in plasma or in whole blood an enzyme that rapidly inactivates TRF *in vitro* (Redding and Schally, 1969a,b). We have reported various means of inactivation of this enzymatic mechanism that destroys TRF *in vitro*. The enzymatic system that destroys TRF *in vitro* appears to have some specificity for TRF since it destroys various synthetic analogs of TRF at rates which are different from those observed when TRF is used as the substrate (Vale et al., 1971a). While these results are undoubted and have been seen in several laboratories, the physiological significance of the plasma enzyme that destroys TRF *in vitro* remains open to question: Indeed recent studies have shown that in rats as much as 75% of a dose of TRF administered as a single intravenous injection (from 1 to 5 μg) is recovered in the urine as a biologically active material within 2 hours of its administration (i.e., it can be extracted from the urine and shown to possess full TRF activity in bioassays). The urinary excretion appears to follow very closely that of inulin in studies using separate as well as concomitant administration of inulin-^{14}C and TRF-[3]H (Braudo et al., 1971), thus suggesting that TRF is filtered freely with little tubular reabsorption. Thus, an alleged physiological role of a plasma enzyme inhibiting TRF is difficult to understand in view of the results obtained in studies of the urinary excretion of TRF.

TRF can stimulate the secretion of TSH when injected intravenously, acutely or as an infusion, when administered intraperitoneally, or orally (Vale et al., 1970). Also we have shown, in collaboration with Porter, that administration of TRF directly into one single portal vessel going to the anterior lobe of the pituitary leads to dramatically increased secretion of TSH (Porter et al., 1971).

The ability of TRF to stimulate the secretion of TSH has been demonstrated not only by indirect methods for TSH secretion based on measurement of thyroid hormone levels, labeled with ^{125}I or ^{131}I in the plasma of the animal administered TRF [usually rats or mice as bioassay animals (Yamazaki et al., 1963a; Bowers and Schally, 1970)] but also directly by measuring actual levels of plasma TSH by radioimmunoassays (Martin and Reichlin, 1970) or bioassays (Ducommun et al., 1965). Methods of direct measurement of plasma TSH concentrations either by radioimmunoassays or bioassays have yielded identical results: TRF indeed stimulates secretion of TSH as demonstrated by increased levels of plasma TSH as early as 60 seconds after administration of a single dose of TRF into a peripheral vein. The curve describing plasma TSH level as a function of time following intravenous injection of a single dose of TRF is very similar to that obtained for plasma TSH after electrical stimulation of the preoptic area of the hypothalamus (Martin and Reichlin, 1970). This suggests indeed that the acute elevation of plasma TSH observed following hypothalamic electrical stimulation is due to endogenous release of TRF.

Perhaps one of the most salient features of the physiology of TRF is its remarkable specificity of action. In both in vivo and in vitro experiments, TRF has been shown to stimulate specifically the secretion of the pituitary hormone TSH and only of that hormone. Our early observations on this point had led us to conclude (Guillemin, 1964) that the TSH-activity observed at that time in highly purified preparations of LH was most likely due to contamination of LH by TSH, a problem then of considerable debate between interested biochemists, since we were able to obtain "pure" TSH action devoid of LH action after injection of TRF, and "pure" LH action devoid of TSH action after injection of LRF. These early observations have been amply confirmed with highly purified native TRF or synthetic TRF (Guillemin, 1971a). The specificity of action of TRF for the release of TSH is all the more interesting now that it is known from the recent work of Pierce, Ward and their collaborators that TSH and LH are closely related glycoproteins sharing a common core of peptidic nature (Pierce, 1971). Obviously the high specificity of TRF for stimulating the release of TSH must reside in an exclusive fit between the molecule of TRF and its receptor site. Little is known, at the moment, of the nature of the TRF-receptor site.

At the moment nothing is known of the nature of the CNS transmitter or the intimate mechanism which is responsible for the acute release of TRF such as, for instance, in response to exposure to cold.

The same can be said about the exact anatomical elements in the hypothalamic hypophysiotropic area which are the true secretory cells of the molecule of TRF.

Availability, on the horizon, of method of radioimmunoassays for TRF should greatly facilitate studies of these and other still unanswered questions.

VIII. Mechanism of Action of TRF

There have been, so far, two basic approaches to the investigation of the mechanism of action of TRF. One has been to monitor a metameter presumably specific to thyrotrophs such as TSH secretion or level of incorporation of radioactive amino acids into immunoprecipitable TSH. Another approach has involved measuring a metameter that is not specific to thyrotrophs, for example adenohypophysial cyclic AMP levels or cellular transmembrane potentials as they would be affected by administration of TRF or other stimuli. Thyrotrophs make up only a small percentage of the cells of a normal adenohypophysis; therefore, levels of a nonthyrotroph-specific metameter may be irrelevant to conditions that exist in the thyrotrophs. If it is assumed that TRF and/or thyroxine affect only thyrotrophs, significant changes observed in a nonthyrotroph-specific metameter would yield useful information if large enough to be detected over the "noise" contributed by the other cell types. Similar studies are actually best carried out on cell populations which have a higher percentage of thyrotrophs than normal anterior pituitary tissue such as TSH-secreting tumors (Furth, 1955) or anterior pituitaries obtained from chronically thyroidectomized donors (Goluboff et al., 1970). Anterior pituitary cells can be dispersed by trypsin and can be fractionated on BSA gradients (Hymer and Evans, 1970); morphological evidence indicates that considerable separation of various anterior pituitary cell types is achieved using this method and, therefore, it should be possible to obtain a cell population high in thyrotrophs. The latter method appears very promising for future studies on cellular functions that are not specific to thyrotrophs; it has not been used extensively as such, as the methodology has only very recently been reduced to practice.

It would seem that the major tenets of the mode of action of TRF can be related to secretory phenomena in other systems which to date have been more completely investigated. Douglas and Rubin (1961), reporting on their experiments on secretion of catecholamines by the adrenal medulla, proposed the term "stimulus-secretion coupling" to encompass all the events occurring in the cell exposed to an "adequate stimulus" that eventually lead to the arrival of its characteristic secretory product in the extracellular environment. This term was patterned after the phrase "excitation-contraction coupling" applied to related events occurring in muscle by Sandow (1952). Douglas and co-workers have found that exposure of adrenal chromaffin cells to acetylcholine, elevated extracellular [K^+] or electrical current results in depolarization of the cell membranes (Douglas et al., 1967a,b). This depolarization is associated with an increased uptake of ^{45}Ca (Douglas and Poisner, 1961). Of all of the ions in the external media, only Ca^{2+} was found to be absolutely necessary for the secretion of catecholamines in response to various depolarizing adequate stimuli. Depolarization is not by itself a sufficient stimulus for secretion; elevated [K^+] depolarizes chromaffin cell membranes in the absence of external Ca^{2+} and yet does not induce secretion of catecholamines (Douglas et al., 1967b). The fall in membrane potential across the chromaffin cell membrane is possibly merely the electrical sign of a chemical change in the membrane, one of the consequences being Ca^{2+} entry.

Studies on other secretory processes have indicated that an essential role of calcium in stimulus-secretion coupling may be a general phenomenon. Results similar to those on the adrenal medulla have been obtained on the posterior pituitary (Douglas and Poisner, 1964a,b), the pancreas (Grodsky and Bennett, 1966), salivary glands (Bdolah et al., 1964), mast cells (Mongar and Schild, 1962), polymorphonuclear leukocytes (Woodin and Wienecke, 1964), sympathetic nerve endings (Hukovic and Muscholl, 1962), and cholinergic neurons (Hodgkin and Keynes, 1957). Following these lines of thought and experimentation, we have found that omission of Ca^{2+} from the incubation medium decreases the amount of TSH released in response to TRF ($10^{-10} M$, using rat pituitary glands incubated in vitro for short periods) (Vale et al., 1967b). Addition of Ca^{2+} to pituitary glands previously deprived reinstates the full response to TRF, demonstrating the reversibility of that inhibition. Deletion of Mg^{2+}, K^+, Cl^-, SO_4^{2-}, or PO_4^{3-} from the incubation medium does not decrease the amount of TSH released by TRF (Guillemin et al., 1969). Many secretory responses are inhibited by elevated Mg^{2+} (Douglas and Rubin, 1963, 1964; Mikiten and Douglas, 1965; Milner and Hales, 1967), possibly by virtue of the ability of Mg^{2+} to antagonize Ca^{2+} uptake (Malaisse-Lagae and Malaisse, 1971; Douglas and Poisner, 1964b). In contradistinction to these observations, increasing [Mg^{2+}] of the media to 20 mM does not decrease the response to TRF (Vale, 1968).

Elevating [K^+] of the medium as little as 3- to 4-fold (17.7–23.6 mM) increases the rate of TSH secretion in vitro (Vale and Guillemin, 1967).

Raising media [K^+] also provokes the secretion of LH (Samli and Geschwind, 1968), FSH (Jutisz and de la Llosa, 1968), ACTH (Vale et al., 1967a), and STH (MacLeod and Fontham, 1970). Thus, high [K^+] is a nonthyrotroph-specific stimulus. TRF on the other hand, releases specifically TSH (Guillemin and Vale, 1970); this includes a total lack of effect of TRF on the secretion of LH, a molecule closely related to TSH (Liao and Pierce, 1970). The release of TSH in response to elevated [K^+] is inhibited by pretreatment of the anterior pituitary glands with thyroxine as is the case for TRF (see below). Also, removal of Ca^{2+} from the medium completely inhibits the response to elevated [K^+] (Vale and Guillemin, 1967). Thus, it is tempting to suggest that high [K^+] and TRF act through similar mechanisms involving an increase in cell permeability to Na^+ and Ca^{2+} with concomitant membrane depolarization. However, under similar conditions, a maximal dose of TRF stimulates the secretion of more TSH than does any concentration of [K^+] (from 23.6 to 118 mM); also, TRF further increases the rate of TSH secretion from pituitary glands incubated in elevated [K^+] (Vale and Guillemin, 1971a). This residual effect of TRF in the presence of high [K^+] is analogous to the ability of acetylcholine to release additional catecholamines from chromaffin cells already depolarized by incubation in high [K^+] (Douglas and Rubin, 1963). These observations would seem to indicate that TRF might act on loci additional to those acted upon by high [K^+]. Perhaps TRF can more completely dissociate intracellularly bound calcium or can increase the pool size of readily releasable TSH. The general hypothesis of stimulus-secretion coupling proposed by Douglas and Rubin may thus be applicable to the mechanism by which TRF releases TSH. According to this hypothesis, TRF would alter the permeability or the characteristics of the cell membrane of the thyrotroph and lead to an increase in the intracellular activity of Ca^{2+} ions either through a decrease in intracellular calcium-binding or a positive net influx of extracellular Ca^{2+}. This increased Ca^{2+} activity would then be required for the release of TSH.

Kraicer and Milligan (1970) have found that high extracellular [K^+] causes a reversal of the membrane potential in the majority of cells of rat anterior pituitary glands incubated in vitro. They have also found an increase in the ^{45}Ca space in response to high [K^+] (Milligan and Kraicer, 1970). We have also observed an increase in ^{45}Ca uptake induced by high [K^+] (Guillemin et al., 1968); however, we have been unable to find a significant effect of TRF on the ^{45}Ca space under similar conditions. It is probable that any effect of TRF on ^{45}Ca flux would be obscured due to the small representation of thyrotrophs in the heterogeneous anterior pituitary gland.

The precise role played by Ca^{2+} in the secretory response to TRF is not known. Calcium may be involved in the activation of an enzyme such as a phospholipase which could affect membrane structure and function (Banks, 1966). Thorn (1965) has postulated that Ca^{2+} plays a crucial role in the release of vasopressin from the neurohypophysis by dissociating vasopressin from a complex of the hormone and its carrier, neurophysin. Poisner and Trifaró (1967) in studies on the adrenal medulla and the posterior pituitary, have proposed that Ca^{2+} may serve to link negatively charged groups at the surface of the storage granule and at the inner surface of the cell membrane thereby bringing the two membranes into close apposition. Following the approximation of the granule and plasma membranes, they suggest that the release of granular contents into the medium involves the hydrolysis of ATP by a Mg^{2+}-dependent ATPase. A similar mechanism was proposed by Woodin and Wienecke (1964) to describe the extrusion of enzymes from the polymorphonuclear leukocyte. Lacy et al. (1968) proposed that contraction of a microtubular-microfilamentous system containing actomysin-like material which would connect secretory granules with the plasma membrane might be involved in the secretion of insulin. It is possible that calcium would be required for the contraction of these elements.

In 1967, we reported that the potassium salt of dibutyryl-3′,5′-cyclic AMP released TSH, and that incubation of anterior pituitary glands in theophylline (which, as part of its action, inhibits the cyclic nucleotide phosphodiesterase that degrades cyclic AMP) increased the amount of TSH released in response to TRF (Guillemin, 1967). It was suggested that TRF might act through a mechanism involving an increase in intracellular cyclic AMP. We subsequently found that the preparation of dibutyryl cyclic AMP we were using contained twice as much K^+ (as a K-butyrate contaminant) as would have been expected. In view of the previously mentioned effect of elevated $[K^+]$ on the secretion of TSH, we considered the results with the K salt of dibutyryl cyclic AMP as suspect and investigated the effect of sodium dibutyryl cyclic AMP on TSH release. In our hands, sodium dibutyryl cyclic AMP at doses from 10^{-4} to $10^{-2} M$ is ineffective in stimulating TSH secretion (Guillemin et al., 1968). Other investigators have reported that dibutyryl cyclic AMP releases TSH (Bowers et al., 1969b; Wilbur et al., 1969; Cehovic, 1969). In one of these studies (Cehovic, 1969), dibutyryl cyclic AMP was reported to release TSH at levels of 2.2×10^{-4} to $4.4 \times 10^{-4} M$. Although the salt form was not mentioned, it is unlikely that surplus cation would have been responsible for the reported increased TSH secretion in those experiments, for which we have no explanation that would reconcile their results with our own negative ones.

Reports that crude hypothalamic extracts increase cyclic AMP levels in the anterior pituitary while releasing pituitary hormones are inconclusive at best (Zor et al., 1969; Steiner et al., 1970). Little can be presumed about the level of cyclic AMP in any one cell type on the basis of this type of experiment. However, the studies of Steiner et al. (1970), demonstrated that the increase in cyclic AMP levels which occurred in response to hypothalamic extract was not dependent on the presence of Ca^{2+} in the incubation medium. Rasmussen and Tenenhouse (1968) found that Ca^{2+} was not required for the stimulation of cyclic AMP levels in parotid glands by epinephrine and proposed that Ca^{2+} requirements in secretory processes are not mediated through an effect on cyclic AMP synthesis.

In an abstract, Bowers et al. (1969b) stated that highly purified TRF increases the concentration of cyclic AMP in the pituitary. However, the data and methodology of this experiment have not yet been published. The amount of increase in cyclic AMP levels of thyrotrophs would indeed have to be very great to see an overall increase in the whole gland.

Studies by Butcher and Baird (1968) on fat pads have well demonstrated the problems involved with interpreting data on cyclic AMP in heterogeneous tissues. The prostaglandin PGE_1 increases cyclic AMP in rat epididymal fat pads incubated in vitro (Butcher and Baird, 1968). When fat pad cells were dispersed by treatment with collagenase and separated into two populations, fat cells and stromovascular component, it was found that PGE_1 elevated cyclic AMP levels in the stromovascular component, whereas PGE_1 decreased cyclic AMP levels in isolated fat cells treated with epinephrine and caffeine. Therefore, PGE_1 had opposite effects on the two components of the epididymal fat tissue. A similar if not more complicated situation exists in the anterior pituitary tissue with not only stromovascular components but the various secretory elements contributing to any nonthyrotroph specific metameter.

Prostaglandins have been found to increase the accumulation of cyclic AMP in the thyroid (Kaneko et al., 1969), the ovaries (Kuehl et al., 1970), the anterior pituitary (Zor et al., 1969), and other organs (Ramwell and Shaw, 1970). In addition, prostaglandins have been demonstrated to stimulate secretion by a number of tissues including the thyroid (Onaya and Solomon, 1969), the adrenals (Flack et al., 1969), the ovaries (Pharriss et al., 1968), and the anterior pituitary (MacLeod and Lehmeyer, 1970). Prostaglandins of the PGE_1 series increase the rate of TSH secretion in vitro (Kudo and Beck, 1970; Vale et al., 1971b). In our experiments, as little as $2.8 \times 10^{-6} M$ PGE_1 has been seen to stimulate TSH secretion in vitro. Recently, a prostaglandin analog, 7-oxa-13-prostanoic acid, has been reported to be a prostaglandin antagonist on smooth muscle (Fried et al., 1969) and the ovary (Kuehl et al., 1970). This antagonist inhibits the release of TSH which occurs in response to either high [K$^+$] or TRF (Vale et al., 1971b). Therefore, it appears that stimulation of a prostaglandin receptor might be involved in the TSH secretory process. It is possible that high [K$^+$] and TRF increase the rate of prostaglandin synthesis. Increased prostaglandin efflux from various tissues stimulated to secrete has been observed (see Ramwell and Shaw, 1967, for review).

It is tempting to hypothesize that prostaglandins are acting on adenyl cyclase to increase cyclic AMP levels in the thyrotrophs and that this increase in cyclic AMP somehow mediates the secretion of TSH through a calcium-dependent mechanism. Rasmussen and Tenenhouse (1968) reported that high potassium as well as epinephrine increase the level of cyclic AMP in parotid gland slices. They have suggested that cyclic AMP is an important regulator of the permeability of cellular membranes to calcium or of the binding of this ion to membranes. High potassium has also been reported to increase cyclic AMP in brain slices; however, that phenomenon may be a result of inhibition of cyclic nucleotide phosphodiesterase since the effect is obscured by theophylline (Shimizu et al., 1970).

It is important to emphasize at this point that the involvement of cyclic AMP in the TSH release process is by no means established. When a suitable thyrotroph population is available for study, concomitant measurement of cyclic AMP levels, calcium movements, membrane potentials and prostaglandin synthesis rates in response to various adequate stimuli will yield the information necessary to dissect the TSH secretion mechanism.

Another common denominator of secretory mechanisms in many organs is that they are sensitive to procedures that compromise their energy metabolism (Douglas et al., 1965; Hokin, 1951; Bdolah et al., 1964; Coore and Randle, 1964). The activity of TRF to release TSH from pituitary glands incubated in Krebs-Ringer bicarbonate glucose is not inhibited by a variety of metabolic inhibitors: $10^{-3} M$ cyanide, $10^{-2} M$ 2-deoxyglucose, $10^{-4} M$ ouabain, $3 \times 10^{-3} M$ arsenate, $10^{-2} M$ fluoride, $10^{-4} M$ dinitrophenol or 1 µg tetrodotoxin/ml (Guillemin et al., 1969). However, the release of TSH that occurs in response to TRF is probably an energy-requiring process as it is inhibited by 1 µg of oligomycin per milliliter (Wilber and Utiger, 1968; Guillemin et al., 1968), dinitrophenol in a glucose free medium (Wilber and Utiger, 1968), or incubation without oxygen (under an atmosphere of N_2-CO_2) (Guillemin and Vale, 1970). The release of TSH by TRF or high [K$^+$] is blocked by $10^{-3} M$ N-ethylmaleimide or iodoacetamide (Guillemin et al., 1968). It is not known which aspects of the release process are compromised by any of the above procedures. Adequate ATP levels would be required for cyclic AMP synthesis. However, Bdolah and Schramm (1965), finding that dinitrophenol inhibited secretion from parotid glands even when dibutyryl cyclic AMP replaced epinephrine as the secretagogue, tentatively concluded that the energy requirement is not limited to the synthesis of cyclic AMP in the cell. ATP might be required for an ATPase-mediated mechanism involving contraction of actomyosin-like microfilaments similar to that proposed by Poisner and Trifaró (1967) to explain secretion from the adrenal medulla. Oxygen deprivation may decrease stimulated secretion because of suppression of aerobic metabolism or inhibition might be related to the observation that molecular oxygen is required for prostaglandin synthesis (Samuelsson, 1965). Energy may also be required in order to increase calcium uptake. Malaisse-Lagae and Malaisse (1971) have reported that ^{45}Ca uptake by isolated islets of Langerhans is decreased by incubation at room temperature instead of 37°C. The effects of energy-compromising procedures reported above on the actions of TRF are probably not mediated through an inhibition of TSH synthesis because uninterrupted protein synthesis is not required for the acute response to TRF (see below).

The *in vivo* or *in vitro* secretion of TSH that occurs in response to a single administration of TRF is not impaired by pretreatment with cycloheximide, puromycin or actinomycin D (Vale *et al.*, 1968; Redding and Schally, 1967; Bowers *et al.*, 1968b). Therefore, it would appear, that the acute effect of TRF is to release previously synthesized TSH. These results, of course, do not preclude an effect of TRF on the rate of synthesis of TSH.

Bowers *et al.* (1967) have reported that an appropriate dose of TRF given to mice stimulates TSH secretion (as measured by ^{131}I release from the thyroid) without changing pituitary TSH levels. They suggested on the basis of these data that TRF produced an increase in TSH synthesis as well as release. It is unlikely, however, that a bioassay could have detected the small depletion in pituitary TSH content which would have resulted from a single injection of TRF. There are two reports that hypothalamic extracts or purified TRF increases the total TSH content of anterior pituitary glands plus media maintained in organ culture for several days (Sinha and Meites, 1966; Mittler and Redding, 1969). We have obtained similar results in studies of the effects of synthetic TRF on anterior pituitary cell monolayers kept in tissue culture for up to 8 weeks (Vale and Guillemin, 1971a). However, without information on the relative stability of TSH in the intracellular and extracellular environment, one cannot conclude that TSH synthesis was enhanced in these studies (Smith and Farquhar, 1966).

Solomon and McKenzie (1964) reported that crude hypothalamic extracts increased the rate of incorporation of radioactive amino acids into an anterior pituitary protein which had a distribution coefficient identical with TSH on Sephadex G-100; it is unlikely that this method specifically monitored TSH secretion rate. Another group of investigators has studied the effect of TRF on the incorporation of radioactive glucosamine into immunologically precipitable TSH. In the first report (Wilber and Utiger, 1969) they found no effect of TRF on rate of glucosamine incorporation into TSH. In a later abstract, Wilber (1970) reported that either TRF or high [K+] would increase the rate of glucosamine incorporation into TSH. An effect of high [K+] on rate of TSH synthesis might be interpreted as an indication that the release of hormone represents the stimulus for increased synthesis. A discussion of the explanation of the different results in their two notes will have to await publication of the methodology used in the second study.

Schreiber et al. (review in Schreiber, 1963) have claimed on the basis of questionable methodology that "TRF," in the form of various types of hypothalamic extracts, would increase adenohypophysial acid phosphatase content; these conclusions were not confirmed by Davis et al. (1967) using a highly purified preparation of ovine TRF.

Overwhelming physiological evidence indicates that thyroxine suppresses the secretion of TSH by acting primarily on the appropriate pituitary cells. Thyroxine inhibits the release of TSH in response to TRF in vivo or in vitro (Guillemin et al., 1963; Vale et al., 1967c). The latent period for thyroxine action is 15 minutes in vitro and several hours in vivo. The inhibition of TRF release by thyroxine is not an all-or-none phenomenon; the blockade of a given dose of TRF by a given dose of thyroxine can be overcome by administration of a larger quantity of TRF. Therefore, the amount of thyroxine required to inhibit TSH secretion is a function of the amount of TRF administered (Vale et al., 1967a). This functionally competitive relationship between TRF and thyroxine is not the result of a direct competition for a single site between the two molecules. The actions of two other adequate stimuli on the secretion of TSH, i.e., elevated [K+] (Vale and Guillemin, 1967) and theophylline (Guillemin et al., 1968; Wilber and Utiger, 1968) are also inhibited by thyroxine.

Low doses of actinomycin D can prevent the blockade of TRF action by triiodothyroninine or thyroxine in vitro (Vale et al., 1968) and in vivo (Bowers et al., 1968b). Cycloheximide or puromycin can prevent and reverse the effect of thyroxine in vitro (Vale et al., 1968) or in vivo (Bowers et al., 1968a). One interpretation of these data is that thyroxine acts through a mechanism requiring undisturbed DNA-dependent RNA-synthesis and protein synthesis. It has been postulated (Vale et al., 1968) that, acting through the synthesis of a specific mRNA, thyroxine induces in thyrotrophs the synthesis of a rather labile protein or peptide that is responsible for the inhibition of TSH secretion in response to various stimuli. The interaction of thyroxine with the various adequate stimuli for TSH secretion as they affect thyrotroph levels of cyclic AMP, calcium movements, prostaglandin production and other metameters will be of assistance in further elucidating and hopefully understanding the cellular and subcellular mechanisms of action of TRF in the secretion of TSH.

IX. Clinical Administration and Use of TRF

At the time this review is being written, synthetic TRF has already been administered to several hundred individuals or patients to test pituitary TSH reserve or pituitary TSH reactivity to TRF. The doses injected intravenously have ranged from 250 μg to 1 mg of the pure peptide acetate; TRF has also been administered by mouth in doses ranging from 2 mg to 10 mg (Fleischer et al., 1970; Hall et al., 1970; Hershman and Pittman, 1970). No untoward side effects or reactions have been noted with peripheral administration of even large doses of TRF with the exception of some inconsistent feelings of "light-headedness" or nausea in some individuals. This effect does not appear to be related to the dose administered, is not consistently reported by the subjects, and has not been reported by several subjects (physicians) who have taken relatively large doses of TRF several times for time studies of plasma TSH levels. In humans, normal individuals show the same type of plasma TSH response as that observed in experimental animals in response to a single acutely administered dose of TRF. As in the experimental animals, administration of thyroid hormones, chronically or acutely, can prevent the normal TSH-response to TRF. What is of interest is that administration of TRF permits one to differentiate between pituitary or hypothalamic sites for a functional or organic lesion leading to a deficiency in TSH secretion in a series of patients. Costom et al. (1971), Bartter (1971), and Milhaud et al. (1970) have already reported a series of cases of idiopathic hypopituitarism with hypothyroidism which responded to TRF by elevating plasma levels—thus pointing to a hypothalamic abnormality as the origin of their TSH hypopituitarism. It is of interest that most of these cases, according to Costom et al., respond to TRF (radioimmunoassayable plasma TSH) with a curve (as a function of time) very different from that seen in normal individuals: the elevation of plasma TSH appears to be considerably delayed (up to 30–45 minutes) with a slope of elevation and subsequent decay of plasma TSH concentration quite different from those seen in normal individuals. In some children, the possibility of the chronic administration of TRF has been considered as a replacement therapy. These early clinical studies with a hypothalamic hormone isolated, characterized and synthesized less than one year ago, will no doubt be considerably expanded in the future. The possible availability of an antagonist to TRF also may well be of considerable clinical interest.

REFERENCES

Averill, R. L. W. (1970). *Endocrinology* **87**, 176.
Averill, R. L. W., Salaman, D. F., and Worthington, W. C., Jr. (1966). *Nature (London)* **211**, 144.
Banks, P. (1966). *Biochem. J.* **101**, 18c.
Bartter, F. (1971). Unpublished data.
Baugh, C. M., Krumdieck, C. L., Herschman, J. M., and Pittman, J. A., Jr. (1970). *Endocrinology* **87**, 1015.
Bdolah, A., and Schramm, M. (1965). *Biochem. Biophys. Res. Commun.* **18**, 452.
Bdolah, A., Ben-Zvi, R., and Schramm, M. (1964). *Arch. Biochem. Biophys.* **104**, 58.
Bøler, J., Enzmann, F., Folkers, K., Bowers, C. Y., and Schally, A. V. (1969). *Biochem. Biophys. Res. Commun.* **37**, 705.
Bowers, C. Y., and Schally, A. V. (1970). *In* "Hypophysiotropic Hormones of the Hypothalamus" (J. Meites, ed.), p. 74. Williams & Wilkins, Baltimore, Maryland.
Bowers, C. Y., Schally, A. V., Reynolds, G. A., and Hawley, W. D. (1967). *Endocrinology* **81**, 741.
Bowers, C. Y., Lee, L. L., and Schally, A. V. (1968a). *Endocrinology* **82**, 72.
Bowers, C. Y., Lee, K. L., and Schally, A. V. (1968b). *Endocrinology* **82**, 303.
Bowers, C. Y., Schally, A. V., Enzmann, F., Bøler, J., and Folkers, K. (1969a). *Program 45th Meet. Amer. Thyroid Ass.* p. 15.
Bowers, C. Y., Robison, G. A., Schally, A. V., de Balbian, G., and Verster, F. (1969b). *Proc. Int. Meet. Int. Soc. Neurochem., 2nd, 1969* p. 103.
Bowers, C. Y., Weil, A., Chang, J. K., Sievertsson, H., Enzmann, F., and Folkers, K. (1970a). *Biochem. Biophys. Res. Commun.* **40**, No. 3, 683.
Bowers, C. Y., Schally, A. V., Enzmann, F., Bøler, J., and Folkers, K. (1970b). *Endocrinology* **86**, 1143.
Braudo, M., Vale, W., Dunn, T. F., and Monahan, M. (1971). Unpublished data.
Burgus, R., and Guillemin, R. (1967). *Fed. Proc., Fed. Amer. Soc. Exp. Biol.* **26**, 255.
Burgus, R., and Guillemin, R. (1970). *In* "Hypophysiotropic Hormones of the Hypothalamus" (J. Meites, ed.), p. 227. Williams & Wilkins, Baltimore, Maryland.
Burgus, R., Ward, D. N., Sakiz, E., and Guillemin, R. (1966a). *C. R. Acad. Sci.* **262**, 2643.
Burgus, R., Stillwell, R. N., McCloskey, J. A., Ward, D. N., Sakiz, E., and Guillemin, R. (1966b). *Physiologist* **9**, 149.
Burgus, R., Dunn, T. F., Desiderio, D., Vale, W., and Guillemin, R. (1969a). *C. R. Acad. Sci.* **269**, 226.
Burgus, R., Dunn, T. F., Desiderio, D., and Guillemin, R. (1969b). *C. R. Acad. Sci.* **269**, 1870.
Burgus, R., Dunn, T. F., Ward, D. N., Vale, W., Amoss, M., and Guillemin, R. (1969c). *C. R. Acad. Sci.* **268**, 2116.

Burgus, R., Dunn, T. F., Desiderio, D., Ward, D. N., Vale, W., and Guillemin, R. (1970a). *Nature (London)* **226**, 321.
Burgus, R., Dunn, T. F., Desiderio, D., Ward, D. N., Vale, W., Guillemin, R., Felix, A. M., Gillessen, D., and Studer, R. O. (1970b). *Endocrinology* **86**, 573.
Butcher, R. W., and Baird, C. E. (1968). *J. Biol. Chem.* **243**, 1713.
Cehovic, G. (1969). *C. R. Acad. Sci., Ser. D* **268**, 2929.
Coore, H. G., and Randle, P. J. (1964). *Biochem. J.* **93**, 66.
Costom, B. H., Grumbach, M. M., and Kaplan, S. L. (1971). *J. Clin. Invest.* (in press).
Davis, T. Q., Vale, W., and Guillemin, R. (1967). *Neuroendocrinology* **2**, 330.
Douglas, W. W., and Poisner, A. M. (1961). *Nature (London)* **192**, 1299.
Douglas, W. W., and Poisner, A. M. (1964a). *J. Physiol. (London)* **172**, 1.
Douglas, W. W., and Poisner, A. M. (1964b). *J. Physiol. (London)* **172**, 19.
Douglas, W. W., and Rubin, R. P. (1961). *J. Physiol. (London)* **159**, 40.
Douglas, W. W., and Rubin, R. P. (1963). *J. Physiol. (London)* **167**, 288.
Douglas, W. W., and Rubin, R. P. (1964). *J. Physiol. (London)* **175**, 231.
Douglas, W. W., Ishida, A., and Poisner, A. M. (1965). *J. Physiol. (London)* **181**, 753.
Douglas, W. W., Kanno, T., and Sampson, S. R. (1967a). *J. Physiol. (London)* **188**, 107.
Douglas, W. W., Kanno, T., and Sampson, S. R. (1967b). *J. Physiol. (London)* **191**, 107.
Ducommun, P., Sakiz, E., and Guillemin, R. (1965). *Endocrinology* **77**, 792.
Ducommun, P., Sakiz, E., and Guillemin, R. (1966). *Amer. J. Physiol.* **210**, 1257.
Dunn, T. F. (1971). Unpublished data.
Dunn, T. F., Monahan, M., and Burgus, R. (1971). Unpublished data.
Edsall, J. T. (1943). *In* "Proteins, Amino Acids and Peptides" (W. A. Hamor, ed.), p. 85. Hafner, New York.
Everett, J. W. (1969). *Annu. Rev. Physiol.* **31**, 383.
Fellows, R., Mudge, A., and Burgus, R. (1971). Unpublished data.
Flack, J. D., Jessup, R., and Ramwell, P. W. (1969). *Science* **163**, 691.
Fleischer, N., Burgus, R., Vale, W., Dunn, T. F., and Guillemin, R. (1970). *J. Clin. Endocrinol. Metab.* **31**, 109.
Flouret, G. (1970). *J. Med. Chem.* **13**, 843.
Folkers, K., Enzmann, F., Bøler, J., Bowers, C. Y., and Schally, A. V. (1969). *Biochem. Biophys. Res. Commun.* **37**, 123.
Fried, J., Southanakrishnan, T. S., Himizu, J., Lin, C. H., Ford, S. H., Rubin, B., and Grigas, E. O. (1969). *Nature (London)* **223**, 208.
Furth, J. (1955). *Recent Progr. Horm. Res.* **11**, 221.
Gillessen, D., Felix, A. M., Lergier, W., and Studer, R. O. (1970). *Helv. Chim. Acta* **53**, 63.
Goluboff, L. G., MacRae, M. E., Ezrin, C., and Sellers, E. A. (1970). *Endocrinology* **87**, 1113.
Grodsky, G. M., and Bennett, L. L. (1966). *Diabetes* **15**, 910.
Guillemin, R. (1964). *Recent Progr. Horm. Res.* **20**, 89.
Guillemin, R. (1967). *Annu. Rev. Phys.* **29**, 313.
Guillemin, R. (1968). *In* "Pharmacology of Hormonal Polypeptides and Proteins" (N. Back *et al.*, eds.), p. 148. Plenum Press, New York.
Guillemin, R. (1971a). *Advan. Metab. Disord.* **5**, 1.
Guillemin, R. (1971b). *Neuroscience* (in press).
Guillemin, R., and Sakiz, E. (1965). *Nature (London)* **207**, 297.

Guillemin, R., and Vale, W. (1970). *In* "Hypophysiotropic Hormones of the Hypothalamus" (J. Meites, ed.), p. 21. Williams & Wilkins, Baltimore, Maryland.

Guillemin, R., Yamazaki, E., Jutisz, M., and Sakiz, E. (1962). *C. R. Acad. Sci.* **255,** 1018.

Guillemin, R., Yamazaki, E., Gard, D. A., Jutisz, M., and Sakiz, E. (1963). *Endocrinology* **73,** 564.

Guillemin, R., Sakiz, E., and Ward, D. N. (1964). *C. R. Acad. Sci.* **258,** 6567.

Guillemin, R., Sakiz, E., and Ward, D. N. (1965). *Proc. Soc. Exp. Biol. Med.* **118,** 1132.

Guillemin, R., Burgus, R., Sakiz, E., and Ward, D. N. (1968). *C. R. Acad. Sci.* **262,** 2278.

Guillemin, R., Burgus, R., and Vale, W. (1969). *Proc. Int. Congr. Endocrinol., 3rd, 1968* Int. Congr. Ser. No. 184, p. 577.

Hall, R., Amos, J., Garry, R., and Buxton, R. L. (1970). *Brit. Med. J.* **2,** 274.

Hershman, J. M., and Pittman, J. D. (1970). *J. Clin. Endocrinol. Metab.* **31,** 457.

Hodgkin, A. L., and Keynes, R. D. (1957). *J. Physiol. (London)* **138,** 253.

Hoffmann, K., and Bowers, C. Y. (1970). *J. Med. Chem.* **13,** 1099.

Hokin, L. E. (1951). *Biochem. J.* **48,** 320.

Hukovic, S., and Muscholl, E. (1962). *Naunyn-Schmiedebergs Arch. Exp. Pathol. Pharmakol.* **244,** 81.

Hymer, W., and Evans, W. (1970). *J. Cell. Biol.* **47,** 94a.

Jutisz, M., and de la Llosa, M. P. (1968). *Bull. Soc. Chim. Biol.* **50,** 2521.

Jutisz, M., de la Llosa, P., Sakiz, E., Yamazaki, E., and Guillemin, R. (1963a). *C. R. Soc. Biol.* **157,** 235.

Jutisz, M., Yamazaki, E., Berault, A., Sakiz, E., and Guillemin, R. (1963b). *C. R. Acad. Sci.* **256,** 2925.

Kamm, O., Aldrich, T. B., Grote, I. W., Rowe, L. W., and Bugbee, E. P. (1928). *J. Amer. Chem. Soc.* **50,** 573.

Kaneko, T., Zor, U., and Field, J. B. (1969). *Science* **163,** 1062.

Kraicer, J. V., and Milligan, J. V. (1970). *Program 52nd Meet. Endocrine Soc., 1970* p. 215.

Kudo, C. F., and Beck, J. C. (1970). *Program 52nd Meet. Endocrine Soc., 1970* p. 143.

Kuehl, F. A., Humes, J. L., Tarnoff, J., Grillo, V. J., and Ham, E. A. (1970). *Science* **169,** 883.

Lacy, P. E., Howell, S. L., Young, D. A., and Fink, C. V. (1968). *Nature (London)* **219,** 1177.

Liao, T., and Pierce, J. G. (1970). *J. Biol. Chem.* **245,** 3275.

McCann, S. M., and Porter, J. C. (1969). *Physiol. Rev.* **49,** 249.

McKenzie, J. M. (1958). *Endocrinology* **63,** 372.

MacLeod, R. M., and Fontham, E. H. (1970). *Endocrinology* **86,** 863.

MacLeod, R. M., and Lehymeyer, J. E. (1970). *Clin. Res.* **18,** 366.

Malaisse-Lagae, F., and Malaisse, W. J. (1971). *Endocrinology* **88,** 72.

Martin, J. B., and Reichlin, S. (1970). *Science* **168,** 1366.

Martini, L., and Ganong, W. F., eds. (1967). "Neuroendocrinology," Vol. 2. Academic Press, New York.

Meites, J., ed. (1970). "Hypophysiotropic Hormones of the Hypothalamus." Williams & Wilkins, Baltimore, Maryland.

Meites, J., and Nicoll, C. S. (1966). *Annu. Rev. Physiol.* **28,** 57.

Mikiten, T. M., and Douglas, W. W. (1965). *Nature (London)* **207**, 302.

Milligan, J. V., and Kraicer, J. (1970). *Fed. Proc., Fed. Amer. Soc. Exp. Biol.* **29**, 312.

Milner, R. D. G., and Hales, C. N. (1967). *Diabetologia* **3**, 47.

Milhaud, G., Rivaille, P., Moukhtar, M. S., Job, J. C., and Binet, E. (1970). *C. R. Acad. Sci.* **271**, 1900.

Mitnick, M., and Reichlin, S. (1971). *Science* **172**, 1241.

Mittler, J. C., and Redding, T. W. (1969). *Proc. Int. Congr. Endocrinol., 3rd, 1968* Int. Congr. Ser. No. 157, p. 93.

Monahan, M., Rivier, J., Burgus, R., Amoss, M., Blackwell, R., Vale, W., and Guillemin, R. (1971). *C. R. Acad. Sci. (Paris)* **273**, 205.

Mongar, J. L., and Schild, H. O. (1962). *Physiol. Rev.* **42**, 226.

Nair, R. M. G., Barrett, J. F., Bowers, C. Y., and Schally, A. V. (1970). *Biochemistry* **9**, 1103.

Nicolaides, E. D., Rebstock, B., and Burgus, R. (1971). Unpublished data.

Onaya, T., and Solomon, D. H. (1969). *51st Meet. Endocrine Soc., 1969* p. 54.

Pharriss, B. B., Wyngarden, L. J., and Gutknecht, G. D. (1968). *In* "Gonadotropins" (E. Rosemberg, ed.), p. 121. Geron-X, Los Altos, California.

Pierce, J. G., Liao, T., Carlsen, R. B., and Reiimo, T. (1971). *J. Biol. Chem.* **246**, 866.

Pietta, P. G., and Marshall, G. R. (1970). *Chem. Commun.* p. 650.

Poisner, A. M., and Trifaró, J. M. (1967). *Mol. Pharmacol.* **3**, 561.

Porter, J. C., Goldman, B. D., and Wilber, J. F. (1970). *In* "Hypophysiotropic Hormones of the Hypothalamus" (J. Meites, ed.), p. 282. Williams and Wilkins, Baltimore.

Porter, J. C., Vale, W., Burgus, R., Mical, R. S., and Guillemin, R. (1971). *Endocrinology* (in press).

Ramwell, P. W., and Shaw, J. E. (1967). *In* "Prostaglandins" (S. Bergström and B. Samuelsson, eds.), p. 283. Wiley, New York.

Ramwell, P. W., and Shaw, J. E. (1970). *Recent Progr. Horm. Res.* **26**, 139.

Rasmussen, H., and Tenenhouse, A. (1968). *Proc. Nat. Acad. Sci. U. S.* **59**, 1364.

Redding, T. W., and Schally, A. V. (1967). *Proc. Soc. Exp. Biol. Med.* **124**, 243.

Redding, T. W., and Schally, A. V. (1969a). *Proc. Soc. Exp. Biol. Med.* **131**, 415.

Redding, T. W., and Schally, A. V. (1969b). *Proc. Soc. Exp. Biol. Med.* **131**, 420.

Redding, T. W., Bowers, C. Y., and Schally, A. V. (1966). *Endocrinology* **79**, 229.

Rivaille, P., and Milhaud, G. (1971). *Helv. Chim. Acta* **54**, 355.

Rivier, J., Burgus, R., and Vale, W. (1971). *53rd Annu. Meet. Endocrine Soc., 1971,* page A-86.

Sakiz, E., and Guillemin, R. (1964). *Proc. Soc. Exp. Biol. Med.* **115**, 856.

Sakiz, E., and Guillemin, R. (1965). *Endocrinology* **77**, 797.

Samli, M. H., and Geschwind, I. I. (1968). *Endocrinology* **82**, 225.

Samuelsson, B. (1965). *J. Amer. Chem. Soc.* **87**, 3011.

Sandow, A. (1952). *Yale J. Biol. Med.* **25**, 176.

Schally, A. V., Bowers, C. Y., and Redding, T. W. (1966a). *Endocrinology* **78**, 726.

Schally, A. V., Redding, T. W., Barrett, J. F., and Bowers, C. Y. (1966b). *Fed. Proc., Fed. Amer. Soc. Exp. Biol.* **25**, 348.

Schally, A. V., Bowers, C. Y., Redding, T. W., and Barrett, J. F. (1966c). *Biochem. Biophys. Res. Commun.* **25**, 165.

Schally, A. V., Arimura, A., Bowers, C. Y., Kastin, A. J., Sawano, S., and Redding, T. W. (1968). *Recent Progr. Horm. Res.* **24**, 497.

Schally, A. V., Redding, T. W., Bowers, C. Y., and Barrett, J. F. (1969). *J. Biol. Chem.* **244**, 4077.

Schneider, F. (1963). *Hoppe-Seyler's Z. Physiol. Chem.* **334**, 26.

Schneider, F., and Schaeg, W. (1962). *Hoppe-Seyler's Z. Physiol. Chem.* **327**, 74.

Schreiber, V. (1963). "The Hypothalamo-Hypophysial System," Publ. House Czech. Acad. Sci., Prague.

Shimizu, H., Creveling, C. R., and Daly, J. W. (1970). *Biochem. Psychopharmacol.* **3**, 135.

Sinha, D. K., and Meites, J. (1966). *Endocrinology* **78**, 1002.

Smith, R. E., and Farquhar, M. G. (1966). *J. Cell Biol.* **31**, 319.

Solomon, S. H., and McKenzie, J. M. (1964). *Can. Med. Ass. J.* **90**, 487.

Steiner, A. L., Peake, G. T., Utiger, R. D., Karl, I. E., and Kipnis, D. M. (1970). *Endocrinology* **86**, 1354.

Thorn, N. A. (1965). *Acta Endocrinol. (Copenhagen)* **35**, 379.

Tsuji, S., Sakoda, M., and Asami, M. (1968). *In* "Integrative Mechanisms of Neuroendocrine System" (S. Itoh, ed.), p. 63. Hokkaido Univ. School of Med. Hokkaido, Japan.

Vale, W. (1968). Doctoral Dissertation, submitted to Baylor College of Medicine, Houston, Texas.

Vale, W., and Guillemin, R. (1967). *Experientia* **23**, 855.

Vale, W., and Guillemin, R. (1971). Unpublished data.

Vale, W., Amoss, M., Burgus R., Guillemin, R. (1967a). *Intern. Symp. Pharm. Horm. Polypeptides*, p. 122. Milan, Italy.

Vale, W., Burgus, R., and Guillemin, R. (1967b). *Experientia* **23**, 853.

Vale, W., Burgus, R., and Guillemin, R. (1967c). *Proc. Soc. Exp. Biol. Med.* **125**, 210.

Vale, W., Burgus, R., and Guillemin, R. (1968). *Neuroendocrinology* **3**, 34.

Vale, W., Burgus, R., Dunn, T. F., and Guillemin, R. (1970). *J. Clin. Endocrinol. Metab.* **30**, 148.

Vale, W., Burgus, R., Dunn, T. F., and Guillemin. R. (1971a). *Hormones* **2**, 193.

Vale, W., Rivier, C., and Guillemin, R. (1971b). *Fed. Proc., Fed. Amer. Soc. Exp. Biol.* **30**, 363.

Wilber, J. F. (1970). *Program 52nd Meet. Endocrine Soc., 1970* p. 42.

Wilber, J. F., and Utiger, R. D. (1968). *Proc. Soc. Exp. Biol. Med.* **127**, 488.

Wilber, J. F., and Utiger, R. D. (1969). *Endocrinology* **84**, 1316.

Wilber, J. F., Peake, C. T., and Utiger, R. D. (1969). *Endocrinology* **84**, 758.

Woodin, A. M., and Wieneke, A. A. (1964). *Biochem. J.* **90**, 498.

Yamazaki, E., Sakiz, E., and Guillemin, R. (1963a). *Experientia* **19**, 480.

Yamazaki, E., Sakiz, E., and Guillemin, R. (1963b). *Ann. Endocrinol.* **24**, 795.

Zor, U., Keneko, T., Schneider, H. P. G., McCann, S. M., Lowe, I. P., Bloom, G., Borland, B., and Field, J. B. (1969). *Proc. Nat. Acad. Sci. U. S.* **63**, 918.

The Chemistry of Parathyroid Hormone
and the Calcitonins

JOHN T. POTTS, JR., HENRY T. KEUTMANN,
HUGH D. NIALL, AND GEOFFREY W. TREGEAR

Endocrine Unit, Massachusetts General Hospital, and Department of Medicine, Harvard Medical School, Boston, Massachusetts

I. INTRODUCTION

In the last several years there have been striking advances in our knowledge of the chemistry of parathyroid hormone and calcitonin. The complete amino acid sequence of the major form of bovine and porcine parathyroid hormone has been determined, and, as well, the complete structure of porcine, human, ovine, bovine, and three different isohormonal forms of salmon calcitonin. These advances are potentially of considerable interest and importance to investigators and clinicians concerned with the physiology, mode of action, and clinical significance of parathyroid hormone and calcitonin. The significance of these chemical advances, particularly the availability of highly potent and completely homogeneous preparations of synthetic parathyroid hormone and calcitonin can best be appreciated in terms of a historical perspective. The importance of the secretory product of the parathyroid glands in maintaining a normal serum calcium has been appreciated since the turn of the century. Collip, over 45 years ago, produced the first biologically active extracts of parathyroid hormone from bovine glands (Collip, 1925). Intensive physiological and clinical investigations have established the importance of parathyroid hormone in normal calcium homeostasis and in certain diseases involving disorders of calcium and bone metabolism. The hormone acts to increase rates of bone resorption and to reduce the rate of urinary calcium loss, thereby maintaining serum calcium and preventing hypocalcemia. It has been appreciated that tumors of the parathyroid glands which secrete excessive amounts of parathyroid hormone lead to a well-described clinical syndrome, primary hyperparathyroidism, in which kidney stones, ulcers, and occasionally severe demineralization of bone, accompany the generally deleterious metabolic effects of a high blood calcium. Earlier arguments concerning the possibility that there were two different hormones secreted from the parathyroid gland—one acting on the receptors in kidney to promote increased phosphate clearance, and a second form active on bone to cause increased exit of calcium from the skeleton—have been resolved. It is now clear that a single hormonal polypeptide from the parathyroids is active on both kidney and bone. However, there is still much to be learned about the details of the molecular interaction between parathyroid hormone and the receptor binding sites in kidney and bone, although recent advances have pointed toward a possible mediating role for increased production of intracellular cyclic AMP. The availability of synthetic peptide subfragments of the parathyroid polypeptide as well as analogs of the sequences found in nature, will permit a detailed evaluation of receptor binding requirements in kidney and bone, particularly with regard to whether the binding requirements of receptor sites are identical in the two tissues. The development of radioimmunoassays sufficiently sensitive to detect endogenous parathyroid hormone has already led to great improvements in diagnosis and management of patients with primary hyperparathyroidism. However, recent evidence has indicated that once parathyroid hormone is released into the circulation its metabolic fate is complex. Degradation appears to occur in the periphery, presumably in a discrete extravascular site or in the circulatory bed of an as yet unidentified organ; the cleavage products resulting from degradation of the secreted hormonal polypeptide persist for hours in the circulation. Since it is now appreciated that small fragments of the hormone are biologically active, it is clear that the chemical nature of the active molecular species of circulating endogenous parathyroid hormone is still not established. Detailed physiological and metabolic studies with the intact hormonal polypeptide and smaller peptide subfragments should help to resolve this question. In addition, despite the diagnostic advances made possible by the application of radioimmunoassay techniques for parathyroid hormone, the presence of discrete fragments of the parathyroid hormone polypeptide in the circulation has apparently led to confusion in interpretation of assay results reported from different laboratories. Since the assay of endogenous parathyroid hormone is based on an immunochemical reaction, namely, the displacement of the radioactivity labeled hormone from antiparathyroid antibody prepared by immunization of animals with the intact hormone extracted from glands, it is now apparent that some portion of what is measured as immunoreactive hormone in blood may be biologically inert fragments that are cleared from blood rather slowly. Measurements of immunoreactive hormone based on detection of these fragments would not provide a clear picture of the secretory activity of the gland nor its responsiveness to normal controlling stimuli. Preparation by peptide synthesis of fragments corresponding to different regions of the hormonal polypeptide will make possible development of immunoassay techniques selective for detection of the biologically active amino terminal subfragments of the hormone and thereby improve the accuracy and interpretability of immunoassay studies. Thus, the advances inherent in complete structural characterization of parathyroid hormone and synthesis of biologically active parathyroid hormone peptides, only now completed some 45 years after the pioneering work of Collip with crude gland extracts, has caught up with rapidly advancing physiological, biochemical, and clinical studies involving parathyroid hormone action. The advances in the chemistry of parathyroid hormone should greatly facilitate progress in other areas of research on parathyroid hormones.

Calcitonin is the potent hypocalcemic, hypophosphatemic peptide hormone which, in many ways, acts as the physiological antagonist to parathyroid hormone. Calcitonin reduces bone resorption and has opposing effects to parathyroid hormone on the kidney; calcitonin increases renal calcium clearance. This hormone, whose existence in nature was unsuspected ten years ago has already been the subject of intensive studies of physiological action and the hormone has been extensively evaluated as a therapeutic agent of potential value in skeletal diseases characterized by excessive demineralization. Advances in our chemical knowledge of calcitonin isolated from man and from many animal species have been extremely rapid when considered in relation to the very recent discovery of the hormone or our still inadequate understanding of the hormonal role of this peptide. Although it is appreciated that calcitonin exerts its hypocalcemic, hypophosphatemic action principally by an overall inhibition of bone resorption, the initial step in hormone action or the character or location of the initial target cells influenced by the hormone is not known. For example, calcitonin is found in abundance in fishes, including some species such as the dogfish shark, which has an entirely cartilaginous skeleton. This paradox plus the recent demonstration that calcitonin acts on the kidney to profoundly influence the transport of numerous ions such as sodium and potassium as well as calcium and phosphate have suggested the possibility that the evolutionary significance of calcitonin and the physiological mode of action of the hormone may be ultimately explained in terms of a primary action on ion transport rather than on specific interaction with bone cells.

Much of the great clinical interest in calcitonin has been stimulated by promising reports of its possible therapeutic value in diseases character-ized by excessive bone turnover and mineral loss from the skeleton, such as Paget's disease of bone.

It is interesting to note the contrasts in rate of growth of knowledge of the chemical features of calcitonin and parathyroid hormone. Even at the present time, when many features of the mode of action of calcitonin or its role in human physiology remain quite unclear, we find that the structure of seven different forms of calcitonin from five different species has been determined and that successful large-scale synthesis of highly active porcine, human, and salmon calcitonin has been accomplished, thereby making available large supplies of purified material for detailed clinical, pharmacological, and physiological investigations.

The rapid advances in the chemistry of both polypeptide hormones made in the last few years reflects primarily the striking improvements that have been made in biochemical techniques used in the isolation, sequence analysis, and synthesis of biologically important polypeptides. A multiplicity of refined techniques for achieving fractionation of poly-peptides has been developed along with several sensitive techniques for assessment of the purity of polypeptide or protein fractions. Techniques for structural analysis, particularly those based on sequential degradation by the Edman technique have been developed to a refined state of great sensitivity and speed, and have been reduced to operation in automatic equipment. Finally, in addition to great improvements in the classic approaches for peptide synthesis using fragment condensation methods, there have been introduced solid phase supports and newer techniques for stepwise addition of amino acids during synthesis. These methodological advances have all combined to make possible extremely rapid progress in structural analysis and synthesis of polypeptides or proteins at a pace of accomplishment that would have been impossible five years ago.

This review will list these advances in the isolation, sequence analysis, and synthesis of calcitonin and parathyroid hormone. The emphasis in the studies reviewed will be current and selective, rather than comprehen-sive, in an effort to present a concise, but clear picture of the present state of our knowledge about the chemistry and structure-activity relations in these hormonal polypeptides. Relevant descriptions of the techniques employed will be listed along with references containing fuller treatments of the methods. Finally, the implications and probable new directions of research relating these chemical advances to the broader context of investigation of parathyroid hormone and calcitonin will be examined.

II. Isolation

A. General Considerations in Peptide Hormone Isolation

Experience with efforts to isolate hormonal polypeptides has led to recognition of numerous potential pitfalls in isolation studies, and have made evident the need both for systematic evaluation of yields of biological activity at each step in fractionation and detailed tests of purity of the final product believed to represent the hormonal peptide in a homogeneous form.

Successful purification of parathyroid hormone and calcitonin from tissues of several species has been made possible by a number of important advances in recent years, both in the methods available for extraction and fractionation of the peptides, and in the techniques used for evaluating purity of polypeptide preparations. A wide variety of newer approaches to peptide fractionation have been developed that make it possible to carry out efficient purification of even minute amounts of hormone with accuracy and confidence.

The powerful nature of the many recently developed schemes for fractionation of peptides stems from the wide range of principles upon which these methods are based. Thus, it is possible to subject an extracted peptide to separation on the basis of size through gel filtration, or on the basis of charge through application of ion exchange chromatography. Solvent partition makes use of the differing solubility properties among different peptides. Advantage may be taken of special physical properties by use of various types of adsorption columns, or by employment of special solvents, such as urea or guanidine solutions, in conjunction with any of these systems. These methods have been particularly useful in application to large-scale purification of milligram or even gram quantities of peptide. Additional techniques, including preparative-scale thin-layer chromatography, disc gel electrophoresis, ultracentrifugation, and isoelectric focusing are particularly helpful in isolation of microgram quantities of peptides.

Even when a purified, biologically active hormonal peptide is finally obtained by use of well chosen fractionation methods, and the product satisfies multiple chemical criteria for homogeneity and shows a constant specific biological activity, it is still essential to subject the preparation to further fractionation procedures. When fractionation methods are employed which are based on different principles than those already used, and it is found that biological activity and the polypeptide fraction remain coincident, further assurance is provided that the hormone has been isolated.

However, the conclusion that a given hormone has been isolated in homogeneous form is never definitive until the structure of the peptide believed to be the hormone has been deduced and is followed by the demonstration that a synthetic peptide, prepared on the basis of the structure proposed, has the full biological activity of the natural product (Potts, 1970b).

The importance of a satisfactory means of initial extraction of hormone from tissue is well illustrated by the difficulties encountered in the extraction of parathyroid hormone from bovine glands. The method must be efficient enough to remove the hormone from the tissue in high yield, but not so vigorous as to cause physical or chemical modification of the hormonal polypeptide. Close attention must also be paid to the percentage recovery of biological activity during each extraction step, to avoid the isolation of an inert peptide with biological activity that represents only trace contamination with the actual hormone (this type of error actually occurred during early studies of calcitonin isolation). It is also important to be aware of the possibility that a nonpeptide cofactor, necessary for biological activity, could be removed during the course of the extraction.

Techniques for monitoring the extent of chemical purification during the course of isolation have also undergone considerable refinement and improvement in recent years. Fractions obtained across peaks of polypeptide eluted from columns may be precisely examined for purity and constancy of composition by such sensitive methods as the Edman phenylisothiocyanate procedure (Niall, 1971), analytical scale disc gel electrophoresis, thin-layer chromatography, and amino acid analysis (see, for example, Hirs, 1967).

It is also essential to monitor the recovery of biological activity. Not only must the activity be recovered in satisfactory yield step by step, but a satisfactory increase in biological potency should be demonstrated following each step. Failure to devote adequate attention to activity could result in significant loss of hormone through the use of inappropriate extraction and purification methods, or damage to or destruction of the hormonal peptide. Quantitative bioassay of all fractions across a column elution profile is particularly valuable in providing assurance that complete activity is being recovered from the column. This method was of special importance in several respects during the purification of the calcitonins, permitting definitive localization of the porcine molecule in the first successful gel filtration experiments, and also resulting in the discovery, later, of two isohormones of salmon calcitonin (Keutmann *et al.*, 1970). Such quantitative monitoring is also essential in the evaluation of disc gel electrophoresis and thin-layer chromatography patterns, particularly in providing assurance that the predominating peptide detected by chemical criteria is indeed one and the same as the active peptide desired. Application of the bovine radioimmunoassay as a quantitative measure of hormonal activity proved to be particularly useful during purification of human parathyroid hormone.

Once it can be stated with complete assurance that the active hormone has been isolated in homeogeneous form, meaningful studies of its composition and physical characteristics can be carried out. Fundamental to these compositional studies is the technique of amino acid analysis, which has undergone recent refinements that have made the technique more versatile and senstive. Complete analyses may now be carried out in 2–3 hours, using as little as 2 or 3 nanomoles of peptide, with the use of completely automatic, highly sensitive amino acid analyzers. Peptides are prepared for analysis both by acid hydrolysis and by the newer technique of total enzymatic digestion (Keutmann and Potts, 1969). The latter procedure permits analysis of certain labile residues destroyed by acid hydrolysis, including amino acids with side chain substituents, such as carbohydrates, iodide, or phosphate. Many conventional analytical procedures are also sufficiently sensitive to be applied to the detection of such prosthetic groups. It is also important to ascertain the status of any cysteine residues by application of special techniques for detection of disulfide linkages and free sulfhydryl groups. Sensitive spectrophotometric methods are available for evaluation of the content of aromatic groups such as tryptophan and tyrosine.

Examples of some pitfalls and problems encountered in peptide isolation, and the value of some of the newer methods of fractionation, chemical and biological monitoring, and compositional analysis are well illustrated by the successful approaches, described in the following sections, to the isolation of homogeneous preparations of the parathyroid hormones and calcitonins.

B. PARATHYROID HORMONE

Although the role of the parathyroid glands in the prevention of tetany and maintenance of normal plasma calcium levels has been appreciated since the late 19th century (MacCallum and Voegtlin, 1909), a reliable method for extraction of an active principle from parathyroid tissue was not accomplished for many years afterward. Success in obtaining an active extract was reported by some workers (Berman, 1924; Hanson, 1925), but the failure of others prompted one authority to remark, "It is now generally agreed that the parathyroid secretion produces no acute effect when injected into blood" (Sharpy-Schaffer, 1924).

In 1925, however, Collip provided conclusive evidence that by use of hot hydrochloric acid a potent substance could be extracted from bovine parathyroid glands which corrected hypocalcemia and tetany in para-thyroidectomized dogs. Collip's method employed treatment of defatted glands with 5% hydrochloric acid for 60 minutes at 100°C, followed by isoelectric precipitation at pH 4.8. This substance, thought on the basis of crude compositional studies to be a polypeptide, was at first named para-thyrin, although later the term parathyroxine was suggested (Thompson and Collip, 1932). A commercial extract was subsequently prepared, using the method of Collip, by the Eli Lilly Company and marketed under the name Parathormone.

Although these crude extracts have been and still are useful in both clinical and laboratory applications, the need for a more highly purified product was evident from the beginning. However, attempts to achieve further fractionation of the acid extract met with little success, as many groups reported obtaining multiple active fractions without any improve-ment in overall potency (Handler et al., 1954; Rasmussen and Westall, 1957; Aurbach et al., 1958). In 1959, Aurbach, examining these observa-tions closely (1959a), recognized the probability that these multiple fractions arose as the result of cleavages within the peptide chain during the acid extraction process. The introduction a few years earlier of re-liable biossay methods (Munson, 1955; Davies et al., 1954) also made possible reliable and precise monitoring of hormone recoveries, facilitating the study of alternative extraction procedures. The result of Aurbach's investigation was the introduction of phenol as the extraction solvent. Use of phenol led to extractions of a stable hormone preparation in high yield, with no evidence of cleavages within the peptide chain. The technique consisted of treatment of the gland powder with 90% (weight/volume) phenol, followed by precipitation of the extract with acetone and ether. The precipitate was redissolved in 80% acetic acid, and a second pre-cipitation was carried out with 3% trichloroacetic acid (Aurbach, 1959a). This method found prompt and widespread use, and has been applied on a commercial scale by the Wilson Laboratories. Subsequently, Rasmussen et al. (1964) introduced another efficient extraction method, using urea and cysteine in cold hydrochloric acid.

After further purification of phenol extracts by countercurrent dis-tribution, Aurbach (1959a) obtained a product which was 2800 times as active as the crude gland powder. Rasmussen and Craig (1959, 1961), using a similar approach, isolated a comparably potent peptide, which they reported to contain 76 amino acids. The somewhat cumbersome nature of the countercurrent method led to a search for other efficient means for large-scale purification of the extracts. The result was the introduction of hormone isolation on the basis of peptide size using gel filtration on Sephadex G-50 (Rasmussen and Craig, 1962) and later Sephadex G-100 (Aurbach and Potts, 1964; Rasmussen et al., 1964). In 1965, Potts and Aurbach reported isolation of a highly purified parathyroid polypeptide by means of Sephadex G-100 gel filtration, followed by ion exchange chromatography on carboxymethyl cellulose (CMC). The sequence of steps in the purification, and the recovery of hormone following each step as monitored by a radioimmunoassay, are summarized in Table I.

Compositional study of this product indicated that the polypeptide consisted of approximately 81 amino acids (Potts et al., 1966). When this material was examined by the highly sensitive technique of disc gel electrophoresis, however, several polypeptide bands could still be detected. After these bands were eluted from the gel, at least two of them were found to contain biological and immunological activity. The active bands were isolated by preparative-scale electrophoresis, and found to differ in amino acid composition by only a few residues, including the content of threonine (Potts et al., 1966).

The phenylisothiocyanate end-group procedure (Edman, 1960; Blomback et al., 1966) has undergone continued improvements in recent years and has become one of the most sensitive and useful methods for monitoring peptide purification. The value of this method in the case of parathyroid hormone became particularly evident during the course of preliminary work on sequence determination. Even the best preparations of

TABLE I

PURIFICATION OF BOVINE PARATHYROID HORMONE: RECOVERY OF IMMUNOLOGICAL
ACTIVITY AND INCREASE IN BIOLOGICAL ACTIVITY AFTER
SUCCESSIVE FRACTIONATION STEPS

| | Immunoassay[a] | | Specific biological activity (USP U/mg) |
Step	Efficiency (%)	Cumulative yield (%)	
Phenol extract	—	(100)	20
Acetone/ether precipitate	97	97	—
NaCl supernatant	93	90	—
TCA precipitate	88	79	340
Sephadex G-100	95	75	2500
Carboxymethyl cellulose	81	61	2500

[a] Starting material, phenol extract of 100 gm acetone-dried bovine parathyroid glands. Data from Keutmann et al. (1971a) and Potts et al. (1968b). Efficiency refers to recovery at each step when compared to yield at the previous step.

carboxymethyl cellulose-purified hormone were found to contain 10–20% contamination by two peptides containing amino terminal leucine and valine, respectively. These were felt clearly to be nonhormonal rather than different forms of the hormone with different end groups, since during the first 10–12 cycles of consecutive degradation three distinct amino acid sequences were detected. When the Edman method was used to examine successive fractions across the peak of hormone from carboxymethyl cellulose (CMC) chromatography (Fig. 1), the content of the contaminant end groups leucine and valine, relative to the alanine phenylthiohydantoins from the hormone itself, increased markedly in tubes to either side of the center of the peak. This suggested that even repeated chromatography with more shallow gradients would still not lead to complete purification by this approach.

Thus, despite the progress represented by the CMC purification method,

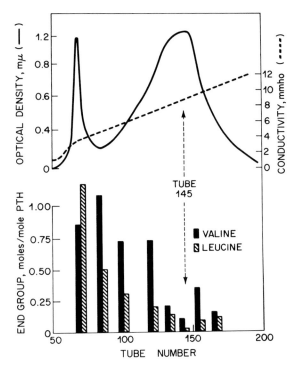

Fig. 1. Elution pattern of bovine parathyroid hormone (PTH) from a carboxymethyl cellulose column developed with a gradient of ammonium acetate buffer. The Edman degradation was used to evaluate the purity of the hormone in selected aliquots across the peptide peak. The vertical bars represent the content of nonhormonal contaminants, as measured by the valine and leucine phenylthiohydantoin end groups. Hormone of better than 90% purity is recovered only at the very center of the peak (tube 145) (Keutmann et al., 1971a).

the presence of several active chemically distinct variants of the hormone, as well as evidence of at least two nonhormonal contaminants spread throughout the hormone peak, called for exhaustive exploration of other means for further purification.

Several approaches to the further purification of hormone following CMC chromatography were investigated. For this work it was extremely helpful to have available the renal-cortical adenyl cyclase assay for parathyroid hormone developed by Marcus and Aurbach (1969). The simplicity, precision, and accuracy of this *in vitro* method make it superior to the rat bioassay (Munson, 1961; Aurbach, 1959b) for screening and evaluating the numerous samples generated during purification efforts. Attempted approaches included Sephadex gel adsorption chromatography in low ionic strength buffer, a method suggested for parathyroid hormone by Hawker *et al.* (1966), and adsorption of parathyroid hormone to hydroxyapatite. These attempts, however, were not successful (Keutmann *et al.,* 1971a).

In the hope of disrupting noncovalent associations between the hormone and contaminants, for example by altering the effective charge of the various peptides, a purification system was evaluated which employed (CMC) chromatography in the presence of 8 *M* urea. This procedure had previously been found useful in the purification of insulin and proinsulin (Steiner *et al.,* 1968). Accordingly, hormone obtained from

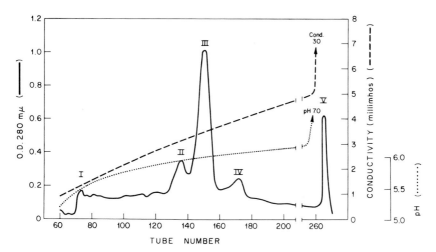

Fig. 2. Final step in the purification of bovine parathyroid hormone by ion exchange chromatography on carboxymethyl cellulose using a linear ammonium acetate gradient in the presence of 8 *M* urea. The predominant form of the hormone (parathyroid hormone I) eluted free from nonhormonal contaminants as peak III. The minor variants of the hormone, parathyroid hormone II and III, eluted in peak II and IV, respectively (Keutmann *et al.,* 1971a).

Sephadex G-100 gel chromatography was applied to a CMC column which had been equilibrated with ammonium acetate buffer containing $8\,M$ urea. The column was then eluted with a linear gradient of the buffer, also containing $8\,M$ urea (Keutmann et al., 1971a). The elution pattern is shown in Fig. 2. Biologically active hormone was found to elute in several components (peaks II, III, and IV), at an ionic strength lower than that previously found for columns run in the absence of urea. The predominant peak (III) was found to contain hormone completely free from nonhormonal contaminants: only a single phenylthiohydantoin, alanine, was detected by end group analysis (Fig. 3). The major, hor-

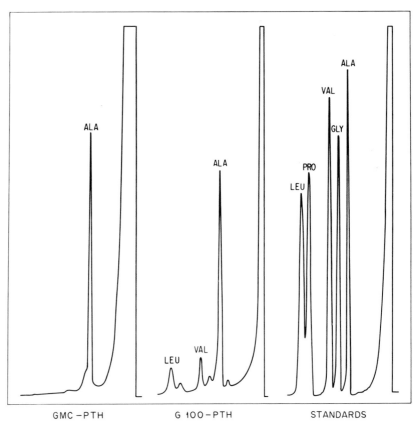

GMC−PTH   G 100−PTH   STANDARDS

Fig. 3. Gas–liquid chromatography of phenylthiohydantoins from Edman amino terminal end group determinations of bovine parathyroid hormone (PTH) from a Sephadex G-100 column, before and after final purification on carboxymethyl cellulose and $8\,M$ urea. The alanine end group is derived from the hormone. Valine and leucine end groups represent contamination by nonhormonal polypeptides, eliminated by the urea CMC chromatography (Keutmann et al., 1971a).

monally active peptide (peak III) contained 84 amino acids in stoichio-
metric yield, but in addition, submolar quantities of threonine were found,
an observation suggesting that small amounts of some additional peptide
were still present. The explanation was found on evaluation of peak II
from urea-CMC chromatography (Fig. 2), which eluted just ahead of the
predominant hormone peak III. The material in this lower-yield peak
also proved to be parathyroid hormone, of comparable biological activity
to the peak III material, but relatively rich in threonine by amino acid
analysis.

When each peak was rechromatographed separately on a urea-CMC
column, completely pure preparations of each hormone variant were obtained free from cross-contamination. On compositional analysis each
variant contained 84 amino acids, and differed only in the content of
threonine and valine. Peak III hormone, termed parathyroid hormone I,
contained 8 residues of valine and no threonine. Peak II, named parathyroid hormone II, contained 1 residue of threonine, and only 7 residues
of valine (Table II). Each migrated as a single band on disc gel, parathyroid hormone II moving slightly slower than the predominating parathyroid hormone I. Each of the isohormones had a specific biological
activity of approximately 1800–2500 units/mg by the rat bioassay
method of Aurbach (1959b), and 1500 units/mg by renal-cortical adenyl
cyclase bioassay (Keutmann et al., 1971a).

The threonine-containing parathyroid hormone II appeared to represent the minor variant, previously recovered from disc gel electrophoresis
by Potts and Aurbach (1966). The peak IV material (Fig. 2) was also
active, although at somewhat lower specific biological activity. Amino
acid analysis of peak IV closely resembled that of parathyroid hormone
II. This component, designated parathyroid hormone III, is currently
undergoing further study to determine whether it is a true isohormone or
an altered form of parathyroid hormone II.

Pure parathyroid hormone I, prepared as described (Keutmann et al.,
1971a) was used in the determination of the complete amino acid sequence of the molecule (Niall et al., 1970).

Applying many of the techniques previously developed for bovine
PTH, Dr. O'Riordan's group at Middlesex Hospital recently has completed the purification of porcine parathyroid hormone (Woodhead et al.,
1971). Their isolation scheme included phenol extraction, trichloroacetic
acid (TCA) precipitation, Sephadex G-100 gel filtration, and, finally,
ion exchange chromatography on CMC. It was not found necessary to use
the additional steps of CMC-chromatography in 8 M urea to obtain a
homogeneous hormonal product.

The radioimmunoassay, using antibody raised against bovine PTH

TABLE II

AMINO ACID COMPOSITION OF BOVINE AND PORCINE PARATHYROID HORMONES

Amino acid	Bovine I	Bovine II	Porcine
Aspartic acid	6	6	5
Asparagine	3	3	3
Threonine	0	1	0
Serine	8	8	8
Glutamic acid	6	6	6
Glutamine	5	5	5
Proline	2	2	2
½-Cystine	0	0	0
Glycine	4	4	5
Alanine	7	7	6
Valine	8	7	9
Methionine	2	2	1
Isoleucine	3	3	3
Leucine	8	8	10
Tyrosine	1	1	0
Phenylalanine	2	2	1
Tryptophan	1	1	1
Lysine	9	9	9
Histidine	4	4	5
Arginine	5	5	5
	84	84	84

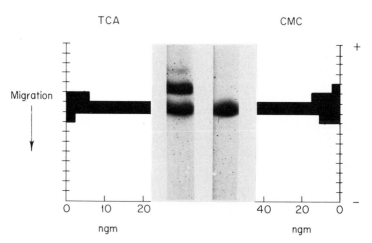

FIG. 4. Disc gel electrophoresis patterns of porcine parathyroid hormone after trichloroacetic acid (TCA) precipitation and after final purification on carboxymethyl cellulose (CMC). The horizontal bars show the distribution of immunologically active hormone after elution of gel slices and measurement by radioimmunoassay. All the activity is seen to coincide with the single peptide band in the CMC preparation (Woodhead et al., 1971).

(O'Riordan and Woodhead, 1970), was used extensively in monitoring the progress of purification. Figure 4 shows the application of this assay method to the assessment of purity by disc gel electrophoresis. The gels containing the peptide bands were split longitudinally; one half was stained, slices were taken from the corresponding portions of the opposite half, and the peptides were eluted and assayed. In the gel containing the partially purified hormone (TCA precipitate), the band containing immunological activity is easily discerned. In the gel containing the CMC purified hormone, the immunological activity is seen to coincide with the single peptide band, confirming that the material purified by the various column steps was indeed parathyroid hormone. The porcine hormone had comparable biological activity to bovine parathyroid hormones I and II.

The porcine hormone also contained 84 amino acids; several interesting differences in the amino acid composition of the porcine hormone were detected, however, including the absence of tyrosine and presence of one methionine residue, rather than two (Table II). The latter difference is of particular interest from the standpoint of structure–activity relationships, since both the bovine (Rasmussen and Craig, 1962; Tashjian et al., 1964) and the porcine (Woodhead et al., 1971) hormones lose biological activity when their methionines are oxidized to the sulfoxide form.

Limited availability of tissue has thus far restricted efforts to isolate and characterize human parathyroid hormone. O'Riordan and co-workers (1971) obtained from pooled adenoma tissue a peptide preparation which is similar in size and charge properties to the bovine and porcine molecules, although several differences in amino acid composition were found. The highly sensitive radioimmunoassay was essential in monitoring the various steps in the human purification, and revealed that the yield of hormone obtained at each stage was lower than that obtained with the other hormones. Thus, at the stage of TCA fractionation the human material was only 2.5% pure, and after Sephadex gel filtration, estimates of specific activity based on immunoassay indicated that the preparations contained only 10% hormone. At corresponding stages, bovine extracts are 30 and 70% pure, respectively. These findings serve to emphasize the fact that definitive purification and characterization of the human hormone may require not only the accumulation of larger amounts of tissue, but the adaptation of many of the current fractionation and chemical methods for use with minute quantities of peptide.

Another area of increasing interest in the parathyroid field, also benefiting from application of the radioimmunoassay, is the possible existence of a "prohormone" in the parathyroid gland. Drawing on observations that plasma hormone behaved differently in the radioimmunoassay from hormone extracted from gland tissue, Arnaud et al. (1971) postulated existence of a larger molecule stored in the gland, and broken down to the 84-residue peptide on secretion, in a similar manner to the proinsulin–insulin system (Steiner *et al.*, 1968). Sherwood *et al.* (1971), obtained similar assay results from *in vivo* tissue-culture systems. Sherwood concluded that a smaller fragment, of molecular weight 6000–7000, was the circulating active form of the hormone *in vivo* while the 84-residue molecule was itself a "prohormone" stored in the gland. Subsequent studies based on actual gel filtration analysis of plasma samples from peripheral blood and parathyroid venous effluent in man and in animals has indicated that the *in vitro* results of Sherwood *et al.* and Arnaud *et al.* are misleading (Habener *et al.*, 1971a; Potts *et al.*, 1971c). There are circulating fragments of parathyroid hormone smaller than the 84 amino acid hormonal peptide extracted from the glands, but these fragments arise from peripheral degradations. However, the search for a true prohormone, larger than the 84 amino acid polypeptide has continued. Cohn *et al.* (1971) have subsequently reported, on the basis of studies of incorporation of radioactive amino acids by gland tissue slices, the presence of a hypercalcemic factor eluting earlier from Sephadex G-100 than the 84 amino acid hormonal polypeptide; this larger peptide has been isolated from CMC and appears, on the basis of preliminary analyses, to contain approximately 100 amino acids. Isolation of these "prohormones" is attended by additional problems beyond that of small quantity; for example, there is the risk of enzymatic breakdown of these potentially labile peptides to smaller forms during extraction and handling. However, the studies of Cohn *et al.* and of Habener *et al.* are certainly consistent with the presence of a prohormone larger than the principal hormonal peptide extracted from human, bovine, or porcine pararthyroids. The use of techniques such as radioactive labeling during biosynthesis in tissue culture systems may be a promising approach in efforts at isolation of this prohormone.

C. CALCITONIN

The existence of a circulating factor capable of lowering plasma calcium was first demonstrated by Copp and his associates at the University of British Columbia in 1962. They named the substance calcitonin, and their discovery was confirmed soon afterward by MacIntyre and his co-workers at Royal Post-graduate Medical School (Kumar *et al.*, 1963). These earlier studies were based upon results of calcium infusions of the isolated thyroparathyroid gland complex in experimental animals, and a brief but lively debate ensued as to the exact site of origin of the new hormone.

Although originally thought to be elaborated by the parathyroid gland (Copp et al., 1962) the factor was extracted by Hirsch et al. (1963) from rat thyroid glands and named thyrocalcitonin to differentiate it from the presumed parathyroid hypocalcemic factor of Copp. Thyroid origin of the hormone in mammalian species was confirmed by studies in the goat by Foster et al. (1964a) and in the rat by Talmage et al. (1964). The superior parathyroid glands of the goat could be perfused separately from the thyroid. Similar perfusion preparations were used in the pig, with the same conclusions, in studies by Care (1965).

The source of calcitonin was further localized by morphologic studies which suggested that the hormone was elaborated not by the follicular cells, but by the interstitial or parafollicular cells of the thyroid (Foster et al., 1964b). Although these cells had been described many years earlier (Nonidez, 1932), no significant function had previously been ascribed to them. By use of fluorescent antibody techniques, Bussolati and Pearse (1967) were able to demonstrate directly the presence of calcitonin in these parafollicular or "C" cells.

It was of particular significance for later work in the field that these cells were recognized to have a different embryonic origin from the follicular cells of the thyroid (Pearse and Carvalhiera, 1967). Arising from the terminal branchial, or ultimobranchial, pouch, these cells merge with the follicular cells during embryonic development in mammals, but remain separate from the thyroid to form the ultimobranchial gland in lower vertebrates (Copp et al., 1967).

The small concentration of calcitonin stored in the thyroid of mammalian species gave rise to numerous difficulties in the course of early efforts to isolate and purify the hormone. In 1965, Tenenhouse et al. introduced an extraction procedure using cysteine, urea, and acetic acid, and reported obtaining a pure calcitonin peptide after Sephadex gel filtration of the extract. This conclusion proved to be incorrect, however, as the claim did not survive the scrutiny of quantitative monitoring by bioassay (Munson et al., 1967).

Such monitoring procedures were made possible by the introduction of several reliable bioassay systems based on hypocalcemia in the rat (Cooper et al., 1967; Copp and Kuczerpa, 1968; Schlueter and Caldwell, 1967). Repeating the Tenenhouse Sephadex gel filtration procedure, Munson et al. (1967) and Potts et al. (1967) bioassayed eluate pools from throughout the column run and found that only 15–20% of the applied activity eluted with the peak originally thought to be calcitonin. Most of the biological activity eluted in later fractions which were shown by analytical disc gel electrophoresis to be extremely heterogeneous. It was thus evident that much work remained to be done before a pure calcitonin peptide could be obtained.

Small quantities of purified peptide, suitable for preliminary compositional studies, were obtained by use of preparative disc gel electrophoresis (Potts et al., 1968a). However, only with the introduction of large-scale extraction and preliminary purification procedures by workers at the Armour, Ciba, and Lederle Pharmaceutical Companies did preparations of calcitonin become available in quantities sufficient to be used by several laboratories to accomplish, by use of different fractionation schemes, the complete purification of the porcine molecule (Brewer et al., 1968a; Bell, 1968; Gudmundsson et al., 1968).

A 44,000-fold purification of Armour extracts was carried out using successive gel filtration steps on Sephadex G-50 and G-25, followed by ion exchange chromatography on CMC (Brewer et al., 1968a). Biologically active hormone eluted from CMC in a double peak. Successive aliquots from across the entire peak were subjected to detailed analysis of both chemical purity and biological activity. Disc gel analysis of these fractions showed the presence of a single gel band throughout, and amino acid analysis after acid hydrolysis revealed a constant composition across the peak. Specific biological activity of the successive fractions was also constant. Despite this evidence of homogeneity, two discrete components, corresponding to the two segments of the double peak from CMC chromatography, were seen when the successive aliquots were examined by thin-layer chromatography. Amino acid analysis of the two components following total enzymatic digestion revealed that one component contained calcitonin with its single methionine oxidized to the sulfoxide form, while the other component comprised the hormone with its methionine in the native, reduced form. The two forms of calcitonin contained, as mentioned, identical specific biological activities.

A summary of the purification scheme for porcine calcitonin, showing the increase in specific biological activity at each successive step, is shown in Table III.

TABLE III
Purification of Porcine Calcitonin[a]

Step	Specific biological activity MRC units/mg
Porcine thyroid powder	0.0045
Partially purified acidic extract	15
Sephadex G-50 (fine)	50
Sephadex G-25 (superfine)	130
CMC gradient elution	200

[a] An overall purification of 44,000-fold was achieved. Data from Brewer et al. (1968b).

Further tests were made by Brewer *et al.* (1968a) to ensure that the homogeneous peptide isolated by CMC chromatography did indeed represent calcitonin. The purified hormone was subjected to refractionation by preparative thin-layer chromatography and disc gel electrophoresis, procedures based upon different principles of fractionation than ion-exchange chromatography. Bioassay of eluates from the thin-layer chromatogram showed that all biological activity was confined to the area occupied by the peptide. Figure 5 shows the results of bioassay studies of successive fractions from disc gel electrophoresis. The protein and all the applied biological activity appeared as a single coincident, symmetrical peak (Fig. 5). These studies provided convincing evidence that the isolated peptide was indeed calcitonin. Furthermore, assurance was obtained that there were no noncovalently bound cofactors in calcitonin important for biological activity, since such a cofactor would be expected to have been separated from the hormone by the denaturing solvents used during the several fractionation procedures applied.

The presence of cysteine in the calcitonin molecule necessitated the use of further procedures designed to evaluate the total content of this residue and the nature of the disulfide linkages, if any. Precise analysis of cysteine content by acid hydrolysis requires conversion of cystine to the more stable cysteic acid by performic acid oxidation, prior to acid hydrolysis where cysteine is destroyed. Alternatively, total enzymatic digestion permits direct analysis of the cystine itself. Both procedures were consistent with the presence of 2 moles of half-cystine per mole of porcine calcitonin. Titration with Ellmans reagent was carried out to determine whether the half-cystine residues were present in the reduced state (cysteine) or formed a cystine disulfide linkage. No free sulfhydryl

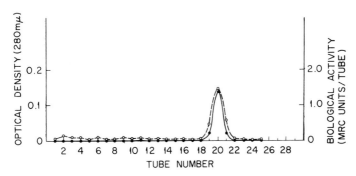

FIG. 5. Bioassay of successive fractions from preparative disc gel electrophoresis of carboxymethyl cellulose purified porcine calcitonin. All the applied biological activity eluted (dashed line) coincident with the single peak of peptide optical density (solid line) (Brewer *et al.*, 1968a).

groups were detected, indicating presence of the disulfide. Performic acid-oxidized calcitonin eluted from Sephadex G-25 in the same position as native calcitonin, providing evidence that the disulfide bridge was intra-chain, rather than joining two or more calcitonin molecules (Brewer et al., 1968).

The content of the labile residue tryptophan was evaluated by amino acid analysis following total enzymatic digestion, as well as by spectro-photometric assay. Direct chemical analysis of the purified product showed that there was no carbohydrate, phosphate, or iodide covalently bound to the calcitonin molecule. These results could be confirmed by demonstration of good agreement between amino acid analyses obtained after acid vs. enzymatic hydrolysis; no unusual amino acids were seen on the analyzer chromatograms after the enzymatic digestion (Brewer et al., 1968a).

Simultaneously, two other laboratories reported the successful isolation of porcine calcitonin. Bell and co-workers at Lederle introduced an ex-traction method similar to that applied earlier to ACTH, employing adsorption to oxidized cellulose. Their extract was purified by use of countercurrent distribution (Bell, 1968; Bell et al., 1968). Investigators at Ciba, in collaboration with the MacIntyre group at Hammersmith, used butanol–water–acetic acid for extraction, followed by purification by partition chromatography (Gudmundsson et al., 1968; Matthews et al., 1968; Neher et al., 1968a). The peptides isolated by all three laboratories were identical; each found a methionine and methionine sulfoxide form of calcitonin with the same specific biological activity.

By use of the method of gel filtration and ion exchange chromatog-raphy, two other ruminant calcitonins—bovine and ovine—were subse-quently purified in high yield from extracts prepared by Armour (Brewer et al., 1970; Potts et al., 1970). The specific biological activity of these two calcitonins and the porcine hormone were found to be closely similar (Table IV), and their amino acid compositions differed by only a few residues (Table V).

The isolation and characterization of human calcitonin was accom-plished by a group of investigators at Ciba in Switzerland, in collabora-tion with the MacIntyre group at the Royal Postgraduate Medical School. Use of normal human thyroid was precluded by the low content of stored calcitonin in the normal gland and difficulty in obtaining suffi-cient quantities of the tissue. Thus, these workers used a medullary carcinoma of the thyroid, a tumor consisting of calcitonin-rich C cells. By use of butanol–acetic acid extraction, gel filtration, and countercurrent distribution, a pure calcitonin polypeptide was isolated from a single tumor (Riniker et al., 1968). Calcitonin peptides of identical amino acid

TABLE IV

SPECIFIC ACTIVITY OF CALCITONINS FROM VARIOUS SPECIES[a]

Species	Mean potency (MRC units/mg)
Salmon I	2700
Salmon II	2400
Porcine	120
Bovine	50
Ovine	60
Human	70

[a] Data from Keutmann et al. (1970); bioassays were performed on lyophilized preparations of the purified polypeptides using the method of Parsons and Reynolds (1968).

composition were subsequently isolated and identified separately from four additional medullary carcinomas (Neher et al., 1968c). Other workers have found peptides with the same composition from separate tumors (Raulais and Keutmann, 1971). Although it is likely that the peptide from tumors is identical to that elaborated by the normal thyroid, the human hormone from normal tissue has still not been isolated in sufficient quantities for definitive characterization.

Two forms of the human peptide were isolated from the medullary carcinoma tissue. The first, calcitonin M, contained the same number of amino acids as the previously identified porcine hormone. The second, calcitonin D, twice as large as calcitonin M, proved to be a dimer of calcitonin M. The dimer could be converted into the monomer form by treatment with ammonium hydroxide (Riniker et al., 1968). Although the dimer was originally described as possessing full biological activity, subsequent evidence has suggested that the human calcitonin dimer is biologically inactive but is converted into the active monomer under the conditions of the bioassay (MacIntyre, 1970). Thus far, no dimer or other polymeric form has been definitively identified for any other species of calcitonin.

The presence of the C cells in a separate ultimobranchial gland in lower vertebrates stimulated interest in study of the calcitonins obtainable from several representative species. Copp and his co-workers demonstrated that calcitonin could be extracted from the ultimobranchial glands of several species of fish, amphibians, and birds (Copp et al., 1967; Copp and Parkes, 1968); this was shown also in the chicken by Tauber (1967). No significant calcitonin activity could be demonstrated in the thyroids of these various species (Copp and Parkes, 1968).

The large-scale extraction of ultimobranchial calcitonin was hindered by lack of a commercial source capable of providing large quantities of glands as a by-product, as was possible with bovine, porcine, and ovine glands obtained from slaughterhouses. The first species to provide such an opportunity was the Pacific salmon, a species not only caught and processed in large numbers commercially, but in which there are easily accessible ultimobranchial glands. In the course of preliminary work with extracts from these species, it was suggested that the salmon hormone was far more potent than any of the calcitonins previously isolated from mammalian species (O'Dor *et al.*, 1969).

Final purification of salmon ultimobranchial calcitonin was achieved by Sephadex gel filtration followed by ion exchange chromatography on

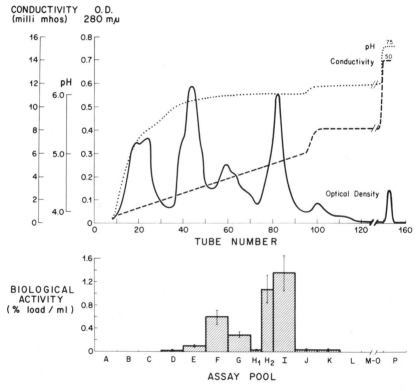

FIG. 6. Elution pattern of the final step in the purification of salmon calcitonin. The peptide was eluted from a carboxymethyl cellulose column using a gradient of ammonium acetate buffer, and the bioassay was performed on 10-tube eluate pools. The percentage of the applied activity recovered in each pool is expressed by the vertical bars. Of the applied activity, 96% was recovered in two active regions. Pools H_2 and I contained pure salmon calcitonin I (specific activity **2700 MRC** units/mg). Pool F contained the still heterogeneous calcitonins II and III (Keutmann *et al.*, 1970).

CMC (Keutmann *et al.*, 1970). The elution pattern from the CMC step is shown in Fig. 6, and illustrates further the usefulness of quantitative bioassay in monitoring column chromatography. Two-thirds of the applied activity eluted in the final peak, which proved to contain the salmon hormone (salmon calcitonin I) in pure form. This calcitonin had a specific biological activity approximately 20 times that of mammalian calcitonins when assayed in the rat (Table IV), and even higher when bioassayed in the mouse. Interest in this hormone was further stimulated by the finding that its amino acid composition differed greatly from that of either the ruminant or human calcitonins (Table V).

The remaining one-third of the biological activity applied to the salmon CMC column (Fig. 6) eluted as a second peak, earlier in the salt gradient than the predominant salmon I peptide. This lower-yield material, while still heterogeneous, appeared to differ by several amino acids from calcitonin I, although its biological potency was estimated to be comparable or perhaps even greater (Keutmann *et al.*, 1970).

Attempts to separate this "minor component" peptide from its con-

TABLE V
AMINO ACID COMPOSITION OF CALCITONINS FROM VARIOUS SPECIES

Amino acid	Porcine	Bovine	Ovine	Human	Salmon I	Salmon II	Salmon III
Lysine	0	1	1	1	2	2	2
Arginine	2	1	1	0	1	1	1
Histidine	1	1	1	1	1	1	1
Asparagine	4	3	3	2	2	2	2
Asparatic acid	0	1	1	1	0	1	1
Serine	4	4	4	1	4	3	3
Threonine	2	2	2	5	5	4	4
Glutamine	0	0	0	2	2	2	2
Glutamic acid	1	1	1	0	1	0	0
Proline	2	2	2	2	2	2	2
Glycine	3	3	3	4	3	3	3
Alanine	1	1	1	2	0	1	1
$\frac{1}{2}$-Cystine	2	2	2	2	2	2	2
Valine	1	1	1	1	1	2	1
Methionine	1	1	1	1	0	0	1
Isoleucine	0	0	0	1	0	0	0
Leucine	3	3	3	2	5	5	5
Tyrosine	1	2	3	1	1	0	0
Phenylalanine	3	2	1	3	0	1	1
Trytophan	1	1	1	0	0	0	0
	32	32	32	32	32	32	32

taminants in the native state by various further fractionation procedures were unsuccessful. Thus, the preparation was subjected to performic acid oxidation, in hopes of changing the charge of the calcitonin relative to the contaminants since oxidation would convert the cystine disulfide group into negatively charged cysteic acid residues. When the oxidation product was passed over an SE-Sephadex ion exchange column, the calcitonin separated readily from the contaminants. Furthermore, this "minor component" hormone was found to consist of two additional calcitonins (salmon calcitonin II and III), differing by four and five amino acids, respectively, from calcitonin I (Table V) (Potts *et al.*, 1971d). Although the biological activity of these calcitonins was lost by conversion to the oxidized state, assays of synthetic calcitonin II, recently prepared (Pless *et al.*, 1971) by Sandoz Pharmaceutical Company on the basis of the amino acid sequence deduced from use of the oxidized preparation, have shown this calcitonin to be of comparable specific activity to calcitonin I (Keutmann *et al.*, 1971c).

The nature of the species microheterogeneity evident in the isolation of these three forms of calcitonin from the salmon has been investigated by Lequin *et al.* (1971). Glands were collected separately from four different species of salmon (Sockeye, Coho, Chum, and Pink). The extracts from the species-selected tissues were purified as done previously (Keutmann *et al.*, 1970). Calcitonin I was found to be the predominant form in all four species. In addition, calcitonin II was found in three of the four species studied (Sockeye, Chum, and Pink). Calcitonin III was found in the fourth species (Coho). The two forms of calcitonin elaborated by each species is reminiscent of the situation encountered with insulin in the rat (Smith, 1966).

The wide differences in amino acid composition among the various calcitonins, and the high potency of the salmon ultimobranchial hormones, has stimulated interest in the isolation—currently underway—of ultimobranchial calcitonin from other species, such as the dogfish shark, trout, and various avian species.

III. Sequence Analysis

A. General Concepts

It is obvious that the determination of the complete amino acid sequence of a hormonal polypeptide must precede any real progress in the study of structure-function relations. Without such detailed structural information, only limited and provisional conclusions may be drawn about the functional groups in the hormone important for biological activity, usually conclusions made on the basis of selective chemical modification. As pointed out later in this review, studies of this kind carried out on calcitonin were shown by subsequent work to be quite misleading. Once the amino acid sequence is known, on the other hand, it it possible to carry out a systematic examination of the structural features involved in the action of the hormone, using both native hormone altered chemically in a controlled fashion, and natural and synthetic hormone fragments. Even during the course of the sequence determination, valuable information of this kind may be obtained, since the strategy used for obtaining the amino acid sequence necessarily involves chemical modification, cleavage, and isolation of fragments of the hormone all of which provide some opportunity for structure-function correlations.

The methods presently used for sequence determination are in a state of transition. The procedures used by protein chemists up to the last two to three years were laborious and expensive in manpower, time, and material. They involved the cleavage of the polypeptide by at least two independent procedures to generate two complete and different steps of small peptide subfragments, adding up to the complete structure. All these peptides had to be isolated, often from mixtures containing 20 to 30 different components, and their amino acid composition, and partial or complete sequence established through the use of a battery of different chemical and enzymatic procedures. The sequence was pieced together on the basis of this combined information, the relative order of the fragments being established by the identification of a sufficient number of overlapping peptides bridging primary cleavage positions.

A dramatic change in this situation came with the development of automated procedures for sequence analysis of proteins (Edman and Begg, 1967) and peptides (Niall et al., 1969a). These methods were based on the degradation devised by Edman (1950) in which the reagent phenylisothiocyanate couples with the terminal alpha amino group of a peptide chain. Under acidic conditions, the terminal amino acid can be selectively cleaved as a heterocyclic derivative (an anilinothiazolinone) thus shortening the chain by one residue. The cleaved amino acid is converted to a more stable isomeric form (a phenyl thiohydantoin) and identified, often by gas chromatography. The peptide chain is then subjected to further cycles of this degradation and identification procedure, establishing the amino terminal sequence.

A long series of investigations of the detailed chemistry of the phenylisothiocyanate degradation by Edman and his collaborators (Edman, 1950, 1956, 1960) established reaction conditions under which the successive removal of amino acids from the amino terminus of a protein could be carried out at close to 100% efficiency. An instrument, the protein sequenator, capable of automated degradation by this method was designed, built, and applied by Edman and Begg. Up to 60 successive amino acids could be determined in a single 4-day run on this instrument. Subsequent modifications of this procedure (Niall *et al.*, 1969a; Sauer *et al.*, 1970) made it possible to carry out effective degradations on shorter peptides not readily handled in the original apparatus. This development was of particular value in establishing the sequences of calcitonins from several different species and of bovine and porcine parathyroid hormone, as discussed below.

As an indication of the rapid improvement in this methodology, it is now possible using special programs for automated peptide degradation in the sequenator to establish the complete sequence of a new calcitonin (32 amino acids) on only 2–4 mg of purified hormone (Niall *et al.*, 1971a). This is less than one-tenth of the material used in the earlier sequence determination of porcine calcitonin by a combination of classical peptide fragmentation and manual Edman degradation only three years ago (Potts *et al.*, 1968c). A reasonable extrapolation of the rate of progress in techniques available for sequence determinations suggests that structural analysis of polypeptides such as pararthyroid hormone and calcitonin may soon be fully automatic, completed in a few days on submilligram amounts of material.

Even before the hormone has been totally purified, its peptide nature can be surmised on the basis of behavior during fractionation, and lability to acid, alkali, or proteolytic enzymes of broad specificity. In these inactivation experiments it is important to include appropriate controls, and to realize that some proteolytic enzymes may split ester as well as amide bonds so that the studies must be interpreted with caution. The approximate molecular weight, amino acid composition, and amino terminal and carboxyl terminal end groups will probably be established during isolation as part of the initial characterization of the peptide, as described above (see Section II). The presence or absence of covalently or noncovalently bound cofactors (e.g., sugar residues, heavy metals, iodide) should also be established before starting the sequence determination.

If the amino terminal alpha amino group of the peptide is available and not blocked by acetylation or pyroglutamyl ring closure, an automated degradation is first carried out on a few milligrams of material. This should establish a large portion of the structure. With a knowledge of the overall composition of the hormone and of the amino terminal sequence, experiments can be planned to provide specific cleavage and isolation of the requisite peptide subfragments for completion of the structure.

These approaches will be illustrated from studies on parathyroid hormone and calcitonin.

B. Parathyroid Hormone

The predominant form of bovine parathyroid hormone (BPTH I) was established to be a single-chain polypeptide with 84 amino acids lacking cysteine and threonine. Two isohormones, containing 1 mole/mole of threonine have also been isolated, as described above. The complete amino acid sequence of the major form of the bovine hormone has recently been determined in our laboratory using the approaches outlined above (Niall et al., 1970; Potts et al., 1971c). An initial degradation on the automated sequenator (Beckman Spinco Model 890) established the sequence of the first 54 amino acids from the amino terminus. The phenylthiohydantoin derivatives of the amino acids split off at each cycle of degradation were identified by gas–liquid chromatography (Fig. 7).

Completion of the sequence in the most rapid and efficient fashion depended upon obtaining a peptide or peptides corresponding to the carboxyl terminal sequence of about 30 amino acids.

From the amino acid composition and the results of the amino terminal degradation, considerable information was available about the distribution of amino acid residues at which specific cleavage could be obtained

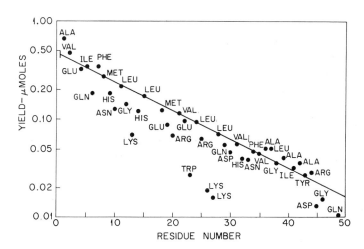

Fig. 7. Yields (in micromoles) of phenylthiohydantoin derivatives obtained during an automated Edman degradation of 54 cycles on bovine parathyroid hormone I. The gradual fall in yield is due to competing reactions occurring to a small extent at each cycle. Some labile derivatives (e.g., serine, tryptophan) are recovered in lower yield.

(Fig. 8). The only two methionine residues were present at positions 8 and 18. Hence cleavage with cyanogen bromide at these residues (though used in confirmatory studies) would not be very helpful in the attack on the carboxyl terminus. Similarly the location of the single tryptophan (position 23) was not advantageous. The single tyrosine residue (position 43) was better placed; however, specific cleavage at tyrosine in good yield is quite difficult to obtain, and this approach was therefore not attempted. However, it was observed that all five arginyl residues in the

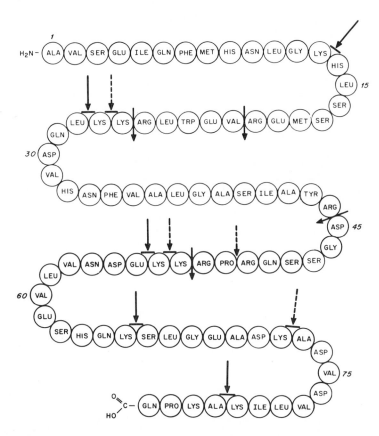

Fig. 8. The amino acid sequence of bovine parathyroid hormone I. The strategy used in the sequence determination is illustrated. After blocking of the lysine side chains with succinic or maleic anhydride, trypsin does not cleave at those residues, as indicated by the "blocked" arrows. Dotted arrows indicate sites where tryptic cleavage does not occur even in native parathyroid hormone, due to the influence of adjacent residues. Arrows which interrupted the sequence show the residual tryptic cleavage sites on lysine blocked hormone. It can be seen that the largest fragment produced by cleavage comprises residues 53–84.

molecule were identified within the first 54 amino acids, the most carboxyl terminal occupying position 52. Hence if the lysine side chains could be specifically blocked, digestion with trypsin should split the chain only at the arginyl residues, so that the fragment 53–84 should be delivered intact. This proved to be possible. The lysine side chains were blocked by reaction with succinic or maleic anhydride, and the resulting derivatized BPTH-I digested with trypsin. The carboxyl terminal fragment consisting of residues 53–84 was isolated in high yield (Fig. 8). An automated degradation carried out on this fragment established the remainder of the amino acid sequence of the hormone (Niall *et al.*, 1970; Potts *et al.*, 1971c). Confirmatory studies were carried out on a variety of fragments isolated after cleavage of the whole molecule with cyanogen bromide and cleavage of the isolated carboxyl terminal fragment with chymotrypsin, and (following removal of maleyl blocking groups from the lysine residues) after cleavage with trypsin. The sequence obtained is in agreement with that established independently in another laboratory (Brewer and Ronan, 1970).

More recently the complete sequence of porcine pararthyroid hormone has been established using similar approaches (Niall *et al.*, 1971a; Potts *et al.*, 1971c). It differs from the bovine hormone in substitutions at positions 1 (serine for alanine), 7 (leucine for phenylalanine), 18 (leucine for methionine), 42 (valine for alanine), 43 (histidine for tyrosine), 47 (glycine for serine), and 74 (alanine for aspartic acid) (Fig. 9).

C. Calcitonin

The amino acid sequence of porcine calcitonin was established in our laboratory in late 1967 (Potts *et al.*, 1968c). Although the molecule is considerably smaller than parathyroid hormone (32 amino acids), the sequence determination in several ways was less straightforward (Potts, 1970a). The carboxyl terminus of the molecule was blocked to carboxypeptidase digestion. An early report also suggested that the amino terminus was blocked (Putter *et al.*, 1967). Although this proved not to be so, the presence of amino terminal half-cystine complicated end group determination since there are difficulties in identifying this residue unless it is first oxidized to the cysteic acid form or alkylated to give a more stable derivative. The molecule as a whole is quite hydrophobic; some of its peptide subfragments particularly from the carboxyl end are markedly so. This causes severe loss of material in the organic solvent extractions used at each step of the phenylisothiocyanate degradation. This caused particular difficulty in the identification of the carboxyl terminal residue as prolinamide rather than proline.

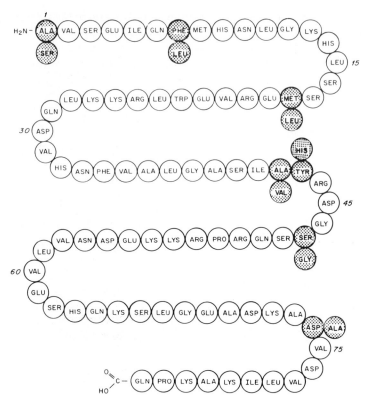

Fig. 9. The structure of porcine and bovine parathyroid hormones. The "back-bone" sequence is that of the bovine hormone. Positions which differ in the porcine structure are shaded, the residue found in porcine parathyroid hormone being shown in apposition.

However, the complete sequence of porcine calcitonin was established by two independent methods. A series of manual Edman degradations were carried out on the intact hormone and on three peptide subfragments produced by cleavage with trypsin and cyanogen bromide. Since the degradations overlapped one another, they established the complete amino acid sequence. The carboxyl terminal prolinamide residue was obtained by stopping the Edman degradation one residue short of the carboxyl terminus, and was identified directly by amino acid analysis in comparison with an authentic prolinamide standard.

An independent solution to the sequence was obtained by isolation and amino acid analysis of over 50 fragments of calcitonin generated by cleavage with dilute and concentrated acid, trypsin, chymotrypsin, pepsin, papain and cyanogen bromide. The sequence obtained was in complete agreement with that established independently in two other laboratories (Neher *et al.*, 1968a; Bell *et al.*, 1968).

Subsequently the sequence of human calcitonin was established by the Ciba group using material isolated from a medullary carcinoma of the thyroid. Similar procedures were used, i.e., manual Edman degradation (using the dansyl method) and isolation of a number of peptide fragments (Neher *et al.*, 1968b).

More recently the sequences of bovine and ovine calcitonin have been obtained in our laboratory (Potts, 1970a; Sauer *et al.*, 1970). The availability of automated equipment for Edman degradation greatly facilitated this work and reduced the requirements of peptide material. In general it has proved possible to obtain the sequence of the amino terminal 25 residues by a single automated degradation. The remainder of the sequence could be established after cleavage at methionyl or arginyl residues usually found toward the carboxyl terminus of the molecule. The structure of the bovine hormone was established independently in another laboratory (Brewer and Ronan, 1969).

The sequence determination on the major form of salmon calcitonin (Niall *et al.*, 1969b) was carried out by a manual Edman degradation of

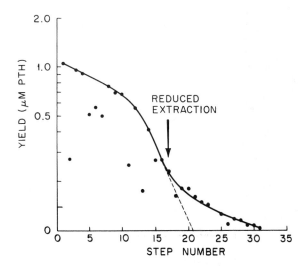

Fig. 10. Repetitive yields (in micromoles) of phenylthiohydantoin derivatives obtained during a complete manual degradation on salmon calcitonin. The extractions were reduced during the degradation to minimize peptide losses. Otherwise the degradation could not have proceeded beyond about cycle 20, as indicated by the dotted line showing the extrapolated yield.

31 cycles (Fig. 10). Reduction in the solvent extractions was effective in reducing peptide losses and allowing the degradation to proceed to the carboxyl terminus. The carboxyl terminal prolinamide was identified directly by amino acid analysis. Much of the sequence was then confirmed by automated Edman degradation. The sequences of porcine bovine, ovine, human, and salmon, calcitonins are shown in Fig. 11. The detailed structure and the significance of the constant and variable residues are discussed below.

Recently the sequences of two variants of salmon calcitonin (calcitonins II and III) have been determined in our laboratory (Lequin et al., 1971; Potts et al., 1971d) using similar approaches involving manual and automated Edman degradation. The structures differ from the predominant form of salmon calcitonin (calcitonin I) in 4 and 5 positions, respectively, as shown in Fig. 12. It appears that each of four separate Pacific coast salmon examined secrete two different calcitonin molecules—the major form and one of the two minor forms.

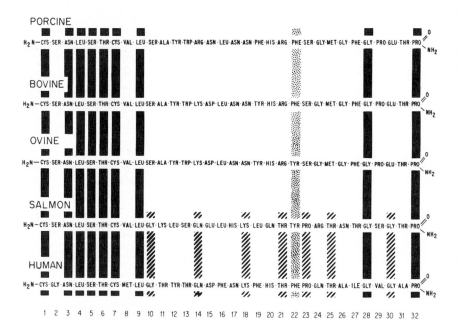

FIG. 11. The amino acid sequences of calcitonins from different species. The salmon sequence shown is that of the predominant or major form. Residues identical in all species are indicated by solid bars. Additional residues common to salmon and human calcitonins are indicated by cross hatched bars. The stippled bar (residue 23) shows a sequence position invariably occupied by an aromatic residue.

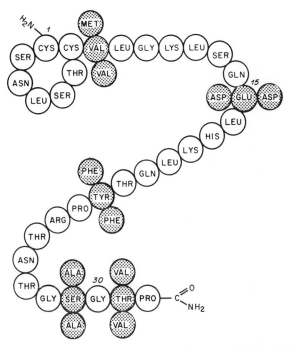

Fig. 12. The amino acid sequence of salmon calcitonins I, II, and III. The main peptide backbone represents the sequence of the predominant form, salmon calcitonin I. The dark circles to the left of the main sequence indicate the four positions in which salmon calcitonin II differs from calcitonin I. In addition to these changes, calcitonin III contains a fifth sequence difference at position 8, as indicated by the dark circles to the right of the main sequence.

IV. STRUCTURE–ACTIVITY RELATIONS

There has always been considerable interest in understanding the biological importance of individual amino acid residues in a hormonal polypeptide as one of the first steps in a systematic analysis of structure activity relations in the hormone. One approach has been the selective chemical modification of single residues or classes of amino acids followed by bioassay of the modified product. Often, however, the results are difficult to interpret or may even be misleading, as loss of activity obtained after selectively modifying a specific amino acid residue may not necessarily prove that that particular residue was vital for biological activity per se. For example, the early work (Brewer, 1969) on the modification of tyrosine and tryptophan in the porcine calcitonin molecule might be interpreted to mean that these residues are essential for hypocalcemic activity. Later work, however, established that neither tryptophan nor tyrosine occur in the highly active salmon calcitonin II and III molecules. An obvious paradox pointing to the limitations of selective modification reactions arose concerning the oxidation of methionine residues. Oxidation of methionine in the human molecule caused complete loss of hypocalcemic activity (Neher *et al.*, 1968c) yet oxidation in the porcine and bovine molecule caused no change in activity (Brewer *et al.*, 1968b). Methionine does not exist at all in the salmon I and III molecules (Fig. 12).

It has always been difficult properly to assess the role of disulfide bonds in determining the biological activity of polypeptide hormones. The disulfide bond can be split by reduction and alkylation or oxidation, but in either case the derivative formed, *S*-carboxymethylcystine or cysteic acid, represents a marked change in the overall chemical topography of the molecule. It is then difficult to conclude whether any observed change in the biological activity results from disruption of the disulfide ring or from the influence of the derivatizing group. Caution must therefore be exercised in interpreting the experimental observation (Brewer *et al.*, 1968b) that reduction and alkylation of the disulfide bridge in the calcitonin molecule caused a complete loss of biological activity. The synthesis of isosteric analogs where, for example, the disulfide bond is replaced by a methylene linkage as was carried out for the neurohypophyseal hormones oxytocin and vasopressin by Schwartz and co-workers (1964) may be a more satisfactory method of establishing the biological importance of the disulfide bridge in the calcitonin molecule.

In the case of oxytocin and vasopressin, reduction and alkylation of the disulfide bridge resulted in a complete loss of biological activity. The synthetic analogs 1,6-djenkolic acid–oxytocin and 1,6-djenkolic acid–vasopressin, in which a methylene group was interposed between the sulfur atoms that form the disulfide bridge in the parent hormone, and deaminocarba[1]-oxytocin, which is derived from oxytocin by omission of the amino group and replacement of one sulfur atom by a methylene group were all found to be biological active. The disulfide group was thus found not to be functionally significant.

Similarly, in the parathyroid hormone field, some of the earlier studies with the bovine molecule indicated that modification of the tyrosine residue with tyrosinase caused a complete loss of biological activity (Potts *et al.*, 1966). However, recent sequence studies (Potts *et al.*, 1971c) have shown that tyrosine does not occur in the porcine molecule and is not contained within the active sequence area of bovine parathyroid hormone (Potts *et al.*, 1971a).

One important chemical modification experiment was the treatment of bovine parathyroid hormone with dilute acid under controlled conditions which gave the clue that only approximately one-third of the molecule from the amino terminal was required for biological activity (Potts *et al.*, 1968b). This experiment combined with the sequence determination of the first forty odd residues, opened the way for synthetic studies enabling the active core region of the molecule to be defined more precisely.

Two important factors have aided considerably in improving the reliability of information that is now evolving on structure–activity relationships in calcitonin and parathyroid hormones; (1) the recent availability of sensitive and specific bio- and immunoassays for monitoring activity and (2) the rapid advances that have occurred in peptide synthesis techniques.

These factors, together with the additional information that can be obtained from a study of the comparative amino acid sequence of the hormones from several different species, will be discussed in more detail in the following sections.

A. CALCITONIN

1. *Synthesis*

The successful chemical synthesis of porcine calcitonin followed shortly after elucidation of the amino acid sequence. Working independently, two Swiss laboratories achieved the synthesis almost simultaneously. The Ciba group of Rittel *et al.* (1968) and Riniker *et al.* (1969) prepared small fragments of the chain by the stepwise approach and by the condensation of suitable small peptides and amino acids, finally assembling the fragments to form the completed chain. The synthetic procedure was noteworthy because of the successful application of the important new biphenylisopropyloxycarbonyl (BPOC) amine-protecting group of Sieber and Iselin (1968a,b) which is expected to find widespread use in peptide synthesis. The Sandoz group (Guttmann *et al.*, 1968) using a different strategy, prepared the protected tridecapeptide amide (20–32) coupled it to a protected central decapeptide (10–19), and allowed the resulting tricosapeptide amide (10–32) to react with the protected (1–9) fragment. Subsequent removal of the protecting groups gave the completed chain. Similar approaches have been used for the synthesis of human calcitonin (Sieber *et al.*, 1968, 1970b; Greven and Tax, 1970) and salmon calcitonin (Guttmann *et al.*, 1969, 1970).

The syntheses of the various calcitonin molecules reported to date have all been achieved by the classical or solution-phase method. While this approach is capable of excellent results, the procedures involved are often difficult and time consuming. The introduction of the solid-phase method by Merrifield (1963, 1969) was a significant advance and greatly simplified the peptide synthesis technique. In this method the peptide chain is assembled in a stepwise manner while anchored at one end to an insoluble support. Removal of excess amino acids and by-products is effected by a simple washing step rather than by the usual tedious recrystallization methods. When the desired sequence has been assembled the peptide is finally cleaved from the insoluble support and purified. Recent advances in this technique, and in particular the development of resins suitable for the formation of carboxyl terminal amides (Pietta and Marshall, 1970) should simplify the synthesis of calcitonins, and indeed such methods are currently under investigation in several laboratories.

2. Structure–Activity Relations

Evaluation of the biological activity of the various synthetic fragments prepared during the course of the porcine calcitonin synthesis was very informative. Figure 13 summarizes some of the results reported by Sieber

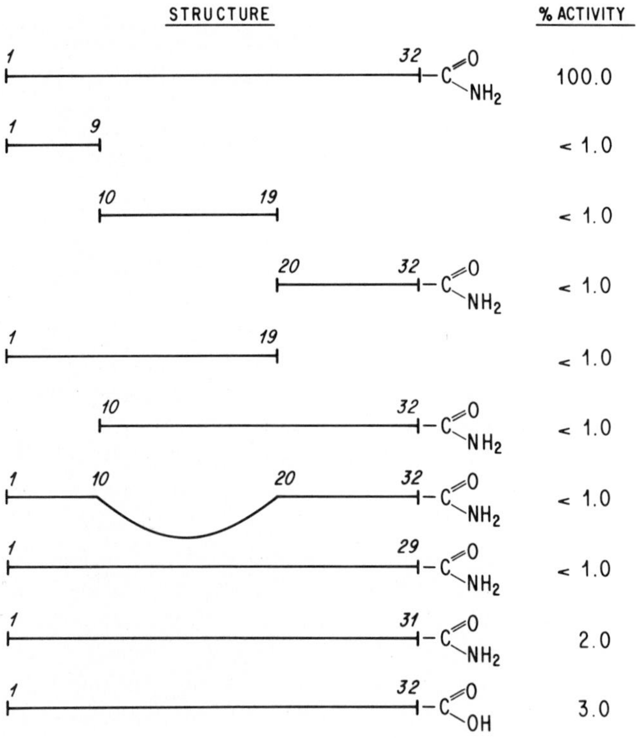

FIG. 13. The relative biological activity of synthetic fragments of the porcine calcitonin molecule (Sieber et al., 1970a; Guttmann et al., 1971).

et al. (1970a) and Guttmann and co-workers (1971). Fragments of the molecule, whether derived from the amino terminal, middle, or carboxyl terminal region are totally inactive. The comparatively long fragments, consisting of residues 10–32, or residues 1–10 joined to residues 20–32 with omission of the central nonapeptide, are similarly inactive. Shortening of the molecule by even one or two amino residues causes almost complete loss of biological activity even if the carboxyl terminal proline amide residue is retained. In fact, even removal of the N-terminal amino group or the C-terminal amide results in a dramatic decrease of hypocalcemic activity.

Thus in contrast to our current knowledge of many other pepide hormones, calcitonin does not contain an "active" core, the entire 32 amino acid chain together with the C-terminal amide being required for full biological activity.

Although small variations in the length of the calcitonin molecule profoundly alter the biological activity, substitution, or modification of various amino acids within the chain are far less critical. Guttmann and co-workers (1971) have described several synthetic analogs of porcine calcitonin, some of which are included in Fig. 14.

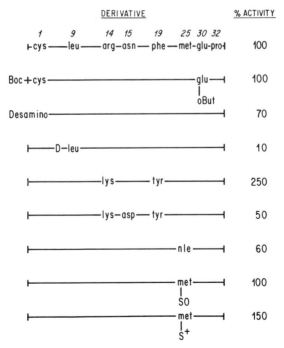

Fig. 14. The relative biological activity of synthetic analogs of porcine calcitonin (Guttmann *et al.,* 1971).

Masking the only acidic residue, the glutamic acid at position 30, by forming the t-butyl ester gave virtually no change in the activity. On the other hand, total suppression of the basicity by masking the side-chain amino functions resulted in a complete loss of activity. Blocking the N-terminal amino function with the tertiary butyloxycarbonyl (BOC) group did not affect the activity.

Replacement of the leucine at position 9 by its D-isomer gave rise to a derivative of very low activity; however, addition of the BOC group to the amino terminal of this molecule doubled its activity. Replacing the arginine at position 14 with lysine and phenylalanine at 19 with tyrosine resulted in a 2.5-fold increase in activity and the duration of its activity was found to be longer. Note, however, that if in addition to these changes the asparagine at position 15 is simultaneously changed to aspartic acid, which in fact is the sequence of bovine calcitonin, the activity falls dramatically to approximately one-half of the original porcine figure.

Brewer *et al.* (1968b) have shown that oxidation of the methionine at position 25 in either the porcine or bovine calcitonin molecule did not affect biological activity; alkylation with iodoacetic acid caused a slight increase in activity. Similarly, Guttmann's synthetic porcine analog with norleucine replacing methionine retained about 60% of the original biological activity. In contrast, the oxidized form of the human calcitonin molecule in which the methionine is at position 8 rather than at 25 was biologically inactive (Neher *et al.*, 1968c). It is interesting to note that there are no methionines in the highly active salmon calcitonin I and II molecules (Fig. 12).

The published data on synthetic analogs of calcitonin has so far been limited. However, with the recent advances in peptide synthesis techniques, the preparation of additional analogs will become an increasingly important and useful tool in evaluating structure–activity relations in the calcitonin molecule. In choosing such analogs for synthesis, the expanding body of data on the sequences of natural calcitonins should serve as a valuable guide.

We now have amino acid sequence data on 7 calcitonins from 5 different species (see Figs. 11 and 12). Each of the calcitonins consists of a 32 amino acid chain with a 1-7 amino terminal disulfide bridge and carboxyl terminal prolinamide. Only nine sequence positions are completely constant in all structures and seven of these nine are in the amino terminal disulfide loop region. The remaining two constant regions are at the carboxyl end of the chain—the C-terminal prolinamide and the glycine at position 28.

In the porcine bovine and ovine calcitonins, considerable similarity is found in the sequences between positions 10 and 27; however, both the human and salmon molecules differ markedly from these three and from one another. The amino acid substitutions in this region are conservative, however, and in general preserve the overall chemical properties of the molecule. Acidic residues occur only at position 15 or position 30 and basic residues are similarly restricted to only relatively few positions. It is interesting to note that in all the calcitonin molecules, hydrophobic residues are distributed at regular intervals along the peptide chain at positions 4, 9, 12, 16, 19, and 22; although sequence differences are found at these positions, leucine, phenylalanine, or tyrosine are invariably present. A nonpolar amino acid always occupies position 8, in most cases it is valine, in the human and salmon III sequence it is methionine. As indicated above, studies with human calcitonin indicate that oxidation of the methionine to the polar sulfoxide derivative causes total loss of biological activity. In the porcine, bovine, and ovine molecules the methionine occurs at position 25 and oxidation of this residue causes no change in the activity. This is compatible with the observation that the polar residue threonine is found at position 25 in salmon and human calcitonins.

In general, the amino acid substitutions which occur in the calcitonin molecule are consistent with one-step changes in the genetic code, or changes that are favored by natural selection substitution patterns deduced by analysis of sequence homology in peptides or proteins with similar biological functions (Dayhoff and Eck, 1969).

One of the most interesting aspects of structure-function relations in the calcitonins is the extremely high potency of the salmon molecule (O'Dor et al., 1969; Keutmann et al., 1970). The hypocalcemic activity of salmon calcitonin I in the rat bioassay varies from 2500–3000 U/mg, compared to the range of 50–200 U/mg for porcine, bovine, ovine, and human calcitonin (Table IV). Two further calcitonins have been isolated from the various salmon species (designated salmon II and III, see Fig. 12), and these forms of the hormone possess a high biological potency similar to that of the salmon I molecule (Keutmann et al., 1971c).

As salmon calcitonin I has also been found to have a higher potency in man than human or porcine calcitonin (Singer et al., 1970, 1971), there is considerable interest in determining the unique structural characteristics which give rise to this increased potency.

The role of conformation or tertiary structure of calcitonin is not clear at this stage. Studies on several species of calcitonin (Brewer, 1970; Brewer and Edelhoch, 1970) have so far shown little or no helical content or other evidence of highly ordered structure. However, it is known that salmon calcitonin has the highest degree of hydration of the calcitonins so far studied. The consequent change in size of the molecule can be observed by gel filtration, where salmon calcitonin, in spite of its lower molecular weight, emerges earlier than the porcine or human hormone (Guttmann *et al.*, 1970, 1971).

The increased potency of salmon calcitonin could be due to a greater affinity of the molecule for receptor sites in bone and other target tissues, an increased resistance to metabolic destruction, or a combination of these two mechanisms. Recent work (Habener *et al.*, 1971b) carried out in our laboratory on the metabolic fate of salmon calcitonin in animals has in fact indicated that the salmon peptide is more resistant to metabolic degradation than porcine calcitonin. The metabolic clearance rate in the dog is only one-tenth that of the porcine hormone. These results suggest that the higher potency may result from protection against metabolic destruction *in vivo*.

The amino acids in nine of the thirty-two positions in salmon calcitonin I (Fig. 15) are different from the corresponding positions in the sequence of all the calcitonins so far isolated and analyzed. Of the minor components, salmon calcitonin II differs from the major sequence in four positions, as illustrated in Fig. 12. The other minor component, salmon calcitonin III is identical to salmon II except at residue 8, where methionine replaces valine. Most of these changes in the amino acid sequence

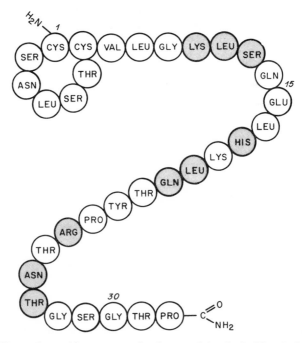

Fig. 15. The amino acid sequence of salmon calcitonin I. The darkened circles indicate those amino acid positions unique to the salmon molecule.

of salmon calcitonin II and III make them resemble more closely human calcitonin.

Comparative chemical studies on calcitonins both from other mammalian species and from other species of fish, the synthesis of further analogs, and additional studies on the metabolic fate of the calcitonins in man and other species may be required before a rational basis for enhanced activity can be established.

B. PARATHYROID HORMONE

1. Synthesis

Earlier work (Rasmussen and Craig, 1962; Potts et al., 1968b) had indicated that the full 84 amino acid sequence of bovine parathyroid hormone was not required for biological activity. Dilute acid hydrolysis studies with the isolated peptide (Potts et al., 1968b) established that the region of biological activity was contained in a 30–40 amino acid fragment at the amino terminal end of the molecule. However, the availability of amino acid sequence data was severely hampered by difficulties encountered in obtaining a pure sample of the hormone free of peptide contaminants, and until recently less than 20% of the sequence was presumed to be established with any degree of confidence.

The first synthesis of a bovine parathyroid hormone fragment was reported by Wang and Merrifield (1969), who used the tryptophan-containing heptapeptide sequence 19–25 as a model for the evaluation of BPOC-amino acid derivatives in the solid-phase procedure. The peptide was not tested for biological activity but more recent studies indicate that it would have been inactive.

As reliable sequence data on the amino terminal region of bovine parathyroid hormone became available, work commenced in our laboratory on the synthesis of amino terminal fragments of the molecule. The solid-phase method was used as it provided a rapid and convenient means of screening selected amino acid sequences for possible biological activity. The general procedure of Merrifield (1969) was modified by the introduction of a new series of synthetic solid-phase supports based on the unique properties offered by graft copolymerization (Battaerd and Tregear, 1967; Tregear, 1969).

The successful synthesis (Potts et al., 1971a) of a biologically active amino-terminal 1–34 fragment of the bovine parathyroid hormone sequence (Fig. 16) confirmed the earlier observation that the entire 84 amino acid sequence was not required for biological activity. The synthetic tetratriacontapeptide was found to possess all the specific physio-

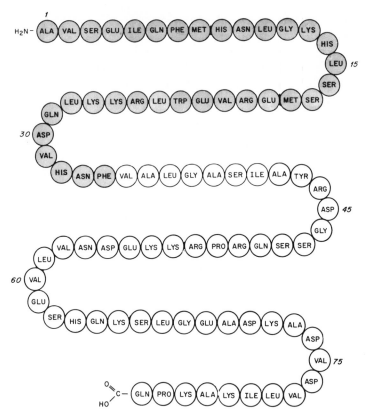

Fig. 16. The amino acid sequence of bovine parathyroid hormone I. The shaded area indicates the sequence of the fragment synthesized by the solid-phase technique. The synthetic peptide was found to be biologically active *in vivo* and *in vitro* on bone and kidney receptors (Potts *et al.*, 1971b).

logical and biochemical properties associated with native parathyroid hormone. In addition to stimulating adenyl cyclase in both bone and kidney cells, the synthetic peptide elevated blood calcium in rats and dogs and caused an increase in renal excretion of both cyclic-AMP and phosphate in the rat.

Evaluation of the *in vitro* biological potency of the synthetic peptide indicated a potency of from 400 to 600 USP units/mg compared to an activity of 1600 USP units/mg for the native 84 amino acid polypeptide. However, the actual intrinsic potency of the linear 1–34 sequence is difficult to assess because the synthetic material was necessarily exposed to chemicals such as hydrogen fluoride and piperidine which in controlled studies were shown to cause a significant reduction of biological activity in the native hormone. Thus the true potency of the synthetic fragment may be higher.

The *in vivo* activity of the synthetic preparation as measured by rat bioassay (Aurbach, 1959b) was found to be only 100 to 150 USP units/mg. The potency of the synthetic peptide relative to that of the natural peptide is therefore less *in vivo* than *in vitro*. This finding suggests that the biological role of at least some portion of the carboxy-terminal two-thirds of the structure of the native molecule may be to protect the active region of the hormone from accelerated metabolic degradation in the circulation. (See discussion concerning the peripheral metabolism of the hormone, below.)

2. Structure–Activity Relations

Progress in the evaluation of structure–activity relations in parathyroid hormone has been greatly aided by the availability of the *in vitro* kidney adenyl cyclase bioassay. This technique, developed by Marcus and Aurbach (1969), provides a rapid and sensitive method for screening the biological activity of natural and synthetic fragments. This assay is much more convenient than previously existing assay methods. Other important tests for biological activity include the classic rat bioassay which measures the increase in serum calcium stimulated by parathyroid hormone (Munson, 1961) measurement of its effect on urinary excretion of phosphate and cyclic-AMP (Chase and Aurbach, 1970) and on cyclic-AMP production in fetal-rat calvaria (Chase and Aurbach, 1970). Evaluation of the synthetic amino terminal 1–34 peptide in these assay systems established that all the structural information required for binding to biological receptors in both bone and kidney cells were contained in the same limited region of the amino-terminal sequence of the hormone.

Recent studies in our laboratory (Keutmann *et al.*, 1971b) with fragments of the native molecule indicate that the sequence 1–29 is in fact sufficient for biological activity. However, the fragment 1–20 was found to be completely inactive in the adenyl cyclase assay. Similarly, the synthetic fragments 1–13, 14–34, 19–34, and 25–34 were biologically inactive. An interesting finding was that deletions of the amino-terminal residue alanine, as in the synthetic fragment 2–34, led to a complete loss of biological activity. In addition, carboxyl-terminal fragments 26–45, 46–52, and 53–84 derived from tryptic digestion of ε-aminolysine-blocked native parathyroid hormone were completely devoid of biological activity. These findings taken together (Fig. 17) define the minimum requirements for expression of the biological effects of parathyroid hormone as being present in a continuous sequence that extends from the amino terminal

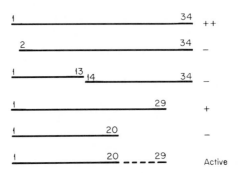

Fig. 17. The biological activity of fragments of the bovine parathyroid hormone molecule. Studies to date indicate that the minimum requirements for activity are included in a continuous sequence that extends from the amino terminal alanine, residue 1, at least 20 residues to a point somewhere between arginine, residue 20, and glutamine, residue 29.

alanine residue 1, at least 20 residues to a point somewhere between arginine, residue 20, and glutamine, residue 29.

An obvious extension to these studies will be the synthesis of analogs of the active fragment. The choice of amino acid substitutions will be simplified as comparative structural information from other species of the hormone becomes available. For example, the finding that there is only one methionine (at position 8) in the active region of the porcine hormone, compared with two in the bovine sequence, has stimulated interest in the synthesis of the norleucine[8]-porcine fragment to define more closely the role of the methionine residues. A systematic synthesis of amino-terminal fragments will also be required to define more precisely the minimum sequence requirements for biological activity and to investigate possible structural modifications to retard metabolic degradation. The availability of these fragments will also be of great practical importance in refining the radioimmunoassay technique for the measurement of circulating levels of parathyroid hormone in man.

V. SUMMARY

We now have available a large body of structural data on parathyroid hormone and calcitonin from several species. In addition to the complete sequence of the major bovine hormone and the closely similar 84 amino acid polypeptide isolated from the porcine species, there is detailed compositional and partial structural information on the two other molecular variants of the bovine hormone, bovine parathyroid isohormones II and III. The validity of the proposed structure of parathyroid hormone, that is, a linear arrangement of unsubstituted amino acids in a simple polypeptide chain, has been confirmed by peptide synthesis and demonstrated biological potency of the amino terminal sequences 1–34 and 1–29. Since the synthetic peptides are active on both kidney and bone *in vivo* and *in vitro*, it can be concluded that receptor binding requirements in the two tissues are at least closely similar.

The structure of 7 calcitonin molecules from 5 different species is now known. In addition, the human, porcine, and salmon hormones have been synthesized as well as many analogs of the naturally occurring sequences. We thus have a rather detailed picture of structure–activity relations in these two peptide hormones, parathyroid hormone and calcitonin.

There are interesting contrasts in the relation of structure to activity when pararthyroid hormone is compared to calcitonin. Parathyroid hormone is a considerably larger polypeptide with a chain length approximately two and one half times greater than that of calcitonin. However, only the amino terminal 29 residues, as a maximum, of the 84 amino acid polypeptide is required for expression of biological activity *in vivo* or *in vitro*. By contrast, the biological activity of calcitonin polypeptides requires essentially the entire sequence of 32 amino acids. At least, no synthetic fragment nor analog shortened by even one residue has been shown to possess significant biological activity. Hence, the size of the minimum active molecular species of the two hormonal peptides is similar, the minimum active fragment of pararthyroid hormone, is in fact smaller than that of calcitonin.

There is not as yet any direct information about the amino acid sequence of human parathyroid hormone. However, the studies of O'Riordan *et al.* (1971), have suggested that the human hormone is closely similar to that of the bovine and porcine hormones in overall size, charge, and amino acid composition. In view of the close similarity now known in the amino acid sequence of bovine and porcine parathyroid hormones, it seems very probable that in the mammalian species, at least, there may be a very restricted number of changes in amino acid sequence of parathyroid hormone from one species to another. Calcitonin, on the other hand, is a polypeptide in which surprisingly wide variations in amino acid sequence have been permitted even within the mammalian species; there are marked differences between human and porcine calcitonin (bovine and ovine are similar to porcine).

Although only 9 of 32 sequence positions are homologous in the calcitonins, the sequence changes that have occurred are generally conservative and preserve a similar chemical topography in each of the calcitonins. On the other hand, the importance of these variations in the amino acid sequence is seen in the unusual biological and metabolic properties of the salmon hormones. There are 11 unique amino acid sequence changes in salmon calcitonin I (see Fig. 15). Since in salmon II and III the Glu at 15 is replaced by Asp as in human, there are, in fact, only 10 amino acid positions unique to the salmon species. One or more of these changes must account for the unusual resistance of the salmon hormone to metabolic destruction.

These findings have therefore stimulated interest in investigation of the amino acid sequence of calcitonins from other species, particularly submammalian vertebrate forms. The studies of Habener *et al.* (1971b) suggest that the rapid metabolic clearance of calcitonin from the circulation is due to cleavage by a proteolytic enzyme not present in plasma but in some discrete extravascular site or fixed to the capillary wall of a given organ, such as liver or kidney. It may be possible to identify the nature of this cleavage. Use of perfusion studies *in vivo* with antisera prepared against the intact salmon, porcine, and human hormones and its peptide subfragments coupled with measurements, through use of indwelling catheters, of arteriovenous gradients in immunoassayable calcitonin across different organs such as liver and kidney may aid in identifying the site of initial cleavage of the peptide chain.

It should then be possible to prepare a series of synthetic analogs in which there is a systematic variation of the amino acid residues immediately adjacent to the initial cleavage site and thereby retard cleavage efficiency. Since enhanced potency seems correlated with resistance to metabolic destruction, investigation of the relation of structure to activity based on naturally occurring sequence changes in calcitonin coupled with a continued program of synthesis of peptide analogs may lead to preparation of even more potent forms of calcitonin than salmon calcitonin.

The recent evidence that the peripheral metabolism of parathyroid hormone, calcitonin, and probably many other peptide hormones is quite complex has added an exciting new dimension to investigation of the mode of action of peptide hormones and as well to the general efforts to measure endogenous hormone concentration in plasma. As already discussed, this rate of peripheral metabolism of calcitonin seems critical in determining relative potency of different calcitonin peptides.

The possible significance of these recent findings concerning hormone metabolism is even greater with respect to parathyroid hormone than with calcitonin. Despite the recent advances in structural characterization and synthesis of parathyroid hormone (based on studies of hormone extracted from the parathyroids), present data based on radioimmunoassays have suggested that the biosynthesis and secretion as well as metabolism of endogenous parathyroid hormone in man and animals is quite complex and that, in fact, the exact chemical nature of the active circulating form of the hormone is not yet known.

Several conclusions can be drawn from these recent studies (Potts *et al.*, 1971c; Habener *et al.*, 1971a) about the physical and immuno-chemical properties of endogenous pararthyroid hormone circulating in peripheral blood as well as the hormone released from the gland in both man and animals. The hormone circulating in peripheral blood is smaller in size than the 1–84 amino acid hormonal polypeptide extracted from glands, whereas the hormone released from the parathyroids *in vivo* is larger than the hormone found in peripheral plasma and is similar in size to the hormone extracted from the glands. Cleavage of the secreted hormone to smaller fragments must occur exclusively in peripheral sites after release from the gland, and not—as has been proposed by Sherwood *et al.* (1971) and Arnaud *et al.* (1971) from their *in vitro* studies—by cleavage in the parathyroid gland concomitant with release. However, since there are circulating fragments of the hormone it is not clear whether the principal active molecular species of endogenous parathyroid hormone is one or more peptide subfragments or the originally biosynthesized 1–84 amino acid polypeptide. Kinetic studies employing serial radioimmunoassays after infusions of intact native hormone or synthetic fragments in animals may be helpful in resolving these various possibilities concerning the active molecular species of endogenous hormone. If the rate of fragmentation of the 1–84 polypeptide is much slower than the rate of degradation of biologically active N-terminal subfragments, then it is likely that the 1–84 polypeptide is the principal active species. If, on the other hand, the kinetic evidence suggests that the concentration of active fragments is high relative to the 1–84 polypeptide released from the gland, the findings will be consistent with a model of hormone action in which peripheral metabolism of the hormone is equivalent to an activation step, that is, that the principal active form of the hormone is generated in peripheral sites after release.

Eventual resolution of these uncertainties concerning the nature of circulating immunoreactive hormone should also open the possibility for considerable refinement in immunoassay studies. It should be possible by any of a variety of approaches to develop antisera that exclusively recognize limited regions of the polypeptide sequence. The chemical advances, particularly availability of synthetic fragments of parathyroid hormone, are essential in these studies. Preparation of such region-specific antisera is currently being investigated by use of several methods:

1. Tests with antisera already available have indicated that they contain antibodies that react with two or more regions of the sequence. Adsorption experiments using fragments from one end or the other of the polypeptide, already seem to provide a rapid method of preparation of exclusively N-terminal or C-terminal reactive antisera.

2. Chromatographic purification of complex mixtures of antisera by coupling discrete fragments of parathyroid hormone to immunoadsorbent columns. Considerable purification of antibody can be achieved by these methods.

3. Immunization with discrete fragments that are prepared synthetically and injected either alone or after coupling to immunologically inert polypeptides such as polylysine.

4. Finally, preparation of peptide subfragments with substitution of tyrosine in the sequence to provide a site for incorporation of radioactive iodine. Such fragments will react only with the antisera that recognize the portion of the molecule identical in sequence to the synthetic fragment and again will provide specificity of measurement of different regions of the molecule.

It seems quite plausible that the considerable discrepancies reported from different laboratories involved in clinical studies with the parathyroid radioimmunoassay may be due to differential rates of clearance of discrete, immunoreactive fragments of parathyroid hormone. These differences may explain much of the present confusion concerning immunochemical and metabolic heterogeneity of plasma parathyroid hormone (Potts *et al.*, 1971c). Ultimately, it should be possible to measure exclusively the biologically active portions of the molecule and thereby provide a much more reliable index of true glandular secretory activity.

Resolution of these questions concerning the chemical nature and significance of circulating hormone fragments will take considerable time particularly in development of the methods required for the appropriate metabolic studies. However, the recent advances in the chemistry of parathyroid hormone at least make possible these very important studies concerning the significance of hormone metabolism, studies which could not even have been initiated prior to this time.

REFERENCES

Arnaud, C. D., Sizemore, G. W., Oldham, S. B., Fischer, J. A., Tsao, H. S., and Littledike, E. T. (1971). *Amer. J. Med.* **50**, 630.
Aurbach, G. D. (1959a). *J. Biol. Chem.* **234**, 3179.
Aurbach, G. D. (1959b). *Endocrinology* **64**, 296.
Aurbach, G. D., and Potts, J. T., Jr. (1964). *Endocrinology* **75**, 290.
Aurbach, G. D., Beck, R. N., and Astwood, E. B. (1958). *Fed. Proc., Fed. Amer. Soc. Exp. Biol.* **17**, 7.
Battaerd, H. A. J., and Tregear, G. W. (1967). "Graft Copolymers." Wiley (Interscience), New York.
Bell, P. M. (1968). *In* "Calcitonin: Symposium on Thyrocalcitonin and the C Cells" (S. F. Taylor, ed.), p. 77. Heinemann, London.
Bell, P. M., Barg, W. R., Jr., Colucci, D. F., Davies, C. M., Dziobkowski, C., Englert,

M. E., Heyder, E., Paul, R., and Snedeker, E. H. (1968). *J. Amer. Chem. Soc.* **90**, 2704.

Berman, L. (1924). *Proc. Soc. Exp. Biol. Med.* **21**, 465.

Blomback, B., Blomback, M., Edman, P., and Hessel, B. (1966). *Biochim. Biophys. Acta* **115**, 371.

Brewer, H. B., Jr. (1969). *Fed. Proc., Fed. Amer. Soc. Exp. Biol.* **28**, 383.

Brewer, H. B., Jr. (1970). *In* "Calcitonin 1969. Proceedings of the Second International Symposium" (S. F. Taylor and G. Foster, eds.), p. 14. Heinemann, London.

Brewer, H. B., Jr., and Edelhoch, H. (1970). *J. Biol. Chem.* **245**, 2402.

Brewer, H. B., Jr., and Ronan, R. (1969). *Proc. Nat. Acad. Sci. U. S.* **63**, 862.

Brewer, H. B., Jr., and Ronan, R. (1970). *Proc. Nat. Acad. Sci. U. S.* **67**, 1862.

Brewer, H. B., Jr., Keutmann, H. T., Potts, J. T., Jr., Reisfield, R. A., Schlueter, R., and Munson, P. L. (1968a). *J. Biol. Chem.* **243**, 5739.

Brewer, H. B., Jr., Keutmann, H. T., Reisfield, R. A., Munson, P. L., Schlueter, R. J., and Potts, J. T., Jr. (1968b). *Fed. Proc., Fed. Amer. Soc. Exp. Biol.* **27**, 690.

Brewer, H. B., Jr., Schlueter, R. J., and Aldred, J. P. (1970). *J. Biol. Chem.* **245**, 4232.

Bussolati, G., and Pearse, A. G. E. (1967). *J. Endocrinol.* **37**, 205.

Care, A. D. (1965). *Nature (London)* **205**, 1289.

Chase, L. R., and Aurbach, G. D. (1967). *Proc. Nat. Acad. Sci. U. S.* **58**, 518.

Chase, L. R., and Aurbach, G. D. (1970). *J. Biol. Chem.* **245**, 1520.

Cohn, D. V., MacGregor, R. R., Chu, L. L. H., and Hamilton, J. W. (1971). *Proc. Parathyroid Conf., 4th, 1970* (in press).

Collip, J. B. (1925). *J. Biol. Chem.* **63**, 395.

Cooper. C. W., Hirsch, P. F., Tovervd, S. U., and Munson, P. L. (1967). *Endocrinology* **81**, 610.

Copp, D. H., and Kuczerpa, A. V. (1968). *In* "Calcitonin: Symposium on Thyrocalcitonin and the C Cells" (S. F. Taylor, ed.), p. 18. Heinemann, London.

Copp, D. H., and Parkes, C. O. (1968). *In* "Parathyroid Hormone and Thyrocalcitonin (Calcitonin)" (R. V. Talmage and L. F. Bélanger, eds.), p. 74. Excerpta Med. Found., Amsterdam.

Copp, D. H., Cameron, E. C., Cheney, B. A., Davidson, A. G. F., and Henze, K. G. (1962). *Endocrinology* **70**, 638.

Copp, D. H., Cockroft, D. W., and Kueh, Y. (1967). *Science* **158**, 924.

Davies, B. M. A., Gordon, A. H., and Munsett, M. V. (1954). *J. Physiol. (London)* **125**, 383.

Dayhoff, M. D., and Eck, R. V. (1969). "Atlas of Protein and Structure." Nat. Biomed. Res. Found., Silver Spring, Maryland.

Edman, P. (1950). *Acta Chem. Scand.* **4**, 283.

Edman, P. (1956). *Acta Chem. Scand.* **10**, 761.

Edman, P. (1960). *Ann. N. Y. Acad. Sci.* **88**, 602.

Edman, P., and Begg, G. (1967). *Eur. J. Biochem.* **1**, 80.

Foster, G. V., Baghdiantz, A., Kumar, M. A., Slack, E., Soliman, H. A., and MacIntyre, I. (1964a). *Nature (London)* **202**, 1303.

Foster, G. V., MacIntyre, I., and Pearse, A. G. E. (1964b). *Nature (London)* **203**, 1029.

Greven, H. M., and Tax, L. J. W. M. (1970). *In* "Calcitonin 1969. Proceedings of the Second International Symposium" (S. F. Taylor and G. Foster, eds.), p. 34. Heinemann, London.

Gudmundsson, T. V., Byfield, P. G. H., Galante, L., and MacIntyre, I. (1968). *In* "Calcitonin: Symposium on Thyrocalcitonin and the C Cells" (S. F. Taylor, ed.), p. 51. Heinemann, London.

Guttmann, S., Pless, J., Sandrin, E., Jaquenoud, P. A., Bossert, H., and Willems, H. (1968). *Helv. Chim. Acta* **51**, 1155.

Guttmann, S., Pless, J., Huguenin, R. L., Sandrin, E., Bossert, H., and Zehnder, K. (1969). *Helv. Chim. Acta* **52**, 1789.

Guttmann, S., Pless, J., Huguenin, R. L., Sandrin, E., Bossert, H., and Zehnder, K. (1970). *In* "Calcitonin 1969. Proceedings of the Second International Symposium" (S. F. Taylor and G. Foster, eds.), p. 74. Heinemann, London.

Guttmann, S., Pless, J., Huguenin, R., Sandrin, E., and Zehnder, K. (1971). *Proc. Amer. Peptide Symp., 2nd, 1970* (in press).

Habener, J. F., Murray, T. M., Powell, D. V., Mayer, G. P., and Potts, J. T., Jr. (1971a). *Proc. Nat. Acad. Sci. U. S.* (submitted for publication).

Habener, J. F., Singer, F. R., Deftos, L. J., Neer, R. M., and Potts, J. T., Jr. (1971b). *Nature (London)* **232**, 91.

Handler, P., Cohn, D. V., and Dratz, A. F. (1954). *In* "Metabolic Interrelations with Special Reference to Calcium" (E. C. Reifenstein, ed.), p. 320. Progress Associates, Inc., Caldwell, New Jersey.

Hanson, A. M. (1925). *Proc. Soc. Exp. Biol. Med.* **22**, 560.

Hawker, C. D., Glass, J. D, and Rasmussen, H. (1966). *Biochemistry* **5**, 344.

Hirs, C. H. W. (1967). *Methods Enzymol.* **11**.

Hirsch, P. F., Gauthier, G. F., and Munson, P. L. (1963). *Endocrinology* **73**, 244.

Keutmann, H. T., and Potts, J. T., Jr. (1969). *Anal. Biochem.* **29**, 175.

Keutmann, H. T., Parsons, J. A., Potts, J. T., Jr., and Schlueter, R. J. (1970). *J. Biol. Chem.* **245**, 1491.

Keutmann, H. T., Aurbach, G. D., Dawson, B. F., Niall, H. D., Deftos, L. J., and Potts, J. T., Jr. (1971a). *Biochemistry* **10**, 2779.

Keutmann, H. T., Niall, H. D., Tregear, G. W., Murray, T. M., O'Riordan, J. L. H., Aurbach, G. D., and Potts, J. T., Jr. (1971b). *Proc. 53rd Meet. Endocrine Soc.* Abstract No. 41.

Keutmann, H. T., Lequin, R. M., Habener, J. F., Singer, F. R., Niall, H. D., and Potts, J. T., Jr. (1971c), *In* "Endocrinology 1971: Proceedings of the 3rd International Symposium" (S. F. Taylor, ed.), Heinemann, London (in press).

Kumar, M. A., Foster, G. V., and MacIntyre, I. (1963). *Lancet* **2**, 480.

Lequin, R., Keutmann, H. T., Niall, H. D., and Potts, J. T., Jr. (1971). In preparation.

MacCallum, W. G., and Voegtlin, C. (1909). *J. Exp. Med.* **11**, 118.

MacIntyre, I. (1970). *In* "Calcitonin 1969. Proceedings of the Second International Symposium" (S. F. Taylor and G. Foster, eds.), p. 1. Heinemann, London.

Marcus, R., and Aurbach, G. D. (1969). *Endocrinology* **85**, 801.

Matthews, E. W., Moseley, J. M., Breed, R. H., Gudmundsson, T. V., Byfield, P. G. H., Galante, L., Tse, A., and MacIntyre, I. (1968). *In* "Parathyroid Hormone and Thyrocalcitonin (Calcitonin)" (R. V. Talmage and L. B. Bélanger, eds.), p. 68. Excerpta Med. Found., Amsterdam.

Merrifield, R. B. (1963). *J. Amer. Chem. Soc.* **85**, 2149.

Merrifield, R. B. (1969). *Advan. Enzymol.* **32**, 221.

Munson, P. L. (1955). *Ann. N. Y. Acad. Sci.* **60**, 776.

Munson, P. L. (1961). In "The Parathyroids" (R. O. Greep and R. V. Talmage, eds.), p. 94. Thomas, Springfield, Illinois.

Munson, P. L., Hirsch, P. F., Brewer, H. B., Jr., Reisfeld, R. A., Cooper, C. W., Orimo, H., and Potts, J. T., Jr. (1967). Recent Progr. Horm. Res. 24, 589.

Neher, R., Riniker, B., Zuber, H., Rittel, W., and Kahnt, F. W. (1968a). Helv. Chim. Acta 51, 917.

Neher, R., Riniker, B., Rittel, W., and Zuber, H. (1968b). Helv. Chim. Acta 51, 1900.

Neher, R., Riniker, B., Maier, R., Byfield, P. G. H., Gudmundsson, T. V., and MacIntyre, I. (1968c). Nature (London) 220, 984.

Niall, H. D. (1971). J. Agr. Food Chem. 19, 638.

Niall, H. D., Penhasi, H., Gilbert, P., Myers, R. C., Williams, F. G., and Potts, J. T., Jr. (1969a). Fed. Proc., Fed. Amer. Soc. Exp. Biol. 28, 661.

Niall, H. D., Keutmann, H. T., Copp, D. H., and Potts, J. T., Jr. (1969b). Proc. Nat. Acad. Sci. U. S. 64, 771.

Niall, H. D., Keutmann, H. T., Sauer, R., Hogan, M., Dawson, B. F., Aurbach, G. D., and Potts, J. T., Jr. (1970). Hoppe-Seyler's Z. Physiol. Chem. 351, 1586.

Niall, H. D., Keutmann, H. T., Sauer, R., O'Riordan, J. L. H., Dawson, B. F., Hogan, M., and Potts, J. T., Jr. (1971a). In preparation.

Niall, H. D., Sauer, R., and Potts, J. T., Jr. (1971b). In preparation.

Nonidez, J. F. (1932). Amer. J. Anat. 49, 479.

O'Dor, R. K., Parkes, C. O., and Copp, D. H. (1969). Can. J. Biochem. 47, 823.

O'Riordan, J. L. H., and Woodhead, J. S. (1970). J. Horm. Metab. Res. (in press).

O'Riordan, J. L. H., Potts, J. T., Jr., and Aurbach, G. D. (1971). Endocrinology 89, 234.

Parsons, J. A., and Reynolds, J. J. (1968). Lancet 1, 1067.

Pearse, A. G. E., and Carvalhiera, A. G. (1967). Nature (London) 214, 929.

Pietta, P. G., and Marshall, G. R. (1970). Chem. Commun. p. 650.

Pless, J., Bossert, H., Zehnder, K., and Guttmann, S. (1971). Helv. Chim. Acta (in press).

Potts, J. T., Jr. (1970a). Fed. Proc., Fed. Amer. Soc. Exp. Biol. 29, 1200.

Potts, J. T., Jr. (1970b). In "Hypophysiotropic Hormones of the Hypothalamus: Assay and Chemistry" (J. Meites, ed.). Williams & Wilkins, Baltimore, Maryland.

Potts, J. T., Jr., and Aurbach, G. D. (1965). In "The Parathyroid Glands" (P. J. Gaillard, R. V. Talmage, and A. M. Budy, eds.), p. 53. Univ. of Chicago Press, Chicago, Illinois.

Potts, J. T., Jr., Aurbach, G. D., and Sherwood, L. M. (1966). Recent Prog. Horm. Res. 22, 101.

Potts, J. T., Jr., Reisfeld, R. A., Hirsch, P. F., Wasthed, A. B., Voelkel, E. F., and Munson, P. L. (1967). Proc. Nat. Acad. Sci. U. S. 58, 328.

Potts, J. T., Jr., Reisfeld, R. A., Hirsch, P. F., Wasthed, A. B., and Munson, P. L. (1968a). In "Calcitonin: Symposium on Thyrocalcitonin and the C Cells" (S. F. Taylor, ed.), p. 63. Heinemann, London.

Potts, J. T., Jr., Keutmann, H. T., Niall, H., Deftos, L., Brewer, H. B., and Aurbach, G. D. (1968b). In "Parathyroid Hormone and Thyrocalcitonin (Calcitonin)" (R. V. Talmage and L. F. Bélanger, eds.), p. 44. Excerpta Med. Found., Amsterdam.

Potts, J. T., Jr., Niall, H. D., Keutmann, H. T., Brewer, H. B., Jr., and Deftos, L. J. (1968c). Proc. Nat. Acad. Sci. U. S. 59, 1321.

Potts, J. T., Jr., Niall, H. D., Keutmann, H. T., Deftos, L. J., and Parsons, J. A.

(1970). *In* "Calcitonin 1969: Proceedings of the Second International Symposium" (S. F. Taylor and G. Foster, eds.), p. 56. Heinemann, London.

Potts, J. T., Jr., Tregear, G. W., Keutmann, H. T., Niall, H. D., Sauer, R., Deftos, L. J., Dawson, B. F., Hogan, M. L., and Aurbach, G. D. (1971a). *Proc. Nat. Acad. Sci. U. S.* **68**, 63.

Potts, J. T., Jr., Murray, T. M., Peacock, M., Niall, H. D., Tregear, G. W., Keutmann, H. T., Powell, D., and Deftos, L. J. (1971b). *Amer. J. Med.* **50**, 639.

Potts, J. T., Jr., Keutmann, H. T., Niall, H. D., Habener, J. F., Tregear, G. W., Deftos, L. J., O'Riordan, J. L. H., and Aurbach, G. D. (1971c). *Proc. Parathyroid Conf., 4th, 1970* (in press).

Potts, J. T., Jr., Niall, H. D., Keutmann, H. T., and Lequin, R. M. (1971d). *Proc. Parathyroid Conf., 4th, 1970* (in press).

Putter, I., Kaczka, E. A., Harman, R. E., Rickes, E. L., Kempf, A. J., Chaiet, L., Rothrock, J. W., Wase, A. W., and Wolf, F. J. (1967). *J. Amer. Chem. Soc.* **89**, 5301.

Rasmussen, H., and Craig, L. C. (1959). *J. Amer. Chem. Soc.* **81**, 5003.

Rasmussen, H., and Craig, L. C. (1961). *J. Biol. Chem.* **236**, 759.

Rasmussen, H., and Craig, L. C. (1962). *Biochim. Biophys. Acta* **56**, 332.

Rasmussen, H., and Westall, R. (1957). *Nature (London)* **180**, 1429.

Rasmussen, H., Sze, Y. L., and Young, R. (1964). *J. Biol. Chem.* **239**, 2852.

Raulais, D., and Keutmann, H. T. (1971). Unpublished observations.

Riniker, B., Neher, R., Maier, R., Kahnt, F. W., Byfield, P. G. H., Gudmundsson, T. V., Galante, L., and MacIntyre, I. (1968). *Helv. Chim. Acta* **51**, 1738.

Riniker, B., Brugger, M., Kamber, B., Sieber, P., and Rittel W. (1969). *Helv. Chim. Acta* **52**, 1058.

Rittel, W., Brugger, M., Kamber, B., Riniker, B., and Sieber, P. (1968). *Helv. Chim. Acta* **51**, 924.

Sauer, R., Niall, H. D., and Potts, J. T., Jr. (1970). *Fed. Proc., Fed. Amer. Soc. Exp. Biol.* **29**, 728.

Schleuter, R. J., and Caldwell, A. L., Jr. (1967). *Endocrinology* **81**, 854.

Schwartz, I. L., Rasmussen, H., and Rudinger, J. (1964). *Proc. Nat. Acad. Sci. U. S.* **52**, 1044.

Sharpey-Schafer, E. (1924). "The Endocrine Organs," 2nd ed. London.

Sherwood, L. M., Rodman, J. S., and Lundberg, W. B., Jr. (1970). *Proc. Nat. Acad. Sci. U. S.* **67**, 1631.

Sherwood, L. M., Lundberg, W. B., Jr., Targovik, J. H., Rodman, J. S., and Seyfer, A. (1971). *Amer. J. Med.* **50**, 658.

Sieber, P., and Iselin, B. (1968a). *Helv. Chim. Acta* **51**, 614.

Sieber, P., and Iselin, B. (1968b). *Helv. Chim. Acta* **51**, 622.

Sieber, P., Brugger, M., Kamber, B., Riniker, B., and Rittel, W. (1968). *Helv. Chim. Acta* **51**, 2057.

Sieber, P., Brugger, M., Kamber, B., Riniker, B., Rittel, W., Maier, R., and Staehelin, M. (1970a). *In* "Calcitonin 1969: Proceedings of the Second International Symposium" (S. F. Taylor and G. Foster, eds.), p. 28. Heinemann, London.

Sieber, P., Riniker, B., Brugger, M., Kamber, B., and Rittel, W. (1970b). *Helv. Chim. Acta* **53**, 2135.

Singer, F. R., Neer, R. M., Krane, S. H., Parsons, J. A., and Potts, J. T., Jr. (1970). *J. Clin. Invest.* **49**, 87a.

Singer, F. R., Keutmann, H. T., Neer, R. M., Potts, J. T., Jr., and Krane, S. M. (1971). *Proc. Parathyroid Conf., 4th 1970* (in press).

Smith. L. F. (1966). *Amer. J. Med.* **40**, 662.

Steiner, D. F., Hallund, O., Rubenstein, A., Cho, S., and Bayliss, C. (1968). *Diabetes* **17**, 725.

Talmage, R. V., Neuenschwander, J., and Kraintz, L. (1964). *Fed. Proc., Fed. Amer. Soc. Exp. Biol.* **23**, 204.

Tashjian, A. H., Ontjes, D. A., and Munson, P. L. (1964). *Biochemistry* **3**, 1175.

Tauber, S. D. (1967). *Proc. Nat. Acad. Sci. U. S.* **58**, 1684.

Tenenhouse, A., Arnaud, C., and Rasmussen, H. (1965). *Proc. Nat. Acad. Sci. U. S.* **53**, 818.

Thompson, D. L., and Collip, J. B. (1932). *Physiol. Rev.* **12**, 309.

Tregear, G. W. (1969). PhD. Thesis, Monash University, Victoria, Australia.

Wang, S. S., and Merrifield, R. B. (1969). *Int. J. Protein Res.* **1**, 235.

Woodhead, J. S., O'Riordan, J. L. H., Keutmann, H. T., Stoltz, M. L., Dawson, B. F., Niall, H. D., Robinson, C. J., and Potts, J. T., Jr. (1971). *Biochemistry* **10**, 2787.

Protein-Polypeptide Hormones of the Human Placenta

BADRI N. SAXENA

*Department of Medicine Firm II, Christian Medical College Hospital,
Vellore-4 (Tamil Nadu), India*

To every thing there is a season, and a time to every purpose under the heaven.

Ecclesiastes 3:1

I. Introduction

The capacity of the placenta to act as an endocrine organ was first postulated by Halban (1905). Later, Selye *et al.* (1933) reported that in hypophysectomized rats the endocrine function of the pituitary gland was not necessary for the continuation of normal pregnancy and parturition. Several investigators (Little *et al.*, 1958; N. M. Kaplan, 1961; Wright and Joplin, 1966) observed that hypophysectomy after the first trimester of gestation had no adverse effect on the course of gestation in human pregnancies. These observations suggest that while the pituitary hormones are necessary for ovulation and successful implantation of the fertilized ova, the placental hormones play an important role in the successful continuation of pregnancy.

Human chorionic gonadotropin (HCG) was the first protein hormone isolated from the placenta. It is established that HCG is synthesized by the chorionic tissue. At the beginning of the 1960's, another hormone—human chorionic somatomammotropin, or HCS (originally designated as human placental lactogen)—was isolated, and its synthesis by human chorionic tissue has been confirmed. The presence of other substances whose hormonal activities resemble those of the pituitary gland, like ACTH, TSH, MSH, and oxytocin, has been demonstrated in the human placenta; also the presence of relaxin, acetylcholine, and other substances with uterotropic and pressor activities has been reported.

Earlier, this subject was reviewed by Newton (1938) and Levin (1944). Later, Diczfalusy and associates (Diczfalusy, 1953; Diczfalusy and Troen, 1961) extensively reviewed the endocrine functions of the human placenta. More recent reviews related to this subject have been published by Solomon and Friesen (1968), Brody (1969), and Villee (1969a,b).

In the present review, the following hormonal activities of the human placenta will be considered:

1. Human chorionic gonadotropin (HCG)
2. Human chorionic somatomammotropin (HCS)
3. Human chorionic thyrotropin (HCT)
4. Adrenocorticotropic hormone (ACTH)
5. Melanocyte-stimulating hormone (MSH)

6. Oxytocin
7. Insulin
8. Pressor factors:
   a. Vasopressin (antidiuretic hormone)
   b. Renin
   c. Norepinephrine and epinephrine
   d. Other factors; "hysterotonin," serotonin
9. Acetylcholine
10. Placental uterotropic hormone (PUH)
11. Relaxin
12. Juvenile hormone

II. Human Chorionic Gonadotropin (HCG)

Since the early reports of Fellner (1913) and Aschner (1913), there is now conclusive evidence that the placenta is capable of synthesizing large quantities of a gonadotropic hormone, designated as human chorionic gonadotropin (HCG). Brody (1969) has recently reviewed the literature on this hormone.

A. Proof of Production of HCG by the Placenta

1. Several investigators (Little et al., 1958; N. M. Kaplan, 1961) have reported normal urinary HCG levels throughout gestation in pregnant women who had undergone hypophysectomy during early pregnancy. These observations indicate that the maternal pituitary is not a source of HCG during pregnancy.

2. Human chorionic gonadotropin is found only in the chorionic tissue and body fluids of pregnant subjects and patients having trophoblastic disease or embryonic testicular or ovarian tumors (Brody, 1969).

3. After the delivery of the placenta, HCG disappears from the maternal circulation (Faiman et al., 1968; Midgley and Jaffe, 1968; Yen et al., 1968a).

4. It was found that HCG excretion continues for a long time following the surgical removal of the fetus but with the placenta left in situ (Siegler et al., 1959; Friedman et al., 1969). Similar observations of continued HCG excretion were reported following intrauterine death of the fetus, either induced (Cassmer, 1959) or spontaneous (Brody and Carlström, 1965a), with the placenta left in situ. These observations exclude a fetal origin for HCG.

5. Kido (1937) directly proved the placental production of HCG by transplanting chorionic tissue into the anterior chamber of the rabbit's eye, and by demonstrating the typical HCG effects on the host's ovary and the excretion of biologically active HCG in the host's urine. Several

other investigators have confirmed and extended these findings (Canivenc, 1951, quoted by Diczfalusy and Troen, 1961; Stewart, 1951; Grenier and Rebel, 1956; Hertz et al., 1959).

6. Tissue culture studies have also established the synthesis of HCG by normal chorionic tissue (Soma et al., 1961) as well as in the abnormal chorionic tissue from molar pregnancies (Waltz et al., 1954). Gitlin and Biasucci (1969) have confirmed placental synthesis of HCG by introducing a ^{14}C-labeled amino acid mixture into placental tissue incubates and recovering labeled HCG from these incubates by means of immunoelectrophoresis and radioautography.

B. SITE OF PRODUCTION OF HCG IN THE PLACENTA

Brody (1969) has reviewed the results of tissue culture, histochemical, and immunohistochemical studies to localize the site of production of HCG in the placenta. It is now agreed that HCG is produced by the trophoblastic cells, but it is still controversial whether HCG is produced by the cytotrophoblastic cells (Langhans cells) or by the syncytiotrophoblastic cells of the chorionic villi. Using a direct immunofluorescent technique, Midgley and Pierce (1962) could detect positive fluorescence only in the syncytiotrophoblastic cells. However, Thiede and Choate (1963), using a more sensitive indirect immunofluorescent technique, found positive fluorescence in both the Langhans and syncytiotrophoblastic cells. The electron microscopic data of several investigators suggest that syncytiotrophoblastic cells are derived by differentiation from the cytotrophoblastic cells and that the secretory capacity of the Langhans cells is doubtful (Midgley and Pierce, 1962; Stegner, quoted by Berle and Schultze-Mosgau, 1969). In view of these controversial data, it seems reasonable to suggest that HCG production starts in the cytotrophoblastic cells and continues in the syncytiotrophoblastic cells.

C. BIOCHEMICAL NATURE OF HCG

This subject has been recently reviewed by Hellema (1971). It has not yet been possible to achieve the complete purification and structural analysis of HCG, since it is an unstable hormone or a hormone complex, which, in addition, shows physicochemical similarities as well as an immunological cross-reactivity with pituitary gonadotropins—luteinizing hormone (LH) and follicle-stimulating hormone (FSH).

1. *Structure of HCG*

It has been reported that HCG has no N-terminal and no C-terminal amino acids but contains *N*-acetylneuraminic acid and fucose as non-reducing terminal units (Bahl, 1969b). Neuraminic acid may be essential for the biological activity of HCG, since activity was lost after enzyme treatment with neuraminidase or after acid hydrolysis (Schumacher *et al.*, 1960; Goverde *et al.*, 1968; Mori, 1969, 1970). Bahl (1969a,b) has isolated two chromatographically homogeneous glycopeptides and, using specific glycosidases, has determined the sequence of monosaccharides in the carbohydrate part of the HCG molecule. The polypeptide chains of HCG are linked to each other by disulfide bridges (Schlumberger and Blobel, 1969; Bahl, 1969a). The apparent molecular weight of HCG varies with the technique used (Bahl, 1969a). By gel filtration it was estimated as 59,000 ± 4000; by ultracentrifugation, 46,600 ± 3000; and treated HCG (reduced and carboxamidomethylated) appeared to have a molecular weight of 30,000± 2000.

2. Immunological Cross-Reactivity

The immunology of HCG was reviewed earlier by Lunenfeld and Eshkol (1967). The similarities in the immunological properties of HCG, LH, FSH, and TSH are perhaps related to their structural similarities (Schlaff *et al.*, 1968). This creates several problems in the radioimmuno-assays of these hormones, since they cross-react with each other in the assay system and since it is difficult to characterize the specificity of the antisera against these hormones (Schlaff *et al.*, 1968; Odell *et al.*, 1969a,b). A problem related to the cross-reactivity is the existence of an antiserum-neutralizing factor present in different gonadotropin prepara-tions (Petrusz, 1969). The antiserum-neutralizing factor possessing little, if any, biological activity, is immunologically active and reacts exten-sively with antibodies capable of neutralizing the biological activity of gonadotropins. Butt (1967, 1969) has shown that chemical or enzymatic treatment of HCG results in a modification of its biological and immuno-logical properties.

Dixon (1968) has isolated a glycoprotein having high sialic acid and proline content from the urine of pregnant subjects, which showed a cross-reactivity with the antisera prepared against glomerular basement membrane fragments from human kidneys. Canfield and Bell (1969) have also demonstrated the cross-reactivity of both purified and crude HCG with the glomerular basement membrane and suggested that this glycoprotein substance might be present as a contaminant in crude HCG preparations. This cross-reactivity may be an inherent property of the HCG molecule itself, although the occurrence of glomerulonephritis due to HCG injection has not yet been reported.

3. Homogeneity versus Heterogeneity of HCG

It has been observed that HCG is a dimer made up of identical and chromatographically homogeneous subunits which have a molecular weight of 23,000 to 28,000 (Bell et al., 1969; Canfield and Bell, 1969) (see Table I). However, reports by Hamashige and associates (Hamashige et al., 1967; Hamashige and Astor, 1969) support the suggestion that HCG represents a complex of hormones composed of at least three different types of HCG molecules. This conclusion was based on the differences observed in electrophoresis and ion-exchange chromatography, as well as in immunological and biological properties. It has been proposed that the cause of heterogeneity lies in the heterogeneity of the carbohydrate moiety of the HCG molecule (J. J. Bell et al., 1969). Several

TABLE I

AMINO ACID COMPOSITION OF A PURIFIED PREPARATION OF
HUMAN CHORIONIC GONADOTROPIN[a]

Lys	7	Ala	10
His	3	Cys/2	12–14
Arg	11	Val	12–13
Asp	13–14	Met	2
Thr	12–13	Ile	4–5
Ser	15–16	Leu	11
Glu	14	Tyr	4–5
Pro	20–21	Phe	4–5
Gly	10	Trp	1
Nana	8–10	Gal	9
GlcNAc	9–12	Man	9
GalNAc	2–3	Fuc	1

[a] Canfield and Bell (1969). Molecular weight 25,200–27,500.

other investigators have also presented evidence that HCG is either a hormone complex or an unstable hormone with unpredictable behavior (Reisfeld et al., 1963; Mathies and Diczfalusy, 1968; Yogo, 1969). One of the factors affecting the stability of HCG in vivo could be the influence of proteases. Schlumberger and Blobel (1967) showed an increase in the biological activity of HCG when HCG was given in combination with protease inhibitors. Albert (1968) has suggested that "the classical definition of a hormone is implicit in its bioassay." Thus, as stated by Hellema (1971), a general objection to all the studies mentioned here can be made, since most of them did not use a reliable bioassay with proper statistical evaluation. The most frequently used test, that of Parlow (1958, 1961), is considered to be of doubtful value under certain circumstances (Koed and Hamburger, 1968).

D. Biological Properties of HCG

Brody (1969) has reviewed the biological properties of HCG.

1. *Effects on the Internal Genitalia*

a. Interstitial Cell Stimulation. The interstitial cell stimulating effect of HCG, both on the testes and the ovaries of several animal species as well as humans, has been repeatedly demonstrated (Brody, 1969).

b. Gametokinetic Properties. The gametokinetic effect of HCG on the ovaries is debatable. Crooke and Butt (1959) regarded the FSH-like effect of urinary HCG preparations to be due to a contamination with pituitary FSH, whereas Albert and associates (Albert and Kelly, 1958; Albert, 1969; Northcutt and Albert, 1970) suggested that the FSH-like activity is either an inherent property of the HCG molecule or may be due to another placental protein hormone separate from HCG. Robyn *et al.* (1969) reported that HCG preparations contain a specific FSH-like activity; they could completely neutralize this activity with an anti-HCG serum without completely eliminating HCG activity. These investigators suggest that the FSH-like activity may be due to another placental glycoprotein hormone, separate from HCG.

The gametokinetic effect of HCG on the testis is also incompletely understood. Brody (1969), after reviewing the literature, concluded that the effect of HCG on testicular tissue is that of repair and stimulation of interstitial cells. The effect of HCG on the seminiferous tubules may be due to a synergistic action between HCG and pituitary gonadotropins and/or to the androgens produced by the stimulated Leydig cells.

c. Weight Increases of Accessory Reproductive Organs as Secondary Effect of the Testicular Stimulation. The weight increase of accessory male organs in immature rats has been described repeatedly. This effect of HCG is now used as a reliable and sensitive assay for its biological activity (Diczfalusy, 1954).

d. Luteotropic Effect. Earlier studies of Hisaw (1944) and Bryans (1951) suggested the luteotropic effect of HCG in monkeys. However, Short (1969) concludes that there is little, if any, evidence in the literature which supports the view that monkey chorionic gonadotropin (MCG) has any luteotropic effect. As in other species, such as the human, mare, sow, and ewe, the hormonal control of corpus luteum function in the monkey is incompletely understood (Short, 1969). In rats, Velardo (1959) has shown the induction of ovulation and prolongation of the pseudo-pregnant stage with HCG as well as the synergistic effects of HCG with pituitary hormones.

e. Steroidogenic Effect. Rice *et al.* (1964a,b) have shown that HCG stimulates the biosynthesis of progesterone by human corpora lutea and that of testosterone by human ovarian stromal tissue when these tissues are incubated with ^{14}C-labeled acetate. The steroidogenic effects of HCG on the testis of several animal species and humans are now well established (Brody, 1969).

2. Effects on the Adrenals

It is still uncertain whether the action of HCG on the adrenals is direct or indirect. Diczfalusy et al. (1950) could not find any effect of large doses of HCG in the hypophysectomized-gonadectomized rats, whereas Velardo (1959) found that a significant increase in adrenal weights occurred following HCG administration to both intact and hypophysectomized rats. Johannisson (1968) reported that large doses of HCG administered intra-amniotically in mid-pregnancy produced electron microscopic histological changes in the human fetal adrenals, suggesting output of steroids. Recently, Cushman (1970) found no stimulatory effect of HCG on the isolated adrenal gland in perfusion studies using mongrel dogs.

3. Effects on Placental Steroidogenesis

The early reports of G. V. Smith and Smith (1934, 1939, 1948; O. W. Smith and Smith, 1937) suggested that HCG had an influence on the biosynthesis of estrogens by the human placenta. The placental perfusion studies of several investigators (Troen, 1959, 1961; Cédard et al., 1961, 1962, 1964; Varangot et al., 1965) seemed to indicate that HCG stimulated the conversion of estradiol to estriol by the human placenta, as well as accelerated the aromatization of neutral steroids by activating the hydroxylation processes in the placenta. However, it was later reported that the estriol mentioned in the previous studies was in fact, 6α-hydroxyestradiol-17β (Cédard and Knuppen, 1965; Alonso and Troen, 1966). The recent reports of Diczfalusy and associates (Diczfalusy, 1967, 1969; Jackanicz and Diczfalusy, 1968) cast further doubts on the validity of the earlier observations. They reported that at mid-pregnancy the placenta lacks the capacity for 16α-hydroxylation and thus cannot synthesize estriol from estrone or 17β-estradiol.

E. NORMAL CONCENTRATIONS OF HCG IN THE PLACENTA AND IN BODY FLUIDS

1. Placental Content

Diczfalusy (1953) was the first to report placental concentrations of HCG in international units. Using improved methods of bioassay of

HCG (Diczfalusy, 1954) and combining their earlier data, Diczfalusy *et al.* (1958) constructed a curve relating placental HCG concentration and duration of pregnancy. In the first trimester (second and third lunar months) they found high HCG concentrations—up to 600 IU per gram wet weight, which declined abruptly between the third and fourth lunar month. From the fourth month onward, HCG concentrations stayed constant at a level below 20 IU per gram tissue. These data are in agreement with those of Loraine and Matthew (1953).

2. Serum Concentrations

Albert and Berkson (1951) were the first to publish a serum HCG curve in international units using bioassays. Several other investigators have also published serum HCG curves obtained with bioassays (Salvatiera, 1954; Loraine and Bell, 1966). With the immunological methods (radioimmunoassays, hemagglutination-inhibition, and microcomplement fixation method), serum HCG levels during normal pregnancy have also been reported (Wide, 1962; Mishell *et al.*, 1963; Brody and Carlstrom, 1962a,b; Wilde *et al.*, 1965, 1967; Midgley, 1966; Goldstein *et al.*, 1968) (see Figs. 1 and 2). There is general agreement about the shape of the serum HCG curve. However, considerable variation has been noted when the values obtained by bioassays were compared with those ob-

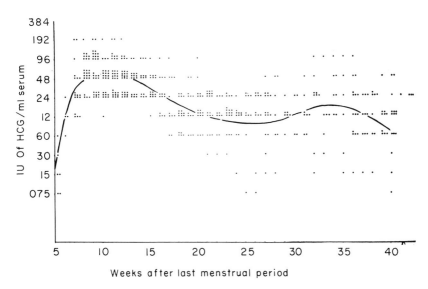

FIG. 1. Serum human chorionic gonadotropin (HCG) levels in normal pregnancy estimated by a micromethod based on complement fixation. According to Brody and Carlström (1962a).

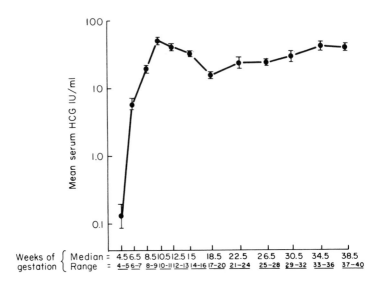

Fɪɢ. 2. Serum human chorionic gonadotropin (HCG) levels in normal pregnancy estimated by a radioimmunoassay method. According to Goldstein *et al.* (1968).

tained by immunoassays (Wide and Hobson, 1967; Baechler *et al.*, 1969). Within 9–12 days after ovulation (Wide, 1969), HCG is detectable in the maternal serum, rising sharply to a peak around day 60 of gestation. By day 80 HCG drops to a lower level, and it remains in the same low range until delivery. Some of the investigators, especially those using immunoassays (Goldstein *et al.*, 1968; Faiman *et al.*, 1968; Parlow *et al.*, 1970) have noted a small rise in HCG just before delivery. Borth *et al.* (1959) found no diurnal variation in serum HCG levels. Thus, the estimation of HCG in maternal serum appears to be as informative as that in 24-hour urine samples.

3. *Urinary Excretion*

Albert and Berkson (1951), using bioassay, and Wide (1962), using immunoassay (see Fig. 3), have constructed time curves for the HCG in pregnancy urine. The general shape of the urinary HCG curve is similar to that of the serum. Variations in the absolute levels of urinary HCG obtained by bioassays and immunoassays have been reported (Wide, 1962; Borth *et al.*, 1965; Wide and Hobson, 1967; E. T. Bell and Loraine, 1967) (see Fig. 4). The reason for this discrepancy is incompletely understood. However, it seems likely that the active sites of the HCG molecule which are responsible for the biological activity differ from those associated with immunological activity.

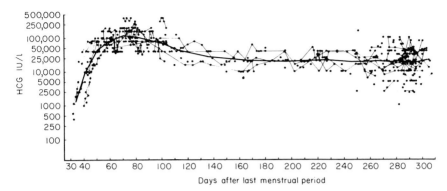

FIG. 3. Urinary human chorionic gonadotropin (HCG) levels in 522 first morning urines collected from 240 women with normal pregnancies. The heavy line represents mean values. The estimations were carried out by the hemagglutination–inhibition technique. According to Wide (1962).

4. Concentrations in Amniotic Fluid

Using bioassay, Berle (1969) has observed that the shape of the HCG curve in amniotic fluid is similar to that in maternal serum and urine (see Fig. 5). Amniotic fluid levels of HCG have also been measured by immunologic methods (McCarthy and Pennington, 1964; Crosignani and Polvani, 1969). It has been suggested that the level of HCG in amniotic fluid is directly proportional to the circulating maternal HCG

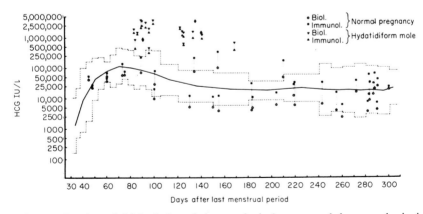

FIG. 4. Results of biological and immunological assays of human chorionic gonadotropin (HCG) activity in 32 urine specimens from 27 women with normal pregnancy and 19 urine specimens from 12 subjects with a hydatidiform mole. The continuous line represents the mean values and the dotted lines the fiducial limits of error $(P = 0.05)$ of the immunological HCG activity in morning urines from women with a normal pregnancy. According to Wide and Hobson (1967).

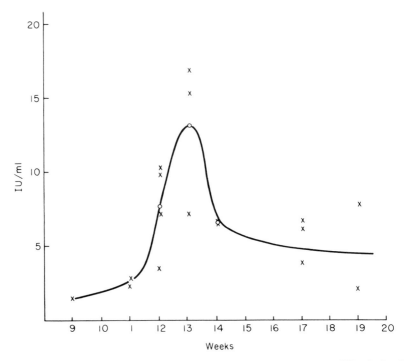

F<small>IG</small>. 5. Concentration of human chorionic gonadotropin (HCG) (IU/ml) in the amniotic fluid during the first 19 weeks of normal pregnancy. According to Berle (1969).

concentrations and that HCG might reach the amniotic fluid by trans-amnial or transchorial passage. The level of HCG in amniotic fluid is lower than that in maternal serum and higher than that in cord blood serum (Crosignani and Polvani, 1969).

5. Umbilical Artery and Vein

Lauritzen and Lehmann (1967) have shown that the concentration of HCG is higher in the umbilical vein than in the umbilical artery, sug-gesting a net uptake by the fetus. Similar findings were reported by Berle and associates (Berle and Schultze-Mosgau, 1968; Berle, 1969).

6. Concentrations in Cerebrospinal Fluid (CSF)

Using bioassay methods, earlier investigators (Ehrhardt, 1931; Zondek, 1942; McCormick, 1954; Tashima et al., 1965) concluded that HCG is found in CSF only when its urinary excretion is high, such as in patients with trophoblastic tumors. This concept of the threshold effect of HCG was challenged by Bagshawe and associates (Bagshawe et al., 1966,

1968; Rushworth *et al.*, 1968). Using a sensitive radioimmunoassay method, they concluded that the concentration of HCG in the spinal fluid of patients with trophoblastic tumors is directly proportional to its concentration in the plasma. Their estimate of the mean plasma: CSF ratio is 177:1.

7. *Other Tissue and Body Fluids*

Human chorionic gonadotropin has also been demonstrated in colostrum (Heim, 1931), vaginal secretions (K. Fukushima, 1934), and saliva (Zondek, 1942). The data reported by Bruner (1951) indicate that almost all the maternal tissues are permeated with HCG.

F. RATE OF SECRETION OF HCG

Earlier studies reported in the literature were based on urinary excretion rates of HCG using bioassay methods (for references, see Diczfalusy and Troen, 1961). Wide *et al.* (1968) have studied the metabolic clearance rate (MCR) of HCG injected into nonpregnant women, using a bioassay and a radioimmunoassay method. They reported an MCR of 4 ml/min. In a similar study using a radioimmunoassay, Rizkallah *et al.* (1969) have found the MCR (l/day) to be 3.38 for men and 3.86 for women. Assuming that the metabolism of HCG is not very different in pregnant and nonpregnant individuals, these investigators have calculated the production rate (PR) of HCG to be 26 mg/day during the peak production period and 1.4 mg/day during the latter half of gestation.

Disappearance rates for HCG have been reported by various investigators. Using both bioassay and radioimmunoassay, Wide *et al.* (1968) have calculated the half-life of injected HCG in nonpregnant women to be about 8 hours. With radioimmunoassay methods (Faiman *et al.*, 1968; Midgley and Jaffe, 1968; Yen *et al.*, 1968a), the disappearance curve for HCG after the delivery of the placenta has been found to consist of two linear components—the first corresponding to a half-life of 8–11 hours and the second corresponding to a half-life of 23–27 hours.

G. CONTROL OF SECRETION OF HCG

There is no conclusive evidence in the literature pointing to a distinct mechanism for the regulation of the production and release of HCG by the human placenta. As discussed previously, there is no evidence to support the suggestion of earlier workers that there is a relationship between HCG production and steroid biosynthesis by the placenta. It was also suggested that there is a placentotropic factor of pituitary origin necessary for the production of HCG by the placenta incubated *in vitro* (Lajos *et al.*, 1959; Lajos, 1960). As far as the *in vivo* synthesis of HCG is concerned, this postulated factor seems to be of little, if any, importance since other investigators (Little *et al.*, 1958; N. M. Kaplan, 1961) have found normal HCG levels throughout gestation in pregnant patients who had undergone hypophysectomy during early pregnancy. Brody and Carlström (1965a,b,c) have suggested that the fetus may have some regulatory influence on the secretion of HCG. Their conclusion was based on the indirect evidence of a relationship between the sex of the fetus and maternal serum HCG levels during the third trimester (see Fig. 6).

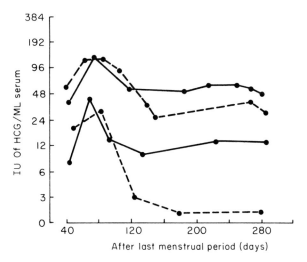

FIG. 6. Range of estimates of serum human chorionic gonadotropin (HCG) levels in women carrying a male fetus (dotted lines) and those with a female fetus (solid lines). Twenty patients were followed throughout pregnancy at intervals of 3–4 weeks. Assays were carried out by complement fixation. According to Brody and Carlström (1965c).

H. FUNCTIONS OF HCG IN PREGNANCY: PHYSIOLOGICAL ROLE

1. *Control of Corpus Luteum Function*

Various studies suggest that an intact corpus luteum is necessary for the continuation of pregnancy for the first few weeks; after that period the endocrine function of the ovaries is not indispensable (Ask-Upmark, 1926; Kulseng-Hanssen, 1951; Tulsky and Koff, 1957; Froewis, 1963). Nelson and Greene (1958) concluded from their histologic studies that the corpus luteum is active during the first 6 weeks of pregnancy and then deteriorates. The luteotropic role of HCG was based on the early reports of several investigators (W. E. Brown and Bradbury, 1947; de Watteville, 1949, quoted by Short, 1969; Bradbury *et al.*, 1950; Segaloff *et al.*, 1951). They all succeeded in postponing menstruation by administering HCG to women during the menstrual cycle. Short (1969) critically reevaluated these studies and found the evidence to be weak. He postulated that menstruation was postponed not because of any intrinsic luteotropic action of HCG, but because in large doses (as used by the earlier investigators), HCG induces the formation of new corpora lutea which in turn inhibit menstruation. Savard *et al.* (1965) showed that HCG is capable of stimulating progesterone synthesis by corpus luteum slices *in vitro.* Measurements of ovarian and peripheral venous progesterone concentrations indicate that the corpus luteum is an important source of progesterone in the first 12 weeks of pregnancy (Mikhail and Allen, 1967). Strott and Lipsett (1968) found that during the luteal phase of the menstrual cycle, both 17-hydroxyprogesterone (17-OHP) and plasma progesterone levels increase. They suggested that the elevated levels of 17-OHP reflect the function of the corpus luteum, since the placenta has either no (Palmer *et al.*, 1966), or only a very limited, capacity (Jungmann and Schweppe, 1957; Telegdy *et al.*, 1970) for 17-hydroxylation. Yoshimi *et al.* (1969) measured plasma levels of progesterone, 17-OHP, and HCG serially after the induction of ovulation by gonadotropins which resulted in single pregnancies (see Fig. 7). They concluded that HCG may play an important role in controlling steroidogenesis by the

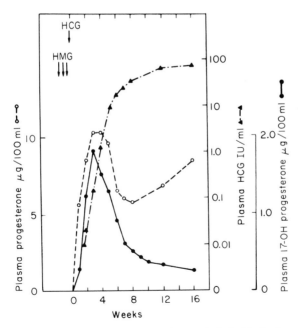

Fig. 7. Mean plasma levels of progesterone (open circles), 17α-hydroxyprogesterone (filled circles) and human chorionic gonadotropin (filled triangles) during early pregnancy. Pregnancy was induced by the sequential administration of human menopausal gonadotropin (HMG) and HCG. According to Yoshimi *et al.* (1969).

corpus luteum during the first 4 weeks of pregnancy since after that period, steroidogenesis declines even though HCG levels are still rising. Recently, LeMaire et al. (1970) reported that the corpus luteum at term pregnancy secretes progesterone, although the amount produced by it is only a fraction of that produced by the placenta. They suggested that HCG and HCS alone or in combination may maintain the functional capacity of the corpus luteum during pregnancy, up to the time of delivery. At any rate, the precise role of HCG as a stimulus for steroidogenesis by the corpus luteum in the early weeks after fertilization remains to be defined.

2. HCG and Placental Steroidogenesis

As discussed earlier, the role of HCG in the regulation of steroidogenesis by the human placenta is not clear.

3. HCG and Maternal Adrenal Steroidogenesis

Although some investigators have found that HCG in large doses causes a rise of 17-ketosteroid (17-KS) excretion in both castrated and menstruating women (Plate, 1952; Borell, 1954; Decio, 1955), others have not observed this effect (Borth et al., 1953). It has also been shown that the administration of HCG to normal, nonpregnant subjects induced a consistent rise in 17-KS but not in 17-hydroxycorticosteroids (17-OH); while ACTH administration stimulated the rise of both types of steroids (Hibbit et al., 1958; Eik-Nes et al., 1959). However, in all these studies, the stimulation of ACTH release and, thus, an ACTH effect on the adrenal cortex could not be ruled out. Therefore, a direct effect of HCG on the maternal adrenals remains to be demonstrated.

4. HCG and Fetal Adrenal Steroidogenesis

Johannisson (1968) has reported on characteristic electron microscopic changes in the fetal adrenals, following the intra-amniotic administration of HCG and ACTH at mid-pregnancy. ACTH treatment produced a depletion of osmiophilic material in the cells of the inner zone, suggesting an increased output of steroids. More prolonged ACTH treatment caused an increase in free ribosomes, indicating an increased synthesis of RNA. Ultrastructural changes of a similar nature were seen in the cells of the fetal zone when high doses of HCG were administered intra-amniotically. When an antiserum to HCG was perfused via the fetal blood circulation, signs of decreased secretory activity of these cells were noted. Benirschke (1956) has suggested that the adrenal gland of anencephalic fetuses develops normally during the first trimester, but after week 20 of gestation the fetal zone undergoes involution comparable to

that seen normally after birth. In view of these findings, it has been suggested that HCG may stimulate adrenal growth during the first few
months of pregnancy (Villee, 1969a). When HCG production decreases
after the 4th month of gestation, the maintenance of the adrenal cortex
is taken over by other hormones which are most probably of fetal pituitary origin. In a recent study, Lauritzen *et al.* (1969) have found that
injections of HCG into male infants stimulate the excretion of dehydroepiandrosterone (DHA). However, the effect is not consistent. No response was obtained in the first three infants studied, and the increase
in the excretion of the remaining four was variable. Further studies are
required to elucidate the role of HCG in the regulation of fetal adrenal
steroidogenesis.

5. HCG and the Fetal Gonads

Morphologic differentiation of the Leydig cells of the interstitial tissue
is seen at about 8 weeks (Niemi *et al.*, 1967). The Leydig cells increase
in number, reaching a maximum in fetuses of 14–16 weeks of age, and
then decline after week 17. Jirasek (1967) has pointed out that the
masculinization of external genitalia is always preceded by differentiation
of Leydig cells. The factor initiating the differentiation of Leydig cells in
the second month of pregnancy is unknown. The earliest period of production of LH by the fetal pituitary is not clear (Levina and Ivanova,
1963, 1964, quoted by Gitlin and Biasucci, 1969; Rice *et al.*, 1968; Gitlin
and Biasucci, 1969). The evidence available at the moment seems to suggest that LH synthesis by the fetal pituitary starts too late to act as a
source by gonadotropic stimulus for the initial differentiation of the
mesenchyme. The pattern of HCG in the amniotic fluid has been found
to be similar to that in the maternal serum (Berle, 1969). Brody and
Carlström (1965a,b) have noted a relationship between the sex of the
fetus and the maternal HCG levels (Fig. 6). Thus, it has been suggested
that the development of fetal Leydig cells may be initiated by HCG
(Villee, 1969b). This suggestion is supported by the increase in histo-
chemically active interstitial tissue (Niemi *et al.*, 1967), coinciding with
the increase of HCG levels in the maternal blood and amniotic fluid. The
decrease in Leydig cell activity after week 17 might be explained in the
same way, since the HCG levels in maternal serum and amniotic fluid
also show a decrease.

The role of the FSH-like activity of HCG is subject to considerable
debate. Whereas Faiman *et al.* (1968) found that FSH levels are high in
pregnancy serum, Jaffe *et al.* (1969) and Parlow *et al.* (1970) did not
find any increase in FSH concentrations. It is not possible to explain the
discrepancy of the data of these investigators; all of them claim to have

used "specific" radioimmunoassays. Albert (1969) has suggested that during the peak period of HCG production (40–90 days), the high amounts of FSH-like activity in HCG may play an important role in the development of fetal ovaries.

I. FUNCTIONS OF HCG IN PREGNANCY: CLINICAL SIGNIFICANCE OF HCG CONCENTRATIONS

This subject has been extensively reviewed by Loraine and Bell (1966), Brody (1969), and Klopper (1970).

1. Multiple Pregnancy

The data of several investigators show a variable picture of HCG levels in twin pregnancies. In some cases abnormally high levels are found, whereas in others the HCG levels were in the upper limit of the normal range. Delfs (1957) and Halpin (1970) have suggested that the high HCG titers may raise some problems in the differential diagnosis of

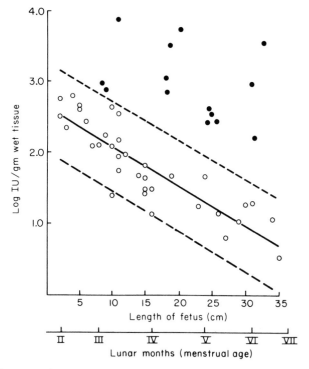

FIG. 8. Concentration of human chorionic gonadotropin in placental tissue from normal pregnant subjects (open circles) and from patients with hydatidiform moles (filled circles). According to Diczfalusy et al. (1958).

twin pregnancy versus molar pregnancy. It seems justifiable to suggest that further investigations should precede any efforts to evacuate a suspected mole.

2. Trophoblastic Disease

Several investigators have reported that the placental concentrations of HCG are quite high in hydatidiform moles (see Fig. 8) (Diczfalusy *et al.*, 1958; Hobson, 1958). Some workers have emphasized the superiority of serum assays (Delfs, 1957; Brody and Carlström, 1926b). Ellegood *et al.* (1969) suggested that although high HCG levels are not always conclusive, the persistence of high HCG levels beyond 15 weeks of gestation should support the diagnosis of a mole or choriocarcinoma. It is now well accepted that HCG estimations are a reliable and sensitive index for monitoring the response of patients to therapy (Hertz *et al.*, 1959, 1961; Saxena *et al.*, 1968b; Yen *et al.*, 1968b). Wide and Hobson (1964, 1967; Hobson and Wide, 1968) reported that the calculation of a B:I ratio of HCG (B = value obtained by bioassay and I = value by immunoassay) in the urine is of considerable diagnostic and prognostic value in trophoblastic tumors. They observed that the urines from pregnant women with a hydatidiform mole have a higher B:I ratio than urines from women with normal pregnancies (see Fig. 9) and suggested that this difference could be used to distinguish between a pregnancy and

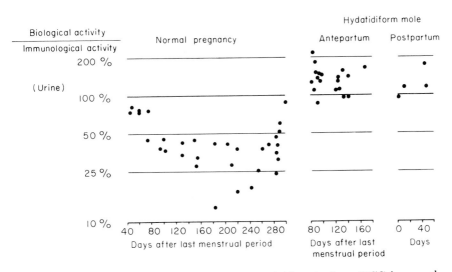

Fig. 9. Ratio of biological and immunological activities of urinary HCG in normal pregnancy and in patients with trophoblastic disease. According to Wide and Hobson (1967).

a hydatidiform mole. However, it is not possible to distinguish between chorioadenoma and choriocarcinoma. They also found a distinct difference between the B:I ratio of urine specimens from women who were still alive and those who had died before the end of the study. A high B:I ratio was associated with a good prognosis and a low B:I ratio with a poor one. Rushworth et al. (1968) suggested that, for diagnosing intracranial metastases of choriocarcinoma, estimations of HCG in the plasma and CSF could be useful. They found the ratio of plasma:CSF to be 100:1 in patients who did not have intracranial metastases and 35:1 in patients who did. There are some reports suggesting that the HCG produced by the normal trophoblast may not be identical with that produced by the abnormal trophoblast (Reisfeld et al., 1959; Schwartz and Mantel, 1963).

3. Diabetic Pregnancy

High levels of HCG have been reported in the maternal serum (White and Hunt, 1943; Samaan et al., 1969; Varma et al., 1970) and the amniotic fluid (Berle, 1969) of pregnant diabetic subjects. However, estimations of HCG appear to be of little value in the management of diabetic pregnancies (Loraine and Bell, 1966; Brody, 1969; Klopper, 1970).

4. Toxemia of Pregnancy

G. V. Smith and Smith (1948) reported high HCG levels in the majority of patients with toxemia, whereas, others have found high levels of HCG only in severe toxemia (Loraine and Matthew, 1950; Lloyd et al., 1951; Loraine and Bell, 1966). It is now generally agreed that estimations of HCG are not useful in the management of a pregnancy complicated with severe toxemia (Loraine and Bell, 1966; Teoh and Sivasamboo, 1968; Samaan et al., 1969; Brody, 1969; Klopper, 1970).

5. Threatened Abortion

It has been suggested that the use of immunoassays for estimating HCG may be more useful than that of bioassays in predicting the outcome of a threatened abortion (Brody, 1969). The published studies do not suggest that HCG assays discriminate clearly between those who are going to abort and those who are not (Klopper, 1970). Since the etiology of abortion is varied, the estimations of HCG may be useful only in those cases when the abortion is due to the pathological condition of the placenta.

6. Rh Isoimmunization

It is now accepted that the measurement of HCG in the maternal serum is not useful in the management of pregnancy complicated by Rh isoimmunization (Goplerud and Bradbury, 1965; Samaan et al., 1969). Berle and Schultze-Mosgau (1969) suggested that HCG estimations in the amniotic fluid might be of some value in determining the severity of Rh-disease.

7. Prolonged Pregnancy

Using immunoassay, Danielsson (1965) found that HCG estimations did not help in the management of prolonged pregnancy.

8. Retarded Fetal Growth

Klopper (1970) found no report which would indicate that HCG estimations are useful in the management of pregnant women with retarded fetal growth and suggested that the subject should be investigated.

III. HUMAN CHORIONIC SOMATOMAMMOTROPIN (HCS)

Ehrhardt (1936) was the first to postulate that prolactin activity is present in the human placenta. After a gap of 25 years, M. Fukushima (1961) isolated a somatotropic substance, and Ito and Higashi (1961) identified a prolactin-like material in the human placenta. About the same time, Josimovich and MacLaren (1962) reported the isolation of a substance which was lactogenic and showed a partial cross-reactivity with antisera to human pituitary growth hormone. They designated this hormonal substance as "human placental lactogen" (HPL). A variety of names have been proposed for this hormone. In order to eliminate the confusion by the use of different terms for the same hormone, it was decided recently to designate this hormone as "human chorionic somato-mammotropin" or HCS (Li et al., 1968). In this report, the term HCS will be used. A number of investigators have published reviews on HCS (Grumbach et al., 1968; Solomon and Friesen, 1968; Selenkow et al., 1969; Spellacy, 1969; Josimovich et al., 1969).

A. PROOF OF PRODUCTION OF HCS BY THE PLACENTA

1. Human chorionic somatomammotropin has been detected in the serum and the placenta of pregnant patients who had undergone hypophysectomy during the first trimester (Josimovich and Brande, 1964). This finding indicating that the maternal pituitary is not the source of HCS during pregnancy was further supported by the observation that no HCS was detected in the pituitary of a pregnant woman (Josimovich and Atwood, 1964).

2. The apparent absence of HCS (less than 1 μg/ml) from fetal serum and fetal pituitaries, as well as its presence in hydatidiform moles and blighted ova with viable trophoblast, suggest that the fetus is not responsible for the synthesis of HCS (Josimovich and Brande, 1964).

3. The chorionic tissue of the placenta appears to be necessary for HCS synthesis since HCS is detectable in the chorionic tissue and body fluids of pregnant subjects and of patients having trophoblastic tumors (Samaan et al., 1966; Spellacy et al., 1966; Grumbach et al., 1968; Saxena et al., 1968a,b). In these studies, it was also found that HCS disappears rapidly from the maternal circulation following delivery of the placenta.

4. Tissue culture studies have confirmed that the placenta not merely stores, but actually synthesizes, HCS. Gusdon and Yen (1967) added a mixture of ^{14}C-labeled amino acids to placental tissue cultures and recovered labeled HCS. Friesen and associates (Friesen, 1968; Suwa and Friesen, 1969a,b) extended these observations and have confirmed the fact that HCS is a major protein synthesized by the term placenta.

B. SITE OF PRODUCTION OF HCS IN THE PLACENTA

Sciarra et al. (1963), using Coon's fluorescent labeled antibody technique, were the first to find the specific fluorescence in the syncytiotrophoblastic villous epithelium. The specific fluorescence in the syncytiotrophoblast was consistently detectable in the placenta from 2 weeks of gestation until term, but no fluorescence could be detected in the cytotrophoblastic layer. These findings have been confirmed recently by J. S. Beck et al. (1969).

C. BIOCHEMICAL NATURE OF HCS

1. *Structure of HCS*

HCS has been obtained in a highly purified form, and its molecular weight has been found to be about 20,000, with a single polypeptide chain (Li et al., 1968). The NH_2 and COOH-terminal residues have been found to be valine and phenylalanine, respectively (Catt et al., 1967; Sherwood, 1967). Recently, Sherwood (1969) reported striking similarities in the location of disulfide bridges of HCS and HGH as well as in the composition of amino acids (see Table II). However, he noted some significant differences, such as 6 histidine and 5 methionine residues in HCS versus 3 of each in HGH. Sherwood also observed striking similarities between HCS and HGH in the sequence of 14 COOH-residues; however, there was a substitution of methionine for isoleucine at position 176 of HGH.

TABLE II
Similarities in the Amino Acid Composition of Human Chorionic
Somatomammotropin (HCS) and Human Growth Hormone (HGH)[a]

Identical peptides of HCS and HGH

HGH 8:	Asp, Ser, Glu, Leu$_3$, Arg	T17a:	Asp, Ser, Glu, Leu$_3$, Arg
HGH 10:	Asp, Thr, Glu$_3$, Gly$_2$, Met, Ile, Leu$_2$, Arg	T8a:	Asp, Thr, Glu$_3$, Gly$_2$, Met, Ile, Leu$_2$, Arg
HGH 13:	Thr, Ser, Glu, Tyr, Lys	T7a:	Thr, Ser, Glu, Tyr, Lys
HGH 15:	Asp, Gly, Cys, Leu$_2$, Tyr$_2$, Phe, Arg	T16a:	Asp, Gly, Cys, Leu$_2$, Tyr$_2$, Phe, Arg
HGH 16:	Lys	T12d:	Lys
HGH 17:	Asp$_2$, Met, Lys	T14a:[b]	Asp$_2$, Thr, Glu, Val, Met, Leu, Phe, Lys, Arg
HGH 18:	Thr, Glu, Val, Leu, Phe, Arg		
HGH 20:	Ser$_2$, Glu, Gly$_2$, Cys, Val, Phe	T5a:	Ser$_2$, Glu, Gly$_2$, Cys, Val, Phe

Similar peptides of HCS and HGH

HGH 1:	Thr, Ser, Pro$_2$, Ile, Leu, Phe, Arg	T18s:	Thr, Ser, Glu, Pro, Val$_2$, Leu, Arg	(3)[c]
HGH 3:	Ser$_2$, Glu$_3$, Pro, Ala, Val, Ile$_2$, Leu$_4$, Phe, His, Try, Arg	T24:	Ser$_2$, Glu$_{2-3}$, Pro, Ala?, Val, Ile$_2$, Leu$_4$, Phe?, Try, Arg	$-$(1)
HGH 4:	Asp, Thr, Glu$_5$, Pro, Ala$_2$, Ile, Leu$_2$, Tyr$_2$, Phe$_2$, His, Lys	T18:	Asp$_{1-2}$, Thr$_2$, Glu$_{4-5}$, Pro, Ala$_2$, Ile$_2$, Leu, Tyr$_2$, Phe, His, Lys	(4)
HGH 5:	Glu$_2$, Lys	T7b:	Asp, Glu, Lys	(1)
HGH 11:	Asp, Ser, Glu, Pro, Gly, Leu, Arg	T9b:	Asp, Ser, Glu, Gly, Leu, Arg	$-$(1)
HGH 12:	Thr, Glu, Gly, Ile, Phe, Lys	T16c:	Thr, Glu, Gly, Ile, Leu, Lys	(1)
HGH 14:	Asp$_5$, Thr, Ser, Ala, Leu$_2$, Phe, His, Lys	T20d:	Asp$_4$, Thr, Ser, Ala, Leu$_2$, Phe, His$_{1-2}$, Lys	(1)
HGH 19:	Glu, Cys, Val, Ile, Arg	T13c:	Glu, Cys, Met, Val, Arg	(1)

[a] Sherwood (1969).
[b] Failure of cleavage at a trypsin-sensitive site produced peptide with composition equal to two adjacent tryptic peptides of HGH.
[c] Number of substitutions or differences from apparently homologous peptides in HGH.

2. *Immunological Cross-Reactivity*

Josimovich and associates (Josimovich and MacLaren, 1962; Josimovich *et al.*, 1963) reported a cross-reaction of partial identity between HCS and HGH in Ouchterlony gel diffusion studies. However, they acknowledged that this reaction of partial identity between HCS and HGH might actually represent a reaction of identity with prolactin superimposed upon growth hormone precipitin lines. In a later study, S. L. Kaplan and Grumbach (1964) supported these observations and suggested that HCS and HGH share certain common antigenic determinants but are separate molecules. Josimovich and Mintz (1968) have further suggested that the lactogenic and mammotropic properties of HCS are associated with different antigenic sites of the molecule. Recently, Gusdon *et al.* (1970) compared the cross-reactivity of anti-HCS sera with HCS and placental proteins from different species like monkey, dog, horse, sheep, rabbit, and cow. They found similar cross-reactivity with HCS and placental proteins (extracted with the same method as that of HCS), a finding that suggests structural and functional similarities between the placental proteins of the species tested. However, Grant *et al.* (1970) observed that monkey chorionic somatomammotropin (MCS) is different from HCS both physicochemically and immunochemically. Sherwood (1969) and Breuer (1969) showed that chemical and enzymatic treatment of HCS results in a modification of its biological and immunological properties.

D. BIOLOGICAL PROPERTIES OF HCS

1. *Somatotropic Activity*

The somatotropic activity of HCS has been repeatedly demonstrated by an increase in the width of costal cartilage, and increased uptake of ^{35}S by the costal cartilage of hypophysectomized rats and body weight gain of intact and hypophysectomized rats (for references, see Selenkow *et al.*, 1969). An increased incorporation of thymidine into rat cartilage or adipose tissue has also been shown (Murakawa and Raben, 1968; Breuer, 1969). The biological (somatotropic) activity of HCS has been found to be about 10% of that of HGH, and a synergistic effect of HCS with HGH has also been demonstrated (Josimovich, 1966; Murakawa and Raben, 1968).

2. *Mammotropic Activity*

When HCS was injected into rats, an increase in the weight of mammary glands (Franchimont, 1965) and the development of mammary alveoli (Turkington and Topper, 1966) was observed.

3. *Lactogenic Activity*

The lactogenic activity of HCS has been shown by various investigators by the pigeon crop sac assay and by the appearance of lactation in pseudopregnant rats (for references, see Selenkow *et al.*, 1969). Turkington and associates found that HCS in combination with insulin and hydrocortisone stimulates the synthesis of milk proteins in mammary epithelial cells in organ culture (Turkington and Topper, 1966; Turkington, 1968, 1970). In 1968, Beck (quoted by Josimovich *et al.*, 1969) observed that HCS causes lactogenesis in rhesus monkeys pretreated with progestins and estrogens.

4. Luteotropic Activity

Luteotropic activity of HCS has been reported by Josimovich and associates (1963; Josimovich, 1968a). They observed that administration of HCS to pseudopregnant rats will maintain an induced endometrial decidual reaction and vaginal mucification for 3 days. They found similar changes with HCG. However, they showed that the administration of HCS in combination with HCG will prolong this effect for 7 days. This was interpreted as a synergistic effect.

5. Metabolic Activity

The increased mobilization of free fatty acids by HCS has been demonstrated in various animal species (for references, see Selenkow et al., 1969). Furthermore, administration of HCS to hypophysectomized rats caused a marked increase in glucose-induced insulin secretion with a less marked increase in the pancreatic insulin content (Malaisse et al., 1969; Martin and Friesen, 1969).

6. Erythropoietic Activity

In normal rodents, HCS increased the red cell mass, plasma volume, and utilization of ^{59}Fe by erythrocytes (Jepson and Lowenstein, 1968a,b). On the basis of their further studies, Jepson and associates suggested that the main action of HCS may be augmentation of the effect of erythropoietin (Jepson, 1968; Jepson and Friesen, 1968).

7. Aldosterone Stimulating Activity

Melby et al. (1966) showed that in adult males and females HCS stimulates aldosterone secretion (for further details, see Section III,H).

E. NORMAL CONCENTRATIONS OF HCS IN THE PLACENTA AND IN BODY FLUIDS

1. Placental Concentrations

The concentration of HCS in the placenta appears to remain at about the same constant level (2–10 mg/100 gm wet weight) throughout the entire period of gestation (Josimovich, 1968b), while the total content of HCS seems to parallel placental growth (Josimovich and Brande, 1964). There is a linearity of increase in placental weight, placental content of HCS, and the concentration of HCS in the maternal plasma from week 12 of gestation until term (Josimovich, 1968b) (see Fig. 10).

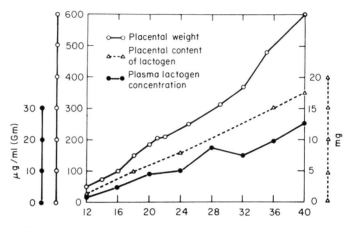

Fig. 10. Linearity of increase in placental weight, placental content of HCS (placental lactogen) and concentration of HCS in maternal plasma from week 12 of gestation to term. According to Josimovich (1968b). The term "lactogen" used in this figure is synonymous with HCS.

2. Serum Concentrations

The serum concentrations have been measured by immunologic methods, mainly by radioimmunoassays (for references, see Selenkow et al., 1969; Leake and Burt, 1969). There is general agreement about the shape of HCS curve. However, considerable differences are noted when values obtained by the different investigators are compared (see Table III). It is likely that this is due to differences in the purity of

TABLE III

MEAN VALUES FOR SERUM HCS IN NORMAL TERM PREGNANCY AND TROPHOBLASTIC
DISEASES REPORTED IN THE LITERATURE BY RADIOIMMUNOASSAY METHODS[a]

Investigators (reference)	Maternal serum IR-HCS (µg/ml)	Cord serum IR-HCS (µg/ml)	Trophoblastic disease (µg/ml)
Kaplan and Grumbach (1965b)	5.6	0.019	—
Beck et al. (1965)	25.0	—	—
Frantz et al. (1965)	2.0–9.0	—	0.001–0.420
Spellacy et al. (1966)	10.8	0.100	—
Samaan et al. (1966)	3.3	0.130	0.02–0.16
Schalch et al. (1967)	5.4	—	—
Beck and Daughaday (1967)	1.15	—	—
Saxena et al. (1968a)	19.8	—	0.014–0.36
Grumbach et al. (1968)	3.7	0.013	0.01–1.0
Selenkow et al. (1969)	6.8	0.053	0.007–0.18

[a] Selenkow et al. (1969).

antigen and potency of antisera. In the maternal serum, HCS is detectable consistently after 6 weeks of gestation and rises progressively to reach a plateau after 34 weeks of gestation (Fig. 11). In cord blood, HCS levels are about 1.4% of the maternal levels, suggesting a limited transplacental flux of HCS from mother to fetus (Selenkow *et al.*, 1969).

3. *Urine Concentrations*

S. L. Kaplan *et al.* (1968) calculated that only about 0.001% of the estimated daily production of HCS is excreted in the urine of pregnant subjects. This may be a result of rapid metabolic degradation.

4. *Amniotic Fluid Concentrations*

The concentration of HCS in the amniotic fluid is about 20% of that seen in the maternal serum (Tallberg *et al.*, 1965; Josimovich, 1968b). S. L. Kaplan *et al.* (1968) observed a very limited transfer of ^{131}I-HCS to the amniotic fluid during term pregnancy. It is still controversial whether HCS reaches the amniotic fluid via the chorioamnion without passing through the fetal circulation (Grumbach *et al.*, 1968) or is directly secreted into the fetal circulation and then excreted by the fetal kidneys into the amniotic fluid (Josimovich, 1968b).

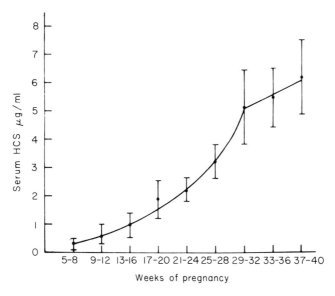

Fig. 11. Serum human chorionic somatomammotropin (HCS) levels in normal pregnancy estimated by a radioimmunoassay method. According to Saxena *et al.* (1969).

F. RATE OF SECRETION OF HCS

S. L. Kaplan *et al.* (1968) found the mean metabolic clearance rate (MCR) of HCS to be 173 liters/day. They also reported that the production rate (PR) of HCS during the third trimester is about 1 gm/day, which is comparable to that reported by P. Beck and Daughaday in 1967, if correction is made for the differences in the immunological potency of HCS standards used in each study. The half-life of circulating HCS has been estimated to be about 29 minutes (Spellacy *et al.*, 1966) or less (P. Beck *et al.*, 1965; S. L. Kaplan and Grumbach, 1965b). In their more recent study, S. L. Kaplan *et al.* (1968) have found that the disappearance curve of plasma HCS consists of two linear components, the first corresponding to a half-life of about 11 minutes and the second component to that of several hours.

G. CONTROL OF SECRETION OF HCS

The production rate of HCS appears to be autonomous, unaffected by maternal exercise, food ingestion, circadian rhythm or maternal hyper- or hypoglycemia (Spellacy *et al.*, 1966; Samaan *et al.*, 1966). Recently, Burt *et al.* (1970) found that HCS tends to decrease significantly in term pregnant subjects during the first 30 minutes of a double intravenous glucose loading test. This finding is in contrast to results of previous investigators, and the discrepancy may be due to differences in sampling or other factors. In their tissue culture studies, Suwa and Friesen (1969b) found no effect of insulin, progesterone, cortisone, or 3',5'-cyclic AMP on the biosynthesis and release of HCS.

H. FUNCTIONS OF HCS IN PREGNANCY: PHYSIOLOGICAL ROLE

1. *Augmentation of Insulin Release and Insulin Antagonism by HCS*

HCS possesses both insulinogenic and diabetogenic actions. In normal subjects given HCS infusion, the insulin secretion is increased but no carbohydrate intolerance occurs after a glucose load (Daughaday and Kipnis, 1966; P. Beck and Daughaday, 1967; Samaan *et al.*, 1968). Kalkhoff *et al.* (1969) reported that an HCS load given in the postpartum period to women who had a normal glucose tolerance test during pregnancy showed minimal effect. However, when the HCS infusion was given to women who had gestational diabetes or to those with subclinical diabetes, it caused impaired carbohydrate tolerance. This observation suggests that HCS is one of the factors associated with the diabetogenic stress of pregnancy.

The progressive decrease in insulin responsiveness parallels the rise in

HCS levels (Spellacy and Goetz, 1963; Yen et al., 1967; Grumbach et al., 1968). The free fatty acids are rapidly mobilized by HCS (Grumbach et al., 1966); therefore, at the peripheral level, the antagonistic action of HCS appears to be due to its lipolytic effect. This suggestion is supported by Turtle and Kipnis (1967), who found specific alterations in glucose and acetate oxidation resulting from the action of HCS on isolated fat-cell preparations. Tyson et al. (1969) found a blunted plasma insulin response to arginine during the first two trimesters, but an exaggerated response was seen in the third trimester. It is not possible to explain the significance of the findings during the first two trimesters. It has been suggested that they might be the result of the arginine stimulus used (Tyson et al., 1969). There is evidence that the circulating glucose level plays a significant role in determining the quantitative release of insulin following arginine infusion (Rabinowitz et al. and Edgar et al., quoted by Tyson et al., 1969). Thus, the poor insulin response observed in the first two trimesters may—at least in part—be due to the lesser degree of hyperglycemia relative to that seen in nonpregnant females (Merimee et al., 1967).

2. Suppression of Anterior Pituitary Growth Hormone (HGH) by HCS

It is now accepted that serum HGH levels throughout the entire period of gestation are within the normal range of nonpregnant individuals (S. L. Kaplan and Grumbach, 1965a; Yen et al., 1967; Spellacy and Buhi, 1969). The HGH response to insulin hypoglycemia and arginine have been found to be blunted during the last trimester of pregnancy and early postpartum period (Spellacy, 1967; Yen et al., 1967; Mintz et al., 1968; Grumbach et al., 1968; Spellacy and Buhi, 1969; Tyson et al., 1969; Katz et al., 1969). However, during early and midpregnancy, HGH response to arginine stimulation is quite different from that seen in insulin hypoglycemia. Tyson et al. (1969) found a normal HGH response to arginine stimulation in the first two trimesters. On the other hand, Spellacy et al. (1970a) and Yen et al. (1970), observed that the HGH response to insulin hypoglycemia is progressively blunted in the first two trimesters. It has been postulated by Katz et al. (1969) that suppression of the HGH response may be a consequence, at least in part, of the high concentrations of HCS during late pregnancy, which may inhibit the hypothalamopituitary growth hormone-releasing mechanism. This suppression persists into early puerperium with a gradual reversal during late puerperium. Animal studies have shown that pituitary growth hormone may inhibit its own secretion by means of a central short-loop feedback mechanism (for references, see Katz et al.,

1969). In humans, Abrams *et al.* (1969) observed that the administration of high doses of HGH suppresses the growth hormone-releasing mechanism. Using a modified staining technique, Goluboff and Ezrin (1969) studied human pituitaries obtained from the autopsies of pregnant and postpartum cases. They found that the somatotropes decreased in number with a concomitant increase of prolactin cells during pregnancy and the early postpartum period. They also postulated that somatotropes may be inhibited by the large amounts of circulating HCS during pregnancy, which may continue for some time after delivery.

However, the actual suppression of growth hormone-releasing factor (GRF) by HCS remains to be demonstrated in clinical experiments. Furthermore, such a thesis of GRF suppression by HCS alone fails to explain the differences in HGH response to arginine and insulin hypoglycemia during the first two trimesters. The disparity in HGH response to arginine and insulin hypoglycemia during early and mid-gestation could be due to a difference in HGH-releasing mechanisms exerted by these two stimuli. It is known that the concentrations of various steroids like free cortisol and progesterone increase during pregnancy. It seems likely that these steroids, along with HCS, may play important roles in regulating the HGH hypothalamopituitary axis during pregnancy (Spellacy *et al.*, 1970a; Yen *et al.*, 1970).

3. Anabolic Activity of HCS

Recent studies in man indicate that HCS causes retention of nitrogen, potassium, and phosphorus as well as an increase in urinary excretion of calcium and hydroxyproline (Catt *et al.*, 1967; Burr *et al.*, 1967; Grumbach *et al.*, 1968). According to Selenkow *et al.* (1969), the most suitable explanation for the net anabolic action of HCS seems to be an increased production of insulin in response to a glucose load. Both these hormones are known to have a powerful effect on protein synthesis and their synergism may result in a more efficient utilization of carbohydrate substrates for the synthesis of proteins. This attractive hypothesis requires experimental verification in human gestation.

4. Lipolytic Activity of HCS

It has been postulated that due to the lipolytic activity of HCS, free fatty acids—a major source of high energy substrate—become available to the mother during pregnancy. As a consequence of this phenomenon, maternal glucose and amino acids could be spared for utilization by the fetus and placenta to meet their metabolic requirements (Grumbach *et al.*, 1968). For the time being, there is no direct evidence to support this hypothesis.

5. Somatotropic Activity of HCS

While animal studies have demonstrated the somatotropic activity of HCS and the synergism of HCS with HGH, such an effect has not yet been demonstrated in human pregnancy. However, such a possibility still exists since recent studies suggest that HCS increases the growth rate of hypopituitary dwarfs (Burr et al., 1967, and Grumbach and co-workers, quoted by Solomon and Friesen, 1968).

6. Lactogenic and Mammotropic Activity of HCS

Despite extensive studies in animals on the lactogenic and mammotropic activities of HCS, little, if anything, is known about these phenomena during human gestation. On the other hand, after treating hypopituitary dwarfs for several months with high amounts of HCS, Grumbach et al. (1968) found no breast enlargement or changes in areola and nipple or galactorrhea.

7. Luteotropic Activity of HCS

In human pregnancy, the luteotropic effect of HCS has not been shown. Recent studies have demonstrated no effect of HCS in stimulating continued progesterone release from the ovary of nonpregnant females once the effect of HCG begins to wane after its administration (Josimovich, 1970).

8. Erythropoietic Activity of HCS

Increased plasma erythropoietic activity has been detected in human pregnancy at the 13 to 16th week of gestation and has been found to rise progressively during the second and third trimesters (Jepson and Lowenstein, 1968b; Jepson, 1968). This pattern parallels the increase of HCS levels in the maternal serum. Thus, the increased erythropoietic activity of pregnancy plasma could be due to the previously demonstrated synergism between HCS and erythropoietin (Jepson and Lowenstein, 1968a,b; Jepson and Friesen, 1968).

9. Aldosterone Stimulation Activity of HCS

Melby et al. (1966) studied the effect of HCS in adult males and females on a normal sodium intake as well as during dietary sodium restriction. HCS induced an average increment of 30% in aldosterone secretion in subjects on a normal sodium intake and stimulated a further increment during sodium restriction. HCS did not increase the excretion of 17-ketosteroids and 17-hydroxycorticosteroids in these subjects. As compared to HCS, HGH did not show a stimulatory effect on aldosterone secretion. Thus, it is possible that one of the contributing factors to the increased secretion of aldosterone in pregnancy may be the stimulatory effect of HCS.

I. FUNCTIONS OF HCS IN PREGNANCY: CLINICAL SIGNIFICANCE OF HCS CONCENTRATIONS

1. Threatened Abortion

Several investigators have suggested that HCS estimations are useful for predicting the outcome of a threatened abortion (Saxena et al., 1969; Selenkow et al., 1969; Genazzani et al., 1969; Singer et al., 1970). In those patients who had a subsequent abortion, low levels of HCS were present about 7 days prior to abortion and remained in that low range. In those patients who had a threatened abortion but did not abort, their HCS levels were either in the normal range or the low levels of HCS rose to reach the normal range within a short period of time. Since the etiology of abortion is varied, the estimations of HCS may be useful only in those instances where the abortion is due to a pathological condition of the placenta.

2. Trophoblastic Disease

Low levels of HCS have been reported in patients having a molar pregnancy (Yen et al., 1968b; Saxena et al., 1968b; Clarks et al., 1970). It has been suggested that in patients clinically suspected of having a molar pregnancy, the finding of low levels of HCS along with normal or high levels of HCG will support the diagnosis (Saxena et al., 1968b). It has also been pointed out that the estimation of serum HCS is not useful in monitoring the response of patients with trophoblastic tumors to the therapy.

3. Retarded Fetal Growth

In patients clinically suspected of having "placental insufficiency" on the basis of retarded fetal growth and constantly low levels of urinary estriol, low but stable levels of HCS have been reported (Saxena et al., 1968a, 1969; Zuckerman et al., 1970).

4. "High-Risk" Pregnancy

In an earlier study (P. Beck et al., 1965), HCS levels in pregnant diabetic women were found to be in the normal range, whereas in later studies (Saxena et al., 1968a, 1969; Zuckerman et al., 1970; Singer et al., 1970; Varma et al., 1970) high levels of HCS and their significant correlation with the bigger placentas were observed.

It has been suggested that a rapid fall (50%) of serum HCS levels in pregnancies complicated with diabetes, toxemia, or postmaturity should alert the obstetrician to consider the possible interruption of gestation (Saxena et al., 1969; Selenkow et al., 1969). Josimovich et al. (1970) found no correlation with fetal outcome and randomly obtained HCS. However, recently Spellacy et al. (1970b) reported that serum HCS estimations are useful in the management of pregnancies complicated by maternal hypertension. They found that fetal deaths occurred in almost all cases whenever maternal HCS levels had entered the "fetal danger zone"—that is, to a level below 4 μg/ml (about 50% less from the normal mean in their radioimmunoassay). On the other hand, Samaan et al. (1969) and Singer et al. (1970) are not impressed by the prognostic value of HCS estimations in diabetic or toxemic pregnancies.

5. Fetal Death

Saxena et al. (1969) reported that after therapeutic abortion by means of intraamniotic saline infusion, no change in serum HCS levels occurred for the next 24–48 hours until labor had started. This observation suggests that in situations in which the fetal death is due purely to a pathological condition of the fetus, like tight-neck cord or fetal infections, serum HCS estimation will be of no value in assessing fetal viability.

6. Rh Isoimmunization

It has been observed that the estimation of HCS levels in maternal serum is of no value in the management of this complication, since no correlation was found between the severity of Rh-disease and the maternal HCS levels (Samaan et al., 1969; Selenkow et al., 1969). However, Josimovich (1970) has suggested that simultaneous measurements of HCS concentrations in the amniotic fluid and maternal serum may be valuable.

Further studies are required to assess the significance of HCS estimation in various types of pathological pregnancies, since in most of the investigations mentioned here, except that of Spellacy et al. (1970b), the number of patients studied was rather small.

IV. Human Chorionic Thyrotropin (HCT)

A number of changes observed during pregnancy, such as the increased activity and, frequently, enlargement of the thyroid gland, are generally ascribed to an increased thyroid-stimulating activity. The observations described below suggest that the human placenta may produce a substance with thyroid-stimulating activity. Hennen et al. (1969) have designated this hormone as human chorionic thyrotropin (HCT), and this term will be used in the present review.

A. PROOF OF PRODUCTION OF HCT BY THE HUMAN PLACENTA

1. It has been shown that plasma TSH (pituitary thyroid-stimulating hormone) concentrations during pregnancy fall within the normal range of nonpregnant females, when measured by radioimmunoassay methods in which HCG is added in excess to the assay system to prevent the cross-reaction with endogenous HCG (Odell *et al.*, 1967; Freychet *et al.*, 1969). These observations suggest that the maternal pituitary is not the source of the increased thyroid-stimulating activity of the maternal serum during pregnancy (Hennen *et al.*, 1969).

2. A thyroid-stimulating substance has been isolated from placental extracts by several investigators (Akasu *et al.*, 1955; Ueda *et al.*, 1964; Hennen, 1965; Hennen *et al.*, 1969; Hershman and Starnes, 1969).

3. The reports of increased thyroid function in patients with chorio-carcinoma and hydatidiform moles (Dowling *et al.*, 1960; Odell *et al.*, 1963; Kock *et al.*, 1966; Galton, 1968), suggest that abnormal tropho-blastic tissue might also secrete a thyroid-stimulating substance.

The observations reviewed above suggest that human placental extracts contain HCT, however, they do not prove that the human placenta elaborates this hormone.

B. BIOCHEMICAL NATURE OF HCT

1. *Physicochemical Properties*

Hennen *et al.* (1969) found that the physicochemical properties of HCT are similar to those of TSH; the active principle appears to be a glycoprotein. They have also reported that the chromatographic and electrophoretic properties of HCT resemble those of TSH, except that HCT seems to have less anionic character. This difference may be due to a different content of sialic acids in HCT and TSH; it has been shown that human TSH has higher amounts of sialic acid compared to those in bovine or porcine TSH preparations (Shome *et al.*, 1968a). Based on the mobility of HCT on Sephadex G-100, Hershman and Starnes (1969) suggested that HCT has the same molecular weight of 25,000 as ^{125}I-labeled human or bovine TSH (Shome *et al.*, 1968b).

2. *Immunological Properties*

Studies of the immunological properties of HCT by Hennen *et al.* (1969) and Hershman and Starnes (1969) indicate that HCT is more closely related to either bovine or porcine TSH than to human TSH.

Hennen *et al.* (1969) have further suggested that TSH from human, bovine, and porcine sources share an antigenic part (or parts) with HCT and have also shown that HCT is immunologically different from HCG.

C. BIOLOGICAL PROPERTIES OF HCT

Hennen *et al.* (1969) have studied the biological properties of HCT using two types of bioassay: (1) bioassay of McKenzie (1958) modified by Rerup and Melander (1965) based on the thyroid release of ^{131}I in mice pretreated with thyroxine; (2) the assay method of Greenspan *et al.* (1956) based on the incorporation of ^{32}P into the thyroid of 1-day-old chicks. They found that HCT is capable of increasing the secretion of thyroid hormones and stimulating the incorporation of ^{32}P into the thyroid and that the activity of HCT is neutralized by specific TSH antisera. Hennen and co-workers hold that the thyroid-stimulating activity of HCT is related to the similarities in the structure of HCT and TSH.

D. CONCENTRATIONS OF HCT IN THE PLACENTA AND IN BODY FLUIDS

It has been reported that the concentration of HCT in the term placenta is about 124 mU/100 gm (Hennen, 1965; Hershman and Starnes, 1969). Using a bioassay method, Hennen *et al.* (1969) found that thyroid-stimulating activity is highest in the maternal serum during the first 2 months of gestation (see Fig. 12); it then shows a progressive

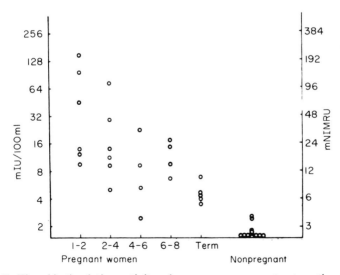

FIG. 12. Thyroid-stimulating activity of pregnancy serum extracts, estimated by a bioassay method. According to Hennen *et al.* (1969).

decline to reach a minimum level at term. However, these levels are higher than the levels found in nonpregnant subjects. Using a radioimmuno-assay method for bovine TSH, Hershman and Starnes (1969) could not detect HCT in maternal serum during labor or in uterine vein blood obtained from women at cesarean section. On the other hand, Hennen et al. (1969) reported that HCT in maternal serum is detectable by either a porcine or a human radioimmunoassay system.

E. PHYSIOLOGICAL ROLE OF HCT IN PREGNANCY

The physiological role of HCT during human pregnancy has not been elucidated. Several investigators have shown that the activity of the thyroid gland increases during pregnancy (Pochin, 1952; Halnan, 1958; Aboul-Khair et al., 1964). The greater incidence of thyroid enlargement during pregnancy has not been satisfactorily explained (Freedberg et al., 1957). Since plasma TSH levels are not elevated during pregnancy, the secretion of HCT could explain the above-mentioned changes. However, Hennen et al. (1969) emphasized that the high circulating thyroid-stimulating activity is not sufficient to produce clinical hyperthyroidism during pregnancy. Hershman and Starnes (1969) also postulated that HCT might be secreted into the fetal circulation and stimulate the fetal thyroid. Gitlin and Biasucci (1969) found that the fetal pituitary begins to synthesize TSH at about 14 weeks of gestation. Since fetal thyroid follicles start forming at about 8 weeks and the iodination of proteins in the fetal thyroid begins at about the 11th week (Shepard, 1967), both these processes might be initiated by HCT. At present, there is no evidence that TSH can cross the human placenta (Ueda et al., 1964).

V. ADRENOCORTICOTROPIC HORMONE (ACTH)

Increased levels of ACTH in maternal plasma during pregnancy have been reported by several investigators (Granirer, 1951; Cassano and Tarantino, 1953; Bromberg et al., 1954). However, other investigators could not detect ACTH activity in peripheral maternal or retroplacental blood (Hunt and McConahey, 1953; Gemzell et al., 1955).

Jailer and Knowlton (1950) were the first to report the successful extraction of an ACTH-like material from the human placenta. After their report, several other investigators supported the finding of ACTH-like material in human placental extracts. Diczfalusy and Troen (1961) reviewed these reports critically. They concluded that there is little or no doubt about the presence of adrenocorticotropic activity in the extracts of human placenta; however, it is not clear whether the ACTH activity is present in the chorionic tissue or in the blood contained by the placenta. Assali and Hammermesz (1954) found that the ACTH activity in the extracts of chorionic tissue is greater than that in extracts from intervillous blood. Schwers and Fanard (1958) could not support this observation and concluded that the source of ACTH activity in placental extracts is either the maternal or fetal pituitary gland. Yamamoto and Morioka (1956) reported that ACTH-like material of the placenta is chromatographically different from pituitary ACTH preparations. On the other hand, Badinand *et al.* (1953) have observed close similarities in the physicochemical properties of pituitary and placental ACTH preparations.

The absence of a significant extrapituitary source for ACTH in human pregnancy has been suggested by the reports of Little *et al.* (1958). A woman hypophysectomized during the 26th week of pregnancy was maintained on cortisone. After 6 weeks of treatment, the abrupt discontinuation of cortisone resulted in the development of the signs of acute adrenal insufficiency within 48 hours. From this observation it appears that there is little, if any, contribution of placental ACTH to the stimulation of steroid synthesis in the maternal adrenal cortex.

VI. MELANOCYTE-STIMULATING HORMONE (MSH)

The cause of hyperpigmentation during pregnancy has been attributed to the elevated MSH activity found in the urine of pregnant women (Konsuloff, 1934; Shizume and Lerner, 1954; Dahlberg, 1960). The studies of several investigators suggest that the MSH activity found in pregnancy urine is different both biologically and electrophoretically from pituitary MSH, and that urinary MSH may be a metabolite of pituitary MSH (Stolte *et al.*, 1952, 1953; Lee and Lee, 1969).

It has been shown that human placental extracts contain MSH activity, and that the MSH activity of the chorionic tissue is greater than that of the intervillous blood (Sulman and Bergmann, 1953; Varon, 1959; Eschbach, 1959). Karkun and Sen (1963) were able to isolate MSH activity from the placenta, but the potency of the extracts was rather low. They pointed out the interfering action of ACTH when present in extracts, since this hormone can also stimulate melanophore changes.

VII. OXYTOCIN

Although the presence of oxytocic activity in human placental extracts has been reported by several investigators (Palmisano, 1948a,b; Bianco and Confalonieri, 1953; Ogier, 1956; Cantone and Martini, 1954), there is no conclusive evidence to indicate that the placenta is able to synthesize oxytocin. However, by means of an inactivating enzyme, oxytocinase, the placenta may play an important role in regulating the circulating level of pituitary oxytocin. The evidence for the placental synthesis of oxytocinase was reviewed by Caldeyro-Barcia in 1960. Semm (1960) was first to introduce the concept of an oxytocin–oxytocinase system, which is supported by the recent data of Klimek and Bieniasz (1969). These investigators have found that the serum oxytocinase levels in women requiring administration of oxytocin for the induction of labor are significantly lower than in parturient women regardless of whether the delivery has been spontaneous or operative. From this observation, they postulate that only that part of oxytocin is effective which represents a difference between the amount of hormone liberated into the circulation and the amount inactivated by oxytocinase.

VIII. INSULIN

The presence of an enzyme, insulinase, which can inactivate insulin has been detected in the term human placenta (Freinkel and Goodner, 1958; Buse et al., 1962; Freinkel, 1964). Adam et al. (1969) suggest that this enzyme activity is not present in the mid-gestational placenta, since they could not find evidence of inactivation or catabolism of injected insulin-[131]I. The transfer of insulin across term placenta is incompletely understood. Buse et al. (1962) have observed no insulin transfer, whereas Gitlin et al. (1965) suggested that it may be transferred in very small amounts. Observations of Adam et al. (1969) indicate that insulin is not transferred across the placenta at mid-gestation.

IX. PRESSOR FACTORS

Motivated to a large extent by a search for factors related to eclampsia, a number of investigators have looked for pressor and antidiuretic factors in the human placenta. Recently, Sims (1970) published a review on pre-eclampsia and related complications of pregnancy.

A. VASOPRESSIN (ANTIDIURETIC HORMONE)

Some investigators were not able to detect pressor activity in placental extracts (Bradshaw, 1946; Chesley and McFaul, 1949) whereas others found varying amounts of pressor and antidiuretic activities (Byron, 1952; Suzuki, 1954). In the serum of normal pregnant subjects, the activity of antidiuretic hormone is not increased (Friedberg et al., 1960). Similar findings in urine were reported by Zuspan et al. (1958). Hence— for the time being—there is no evidence indicating that the placenta can synthesize vasopressin or antidiuretic hormone. However, Hawker (1956) reported that the placenta can inactivate vasopressin by means of the subcellular enzyme vasopressinase, which has been shown to be devoid of oxytocin-inactivating property (Hooper and Jessup, 1959). A similar placental factor which inactivates antidiuretic hormone has been found in pregnancy blood (McCartney et al., 1952).

B. Renin

Plasma renin activity has been found to be elevated during pregnancy although it has been suggested that this activity is primarily of maternal origin (Brown et al., 1966a; Geelhoed and Vander, 1968; Boonshaft et al., 1968). High concentrations of renin are present in the normal human placenta (Hodari et al., 1967; Skinner et al., 1968). Skinner et al. (1968) reported that human chorion contains the highest renin concentration of any tissue other than the adult kidney and suggested that the outward diffusion of renin is limited by the decidua, which would promote its intra-amniotic accumulation. Symonds et al. (1968) have shown in tissue culture studies that the human chorion can synthesize renin. In hypertensive pregnancy, Brown et al. (1966b) found that plasma renin activity is in the same range as normal pregnancy levels. The concentrations of renin in the placentas from preeclamptic pregnancies is not increased (Hodari et al., 1967). The postulated function of renin in the human chorion is that it may act as a contributing source to circulating maternal renin and, thus, influence the sodium homeostasis of pregnancy by regulating the secretion of aldosterone. The latter is known to be increased during pregnancy (Jones et al., 1959; Watanabe et al., 1963).

C. Norepinephrine and Epinephrine

The urinary excretion of norepinephrine (NE) and epinephrine (E) during pregnancy has been estimated by several investigators who used bioassay methods (Burn, 1953; Subrahmanyam, 1959; Castern, 1963). Using a trihydroxyindole chemical method (Zuspan et al., 1967) to measure free urinary NE and E, Zuspan (1970a) has shown that under carefully controlled experimental conditions the antepartum, postpartum, and nonpregnant values are the same for both NE and E. The only significant increase was found in urinary NE in the first 24 hours after delivery, which returned to normal during the second 24 hours. Hence, the increased NE excretion may perhaps reflect the stress of labor and of the delivery process. The earlier bioassay studies of Castern (1963) also support this observation. Sandler and Baldock (1963) found that the placental content of NE and dihydroxyphenylalanine (DOPA) is increased in preeclamptic pregnancies. Barnes and Kumar (1964) concluded that in preeclamptic pregnancy there is no de novo production of pressor substances from the placenta. They consider that the ischemia of the uterus and placenta may diminish the ability of these organs to "detoxify" the pressor substances. Zuspan (1970b) reported that the amniotic fluid of normal pregnancies contains about 3.0 μg/liter of NE and 1.0 μg/liter of E, which are presumably of fetal origin. Because of their extremely small concentrations in the amniotic fluid, the fetal NE and E make a negligible contribution to the maternal NE and E excretion; if so, they can hardly play a significant role in the development of maternal hypertension during pregnancy.

D. OTHER FACTORS

1. Although Hunter and Howard (1960, 1961) reported that the decidua may produce a substance "hysterotonin" which may be responsible for the hypertension in preeclampsia, Gomel and Hardwick (1966) were unable to confirm this finding.

2. Senior et al. (1963) found significantly increased concentrations of serotonin in the placenta of hypertensive pregnancies. Sandler and Baldock (1963) suggested that this finding could be explained on the basis of a monoamineoxidase (MAO) deficiency, since they found reduced metabolism of serotonin, but not of tryptamine, in preeclampsia. They postulated that the placental ischemia resulting from the pressor agent further reduces the activity of the enzyme, thus establishing a vicious cycle.

X. ACETYLCHOLINE

Chang and Gaddum (1933) reported the presence of large amounts of placental acetylcholine equivalents in the human placenta, and Wen et al. (1936, quoted by Goodlin, 1970) suggested that this activity is located in the trophoblastic cells. That acetylcholine is capable of causing myometrial contractions has been shown in vitro by Shabanah et al. (1964) and in vivo by Sala and Fisch (1965). It has been postulated by Torda (1942) that under different experimental and clinical conditions the placental acetylcholine content may depend on placental cholinesterase activity. Goodlin (1970) has found that the amniotic fluid cholinesterase concentration is only a fraction of that present in the maternal blood or placenta and suggests that this low amount of cholinesterase is probably sufficient to inactivate the acetylcholine reaching the amniotic fluid. From his study of patients having therapeutic abortions by intra-amniotic hypertonic saline injections with or without methylene blue, Goodlin (1970) has supported the concept of a positive relationship between uterine contractions and placental acetylcholine activity.

XI. PLACENTAL UTEROTROPIC HORMONE (PUH)

Beas and Flores (1969) isolated a protein from human placental extracts with a molecular weight of approximately 70,000 and have designated it as "placental uterotropic hormone," or PUH. Using zone electrophoresis, immunodiffusion, immunoelectrophoresis, and hemagglutination, these investigators have found that this hormone is not identical with HGH, ACTH, HCS, HCG, TSH, or albumin. In doses of 30 μg/day, PUH produced a significant increase in the uterine weight of young female rats. This effect was completely inhibited by the simultaneous injection of an antiserum prepared against this protein hormone in rabbits. This work has not yet been confirmed independently.

XII. Relaxin

The detection of relaxin in maternal blood and placenta has been reported by several investigators (Pommerenke, 1934; Zarrow et al., 1955). As pointed out earlier by Diczfalusy and Troen (1961), there is no evidence to suggest that relaxin is synthesized by the human placenta and the role of relaxin has not been ascertained during human pregnancy.

XIII. Juvenile Hormone

Since the review of Diczfalusy and Troen (1961), no new information has become available on the chemical nature, placental synthesis, or possible physiological role of juvenile hormone.

XIV. General Summary

1. Human Chorionic Gonadotropin HCG

It has been conclusively proved that the human chorionic tissue synthesizes HCG, but it is still controversial whether it is produced by the cytotrophoblastic cells, the syncytiotrophoblastic cells, or by both. Human chorionic gonadotropin is a glycoprotein, composed of two polypeptide chains, joined by disulfide bridges. The molecular weight of HCG has been estimated to be 47,000 ± 3000 to 59,000 ± 4000, depending upon the technique used. The subject of homogeneity versus heterogeneity of HCG is controversial. One group of investigators suggested that HCG is a dimer, made up of two identical and chromatographically homogeneous subunits (mol. wt. 23,000–28,000), whereas, other investigators have reported that HCG is heterogeneous and is composed of at least three different types of HCG molecules. It has been suggested that the cause of heterogeneity lies in the heterogeneity of the carbohydrate moiety of the HCG molecule. Human chorionic gonadotropin shows immunological cross-reactivity with LH, FSH, and TSH, which are perhaps related to structural similaries. A problem related to the cross-reactivity is the existence of an antiserum neutralizing factor present in different gonadotropin preparations. One group of investigators has shown a cross-reactivity of urinary HCG preparations with the glomerular basement membrane from human kidneys.

In animal studies, the luteinizing (or interstitial cell stimulating) properties of HCG are now well established. The follicle-stimulating property has also been repeatedly demonstrated. However, it is still controversial whether or not the FSH-like activity is a uniformly distributed intrinsic property of the HCG molecule. The stimulation of testicular steroidogenesis by HCG is well documented, but the direct effect of HCG on steroidogenesis in adrenals or placenta has not been shown conclusively.

The placenta synthesizes HCG throughout the entire period of gestation. The placental content of HCG per gram weight is higher during the first trimester, and lower in the second and third trimesters of pregnancy. The pattern of HCG concentration has also been studied during pregnancy in the serum, urine, and amniotic fluid. There is general agreement about the shape of the HCG curve in these body fluids. However, considerable differences have been noted when the values obtained by bioassays were compared with those estimated by immunoassays. Within a fortnight after ovulation, HCG is detectable in serum and urine, and it rises sharply to a peak around day 60 of gestation. By day 80, the HCG concentration in these fluids drops to a lower level but remains at that plateau until delivery. HCG has also been detected in the cerebrospinal fluid; it has been suggested that its concentration is directly proportional to the serum concentrations. Low levels of HCG are present in the umbilical artery and vein.

The disappearance rate of HCG has been studied by various methods. Using both bioassays and radioimmunoassays, one group has calculated the half-life to be 6–10 hours. Using radioimmunoassays only, several other investigators have shown that the disappearance curve consists of two linear components—the first corresponding to 8–11 hours and the second corresponding to a half-life of 23–37 hours. There is no evidence yet available in the literature to point to a distinct mechanism by which the production and release of HCG is controlled.

Estimations of HCG concentrations are useful in the diagnosis and management of trophoblastic disease, but they appear to be of limited value in the management of pregnancies complicated by toxemia, diabetes, Rh isoimmunization, threatened abortion, retarded fetal growth, or prolonged pregnancies.

The precise role of HCG in the regulation of the endocrine changes of human gestation is not clear. However, there seems to be sufficient evidence in the literature suggesting that the physiological functions of HCG during the first trimester of pregnancy include stimulation of steroidogenesis by the corpus luteum during the first 4 weeks, stimulation of fetal adrenal growth, initiation of development of fetal Leydig cells and the development of fetal ovaries. The physiological role of HCG after its peak period of secretion is not clear.

2. Human Chorionic Somatomammotropin (HCS)

The synthesis of HCS by human chorionic tissue is established. There is a consensus of opinion that HCS is produced by the syncytiotrophoblastic cells. The molecular weight of HCS has been shown to be about 20,000 with a single polypeptide chain. The sequence of the amino acids of HCS is similar to that of HGH. A partial cross-reactivity of HCS with HGH has been shown, and it has been suggested that this is due to certain common antigenic determinants in these two molecules.

Animal studies have shown that the biological activity of HCS is considerably weaker than that of HGH. Somatotropic, lactogenic, mammotropic, luteotropic, diabetogenic, and erythropoietic activities of HCS have been demonstrated in various animal species. The synergistic effect of HCS with HGH, HCG and erythropoietin has also been described.

The placenta synthesizes HCS throughout the entire period of pregnancy. The placental concentration of HCS per gram weight remains constant during the entire gestational period. Concentrations of HCS in maternal and fetal body fluids have been measured by immunological methods. There is general agreement about the shape of the HCS curve during pregnancy. However, considerable variation has been noted in the absolute values found. In maternal serum the HCS levels are consistently detectable after 6 weeks of gestation. They rise progressively to a plateau which is reached after 34 weeks of gestation. In earlier studies, following the delivery of the placenta, the half-life of HCS was found to be 29 minutes or less in a single exponential disappearance curve. One recent study suggests two exponential curves—in the first component the half-life of HCS is 11 minutes and in the second component it is of several hours. Low levels of HCS are detectable in pregnancy urine, amniotic fluid, and very small amounts in the umbilical venous blood. The production rate of HCS has been calculated to be about 1 gm/day. For the time being, the mechanism regulating the synthesis and release of HCS during pregnancy is unknown.

The usefulness of the estimation of HCS concentrations in maternal serum in the management of various types of pathological pregnancies is controversial. Recent studies suggest that HCS estimations are useful for the diagnosis of trophoblastic disease and for the prognosis of impending abortion. Opinions vary about the management of high-risk pregnancies on the basis of HCS estimations during the second and third trimesters. One study suggests that a rapid drop of more than 50% in HCS levels in pregnancies complicated with toxemia, diabetes, or post-maturity should alert the obstetrician for possible intervention. The estimation of HCS appears to be valuable in the management of pregnancies complicated with hypertension.

The role of HCS in the regulation of endocrine changes of human gestation is not clear. It has been demonstrated that HCS stimulates insulin release as well as antagonizing insulin activity at the peripheral level. One of the postulated roles of HCS is the hypothalamic suppression of GRF during the third trimester and early postpartum period. The somatotropic effect of HCS has not been demonstrated in pregnancy, although a recent study suggests such an effect in hypopituitary dwarfs. Lactogenic, mammotropic, and luteotropic activities of HCS have not been demonstrated in human gestation. It seems likely that HCS is one of the factors stimulating erythropoiesis, through its synergism with erythropoietin. The effect of HCS has been postulated to be one of the contributory factors to the increased secretion of aldosterone during gestation.

3. Human Chorionic Thyrotropin (HCT)

Extracts of human placentas contain HCT but the placental synthesis of HCT has not yet been demonstrated. The physicochemical properties of HCT resemble those of TSH and the active principle of the hormone appears to be a glycoprotein. It has been shown that immunologically HCT is more related to bovine or porcine TSH, and that it is different from HCG. The molecular weight of HCG appears to be 25,000, the same as that of TSH. In bioassay systems, HCT is capable of increasing the secretion of thyroid hormones and stimulates the incorporation of ^{32}P into the thyroid gland. The biological activity of HCT can be neutralized by antisera which are specific to pituitary TSH. In the term placenta, HCT is estimated to be present in a mean concentration of 124 mU/100 gm. Using bioassay methods, the thyroid-stimulating activity of HCT in the maternal serum was found to be highest during the first 2 months of gestation, progressively declining toward a minimum at term. This pattern resembles that of HCG. The physiological role of HCT in human pregnancy remains to be demonstrated. Plasma levels of TSH have been reported to be normal during pregnancy, although there is an increased activity of the thyroid gland. The secretion of HCT might be responsible for such an activity and for the high incidence of thyroid enlargement observed during normal pregnancy and in pregnancies complicated with trophoblastic disease. It has been suggested that HCT might be secreted into the fetal circulation and stimulate the fetal thyroid growth in the early stages of gestation.

4. Adrenocorticotropic Hormone (ACTH)

Placental extracts contain ACTH-like activity and there is evidence of increased production of ACTH during pregnancy. However, the synthesis of ACTH by placental tissue has not been demonstrated. Also, the physiological role of such a placental ACTH-like material remains to be defined.

5. Melanocyte-Stimulating Hormone (MSH)

There is an increased MSH activity in the urine of pregnant women; it is not clear, however, whether this MSH is of pituitary or extrapituitary origin. Placental extracts contain MSH activity, but the synthesis of MSH by the human placenta has not been demonstrated. It has been suggested that the MSH activity found in pregnancy urine is different from pituitary MSH, and that it might be a metabolite of pituitary MSH.

6. Oxytocin

Oxytocic activity in placental extracts has been reported but actual synthesis of oxytocin by the placenta has not been demonstrated. However, there is a considerable amount of evidence indicating that the placenta may play a role in the regulation of the circulating levels of pituitary oxytocin, by means of an inactivating enzyme, oxytocinase.

7. Insulin

There is evidence to indicate that the placenta at mid-gestation acts as a complete barrier to maternal insulin transfer and does not have the ability to inactivate insulin. However, the ability of the term placenta to inactivate insulin by means of an enzyme, insulinase, has been repeatedly demonstrated. Insulin seems to be transferred across the term placenta, but only in small amounts.

8. Pressor Factors

a. Vasopressin (Antidiuretic Hormone). It has not been demonstrated that the placenta can synthesize vasopressin or antidiuretic hormone. However, it has been shown that the human placenta can inactivate these hormones by specific enzymes.

b. Renin. There is increased plasma renin activity in pregnancy and the concentration of renin in the chorionic tissue is very high. It has been suggested that the decidua limits the outward diffusion of renin and promotes its intra-amniotic accumulation. Tissue culture studies indicate that the human chorion synthesizes renin. The role of renin in the etiology of pregnancies complicated by the hypertension or preeclampsia is not clear.

c. *Norepinephrine* (*NE*) *and epinephrine* (*E*). There is no evidence indicating that in normal pregnancy the placenta or the fetus make any significant contributions to the maternal NE and E excretions. In pregnancies complicated with preeclampsia, increased concentration of NE in the placenta has been reported. It has been suggested that during preeclampsia the placental ability to metabolize the pressor substances is reduced, but there is no placental synthesis of NE and E.

d. *Other Factors.* The existence of a postulated factor "hysterotonin," which would be responsible for hypertension in preeclampsia, has not been confirmed. The serotonin concentration is increased in the placenta in cases of hypertensive pregnancy. It has been suggested that this may be due to a monoamine oxidase (MAO) deficiency. However, the precise role of serotonin or of a MAO deficiency in the etiology of preeclampsia remains to be established.

9. *Acetylcholine*

Large amounts of acetylcholine equivalents have been found in the placenta, and it has been suggested that this activity is located in the trophoblastic cells. It is possible that the acetylcholine content is regulated by a placental cholinesterase activity.

10. *Placental Uterotropic Hormone* (*PUH*)

A placental hormone-PUH-exhibiting uterotropic activity in rats has been detected in human placental extracts. This hormone is not identical with HGH, ACTH, HCS, HCG, TSH, and albumin in immunological studies. The placental synthesis and physiological role of PUH in human pregnancy has not yet been shown.

11. *Relaxin and Juvenile Hormone*

There is no evidence to suggest that relaxin and juvenile hormone are synthesized by the human placenta, and their possible physiological role in human pregnancy has not yet been ascertained.

XV. CONCLUSION

It is established that HCG is synthesized by the human placenta, but it is still uncertain whether HCG is produced by the cytotrophoblastic or the syncytiotrophoblastic cells or perhaps by both. The interstitial cell-stimulating effect of HCG on the ovary and the testis is well documented, but its gametokinetic effect is incompletely understood. Human chorionic gonadotropin cross reacts with FSH, LH, and TSH. The reason for this might be due to certain common antigenic determinants. There is, however, no definite information available as yet on the structure of HCG. Moreover, it is still uncertain whether or not HCG is heterogeneous. The pattern of HCG in body fluids is well established; however, there is a difference in the HCG pattern obtained by bioassay as compared to that found by immunoassay. The reason for this is not clear. The factors regulating HCG secretion are incompletely comprehended and the precise role of HCG in human pregnancy is unknown.

The placental synthesis and syncytiotrophoblastic origin of HCS are established, but no information is available on the mechanism by which this synthesis is regulated. The amino acid sequence of HCS has been shown to be similar to that of HGH; however, the structural differences which may explain the dissimilarities in the biological and immunological activities of HCS and HGH are incompletely understood. There is a general agreement as to the secretion pattern of HCS in maternal serum. This is based on the results of immunoassays. Little, if any information has been obtained by bioassay methods. Despite various types of biological effects of HCS shown in bioassays, the precise physiological role of HCS in human pregnancy is not known.

The presence of other hormonal activities, such as HCT, ACTH, MSH, oxytocin, PUH, and pressor factors in placental extracts has been demonstrated repeatedly; but except for renin, the evidence for their placental synthesis is far from convincing. The physiological roles which these placental activities may play in the regulation of the endocrine changes of human pregnancy remain to be demonstrated.

Thus it is established that the human placenta synthesizes large quantities of HCG, HCS, renin, and perhaps also HCT. On the other hand, ACTH, MSH, oxytocin, PUH, and the pressor factors present in placental extracts may be of fetal and/or maternal origin. Virtually no information is available on the regulating mechanisms and the "raison d'être" for these hormones. However, with the development of improved methods in protein chemistry, biological, and immunological assays and tissue culture techniques, it can be expected that, in this decade of the 1970's, new and useful information about these placental hormones and their functional significance will become available.

REFERENCES

Aboul-Khair, S. A., Crooks, J., Turnbull, A. C., and Hytten, F. C. (1964). *Clin. Sci.* **27**, 195.

Abrams, R. L., Kaplan, S. L., and Grumbach, M. M. (1969), *Program, 51st Annu. Meet. Endocrine Soc.* Abstract, p. 106.

Adam, P. A. J., Teramo, K., Raiha, N., Gitlin, D., and Schwartz, R. (1969). *Diabetes* 18, 409.

Akasu, F., Kawahara, S., Ohki, H., Harano, M., and Tejima, Y. (1955). *Endocrinol. Jap.* 2, 297.

Albert, A. (1968). *J. Clin. Endocrinol. Metab.* 28, 1683.

Albert, A. (1969). *J. Clin. Endocrinol. Metab.* 29, 1504.

Albert, A., and Berkson, J. (1951). *J. Clin. Endocrinol. Metab.* 11, 805.

Albert, A., and Kelly, S. (1958). *J. Clin. Endocrinol. Metab.* 18, 1067.

Alonso, C., and Troen, P. (1966). *Biochemistry* 5, 337.

Aschner, B. (1913). *Arch. Gynaekol.* 99, 534.

Ask-Upmark, M. E. (1926). *Acta Obstet. Gynecol. Scand.* 5, 211.

Assali, N. S., and Hammermesz, J. (1954). *Endocrinology* 55, 561.

Badinand, A., Mallein, R., and Cotte, J. (1953). *C. R. Soc. Biol.* 147, 323.

Baechler, C., Bell, E. T., Borth, R., Brody, S., Carlstrom, G., Kerry, M. G., and Menzi, A. (1969). *Acta Endocrinol. (Copenhagen)* 61, 117.

Bagshawe, K. D., Wilde, C. E., and Orr, A. H. (1966). *Lancet* 1, 1118.

Bagshawe, K. D., Orr, A. H., and Rushworth, A. G. J. (1968). *Nature (London)* 217, 950.

Bahl, O. P. (1969a). *J. Biol. Chem.* 244, 567.

Bahl, O. P. (1969b). *J. Biol. Chem.* 244, 575.

Barnes, A. C., and Kumar, D. (1964). *Mod. Concepts Cardiovasc. Dis.* 33, 841.

Beas, F., and Flores, H. (1969). *Nature (London)* 22, 574.

Beck, J. S., Gordon, R. L., Donald. D., and Melvin, J. M. O. (1969). *J. Pathol.* 97, 545.

Beck, P., and Daughaday, W. H. (1967). *J. Clin. Invest.* 46, 103.

Beck, P., Parker, M. L., and Daughaday, W. H. (1965). *J. Clin. Endocrinol. Metab.* 25, 1457.

Bell, E. T., and Loraine, J. A., eds. (1967). "Recent Research on Gonadotrophic Hormones." Livingstone, Edinburgh.

Bell, J. J., Canfield, R. E., and Sciarra, J. J. (1969). *Endocrinology* 84, 298.

Benirschke, K. (1956). *Obstet. Gynecol.* 8, 412.

Berle, P. (1969). *Acta Endocrinol. (Copenhagen)* 61, 369.

Berle, P., and Schultze-Mosgau, H. (1968). *Acta Endocrinol. (Copenhagen)* 58, 339.

Berle, P., and Schultze-Mosgau, H. (1969). *Arch. Gynaekol.* 207, 460.

Bianco, R., and Confalonieri, C. (1953). *Atti Soc. Lomb. Sci. Med. Biol.* 8, 247.

Boonshaft, R., O'Connell, J. M. B., Hayes, J. M., and Schreiner, G. E. (1968). *J. Clin. Endocrinol. Metab.* 28, 1641.

Borell, U. (1954). *Acta Endocrinol. (Copenhagen)* 17, 13.

Borth, R., Gsell, M., and de Watteville, H. (1953). *Acta Endocrinol. (Copenhagen)* 14, 316.

Borth, R., Lunenfeld, B., Stamm, O., and de Watteville, H. (1959). *Acta Obstet. Gynecol. Scand.* 38, 417.

Borth, R., Ferin, M., and Menzi, A. (1965). *Acta Endocrinol. (Copenhagen)* 50, 335.

Bradbury, J. T., Brown, W. E., and Grey, L. A. (1950). *Recent Progr. Horm. Res.* 5, 151.

Bradshaw, T. E. T. (1946). *Ir. J. Med. Sci.* 6, 235.

Breuer, C. B. (1969). *Endocrinology* 85, 989.

Brody, S. (1969). *In* "Foetus and Placenta" (A. Klopper and E. Diczfalusy, eds.), p. 299. Blackwell, Oxford.

Brody, S., and Carlström, G. (1962a). *J. Clin. Endocrinol. Metab.* **22**, 564.
Brody, S., and Carlström, G. (1962b). *Acta Endocrinol. (Copenhagen), Suppl.* **67**, 19.
Brody, S., and Carlström, G. (1965a). *Acta Obstet. Gynecol. Scand.* **44**, 32.
Brody, S., and Carlström, G. (1965b). *J. Clin. Endocrinol. Metab.* **25**, 792.
Brody, S., and Carlström, G. (1965c). *Ciba Found. Study Group [Pap.]* **22**, 70.
Bromberg, Y. M., Sadowsky, A., and Sulman, F. G. (1954). *J. Amer. Med. Ass.* **154**, 165.
Brown, J. J., Davies, D. L., Doak, P. B., Lever, A. F., and Robertson, J. I. S. (1966a). *J. Endocrinol.* **35**, 373.
Brown, J. J., Davies, D. L., Doak, P. B., Lever, A. F., Robertson, J. I. S., and Trust, P. (1966b). *J. Obstet. Gynaecol. Brit. Commonw.* **73**, 410.
Brown, W. E., and Bradbury, J. T. (1947). *Amer. J. Obstet. Gynecol.* **53**, 749.
Bruner, J. A. (1951). *J. Clin. Endocrinol.* **11**, 360.
Bryans, F. E. (1951). *Endocrinology* **48**, 733.
Burn, G. P. (1953). *Brit. Med. J.* **1**, 697.
Burr, I., Grumbach, M. M., and Kaplan, S. L. (1967). *Program, 49th Annu. Meet. Endocrine Soc.* Abstract, p. 39.
Burt, R. L., Leake, N., and Rhyne, A. L. (1970). *Obstet. Gynecol.* **36**, 233.
Buse, M. G., Robert, W. J., and Buse, J. (1962). *J. Clin. Invest.* **41**, 29.
Butt, W. R. (1967). *In* "The Chemistry of Gonadotrophins" (W. R. Butt, ed.), p. 58. Thomas, Springfield, Illinois.
Butt, W. R. (1969). *Acta Endocrinol. (Copenhagen), Suppl.* **142**, 13.
Byron, F. B. (1952). *Obstet. Surv. (Baltimore)* **7**, 46.
Caldeyro-Barcia, R. (1960). *Acta Endocrinol. (Copenhagen), Suppl.* **50**, 41.
Canfield, R. E., and Bell, J. J. (1969). *In* "Progress in Endocrinology" (C. Gual, ed.), Int. Congr. Ser. No. 184, p. 402. Excerpta Found., Amsterdam.
Cantone, G., and Martini, L. (1954). *Atti Soc. Lomb. Sci. Med. Biol.* **9**, 42.
Cassano, F., and Tarantino, C. (1953). *Folia Endocrinol.* **6**, 319.
Cassmer, O. (1959). *Acta Endocrinol. (Copenhagen), Suppl.* **45**.
Castern, O. (1963). *Acta Pharmacol. Toxicol., Suppl.* **2**, 20.
Catt, K. J., Moffat, B., Nialli, H. D., and Preston, B. N. (1967). *Biochem. J.* **102**, 27c.
Cédard, L., and Knuppen, R. (1965). *Steroids* **6**, 307.
Cédard, L., Yannotti, S., and Varangot, J. (1961). *C. R. Soc. Biol.* **155**, 458.
Cédard, L., Varangot, J., and Yannotti, S. (1962). *C. R. Acad. Sci.* **254**, 3896.
Cédard, L., Varangot, J., and Yannotti, S. (1964). *C. R. Acad. Sci.* **258**, 3769.
Chang, H. C., and Gaddum, J. H. (1933). *J. Physiol. (London)* **79**, 255.
Chesley, L. C., and McFaul, I. E. (1949). *Amer. J. Obstet. Gynecol.* **58**, 159.
Clarks, P. B., Gusdon, J. B., Jr., and Burt, R. L. (1970). *Obstet. Gynecol.* **35**, 597.
Crooke, A. C., and Butt, W. R. (1959). *J. Obstet. Gynaecol. Brit. Emp.* **66**, 297.
Crosignani, P. G., and Polvani, F. (1969). *J. Obstet. Gynaecol. Brit. Commonw.* **76**, 424.
Cushman, P., Jr. (1970). *Amer. J. Obstet. Gynecol.* **107**, 519.
Dahlberg, B. (1960). *Acta Endocrinol. (Copenhagen), Suppl.* **51**, 331.
Danielsson, M. (1965). *Amer. J. Obstet. Gynecol.* **91**, 895.
Daughaday, W. H., and Kipnis, D. M. (1966). *Recent Progr. Horm. Res.* **22**, 49.
Decio, R. (1955). *Acta Endocrinol. (Copenhagen)* **19**, 185.
Delfs, E. (1957). *Obstet. Gynecol.* **9**, 1.
Diczfalusy, E. (1953). *Acta Endocrinol. (Copenhagen), Suppl.* **12**.

144 BADRI N. SAXENA

Diczfalusy, E. (1954). *Acta Endocrinol. (Copenhagen)* **17**, 58.

Diczfalusy, E. (1967). *Proc. Int. Congr. Horm. Steroids, 2nd, 1966* Int. Congr. Ser. No. 132, p. 82.

Diczfalusy, E. (1969). *In* "The Foeto-Placental Unit" (A. Pecile and C. Finzi, eds.), Int. Congr. Ser. No. 183, p. 65. Excerpta Med. Found., Amsterdam.

Diczfalusy, E., and Troen, P. (1961). *Vitam. Horm. (New York)* **19**, 229.

Diczfalusy, E., Nilsson, L., and Westman, A. (1958). *Acta Endocrinol. (Copenhagen)* **28**, 137.

Diczfalusy, E., Holmgren, H., and Westman, A. (1950). *Acta Endocrinol.* **5**, 43.

Dixon, F. J. (1968). *Amer. J. Med.* **44**, 493.

Dowling, J. T., Ingbar, S. H., and Freinkel, N. (1960). *J. Clin. Endocrinol. Metab.* **20**, 1.

Ehrhardt, K. (1931). *Meds. Klin. (Munich)* **27**, 426.

Ehrhardt, K. (1936). *Muenchen. Med. Wochenschr.* **83**, 1163.

Eik-Nes, K. B., Oertel, G. W., Nimer, R., and Tyler, F. H. (1959). *J. Clin. Endocrinol. Metab.* **19**, 1405.

Ellegood, J. O., Mahesh, V. B., and Greenblatt, R. B. (1969). *Postgrad. Med.* **46**, 105.

Eschbach, J. (1959). *Bull. Fed. Soc. Gynecol. Obstet. Lang. Fr.* **11**, 188.

Faiman, C., Ryan, R. J., Zwirek, S. J., and Rubin, M. E. (1968). *J. Clin. Endocrinol. Metab.* **28**, 1323.

Fellner, O. O. (1913). *Arch. Gynaekol.* **100**, 641.

Franchimont, P. (1965). *Ann. Endocrinol.* **26**, 346.

Frantz, A. G., Rabkin, M. T., and Friesen, H. (1965). *J. Clin. Endocrinol. Metab.* **25**, 1136.

Freedberg, I. M., Hamolsky, M. W., and Freedberg, A. S. (1957). *N. Engl. J. Med.* **256**, 505.

Freinkel, N. (1964). *Diabetes* **13**, 260.

Freinkel, N., and Goodner, C. J. (1958). *J. Clin. Invest.* **37**, 895.

Freychet, P., Rosselin, G., and Dolais, J. (1969). *Presse Med.* **77**, 13.

Friedberg, V., Vorherr, H., and Schulte, G. (1960). *Arch. Gynaekol.* **192**, 483.

Friedman, S., Gans, B., Eckerling, B., Goldman, J., Kaufman, H., and Rumnny, M. (1969). *J. Obstet. Gynaecol. Brit. Commonw.* **76**, 554.

Friesen, H. G. (1968). *Endocrinology* **83**, 744.

Froewis, J. (1963). *Wien. Klin. Wochenschr.* **75**, 268.

Fukushima, K. (1934). *Zentralbl. Gynäekol.* **58**, 490.

Fukushima, M. (1961). *Tohoku J. Exp. Med.* **74**, 161.

Galton, V. A. (1968). *Program, Annu. Meet. Amer. Thyroid Ass.* Abstract, p. 35.

Geelhoed, G. W., and Vander, A. J. (1968). *J. Clin. Endocrinol. Metab.* **28**, 412.

Gemzell, C. A., Heijkensjöld, F., and Ström, L. (1955). *J. Clin. Endocrinol. Metab.* **15**, 537.

Genazzani, A. R., Aubert, M. L., Casoli, M., Fioretti, P., and Felber, J. P. (1969). *Lancet* **2**, 1385.

Gitlin, D., and Biasucci, A. (1969). *J. Clin. Endocrinol. Metab.* **29**, 926.

Gitlin, D., Kumate, J., and Morales, C. (1965). *Pediatrics* **35**, 65.

Goldstein, D. P., Aono, T., Taymor, M. L., Jochelson, K., Todd, R., and Hines, E. (1968). *Amer. J. Obstet. Gynecol.* **102**, 110.

Goluboff, L. G., and Ezrin, C. (1969). *J. Clin. Endocrinol. Metab.* **29**, 1533.

Gomel, V., and Hardwick, D. F. (1966). *Amer. J. Obstet. Gynecol.* **94**, 308.

Goodlin, R. C. (1970). *Amer. J. Obstet. Gynecol.* **107**, 429.

Goplerud, C., and Bradbury, J. T. (1965). *Amer. J. Obstet. Gynecol.* **91,** 23.

Goverde, B. C., Veenkamp, F. J. N., and Homan, J. D. M. (1968). *Acta Endocrinol. (Copenhagen)* **59,** 105.

Granirer, L. W. (1951). *J. Amer. Med. Asso.* **146,** 995.

Grant, D. B., Kaplan, S. L., and Grumbach, M. M. (1970). *Acta Endocrinol. (Copenhagen)* **63,** 736.

Greenspan, P. S., Kriss, J. P., Moses, L. E., and Lew, W. (1956). *Endocrinology* **58,** 767.

Grenier, J., and Rebel, A. (1956). *C. R. Soc. Biol.* **150,** 987.

Grumbach, M. M., Kaplan, S. L., Abrams, C. L., Bell, J. J., and Conte, F. A. (1966). *J. Clin. Endocrinol. Metab.* **26,** 478.

Grumbach, M. M., Kaplan, S. L., Sciarra, J. J., and Burr, I. M. (1968). *Ann. N. Y. Acad. Sci.* **148,** 501.

Gusdon, J. P., Jr., and Yen, S. S. C. (1967). *Obstet. Gynecol.* **30,** 635.

Gusdon, J. P., Jr., Leake, N., Van Dyke, A. H., and Atkins, W. (1970). *Amer. J. Obstet. Gynecol.* **107,** 441.

Halban, J. (1905). *Arch. Gynaekol.* **75,** 353.

Halnan, K. E. (1958). *Clin. Sci.* **17,** 281.

Halpin, T. F. (1970). *Amer. J. Obstet. Gynecol.* **106,** 317.

Hamashige, S., and Astor, M. A. (1969). *Fert. Steril.* **20,** 1029.

Hamashige, S., Astor, M. A., Arquilla, E. R., and Van Thiel, D. H. (1967). *J. Clin. Endocrinol. Metab.* **27,** 1690.

Hawker, R. W. (1956). *Quart. J. Exp. Physiol. Cog. Med. Sci.* **41,** 301.

Heim, K. (1931). *Klin. Wochenschr.* **10,** 1598.

Hellema, M. J. C. (1971). *J. Endocrinol.* **49,** 393.

Hennen, G. (1965). *Arch. Int. Physiol.* **73,** 689.

Hennen, G., Pierce, J. G., and Freychet, P. (1969). *J. Clin. Endocrinol. Metab.* **29,** 581.

Hershman, J. M., and Starnes, W. R. (1969). *J. Clin. Invest.* **48,** 923.

Hertz, R., Bergenstal, D. M., Lipsett, M. B., Price, E. B., and Hilbish, T. F. (1959). *Ann. N. Y. Acad. Sci.* **80,** 262.

Hertz, R., Lewis, J., Jr., and Lipsett, M. B. (1961). *Amer. J. Obstet. Gynecol.* **82,** 631.

Hibbit, L. L., Starnes, W. R., and Hill, S. R. (1958). *J. Clin. Endocrinol. Metab.* **18,** 1315.

Hisaw, F. L. (1944). *Yale J. Biol. Med.* **17,** 119.

Hobson, B., and Wide, L. (1968). *Acta Endocrinol. (Copenhagen)* **58,** 473.

Hobson, B. M. (1958). *J. Obstet. Gynaecol. Brit. Emp.* **65,** 253.

Hodari, A. A., Smeby, R., and Bumpus, F. M. (1967). *Obstet. Gynecol.* **29,** 313.

Hooper, H. C., and Jessup, D. C. (1959). *J. Physiol. (London)* **146,** 539.

Hunt, A. B., and McConahey, W. M. (1953). *Amer. J. Obstet. Gynecol.* **66,** 970.

Hunter, C. A., Jr., and Howard, W. F. (1960). *Amer. J. Obstet. Gynecol.* **79,** 838.

Hunter, C. A., Jr., and Howard, W. F. (1961). *Amer. J. Obstet. Gynecol.* **81,** 441.

Ito, Y., and Higashi, K. (1961). *Endocrinol. Jap.* **8,** 279.

Jackanicz, T. M., and Diczfalusy, E. (1968). *Steroids* **11,** 877.

Jaffe, R. B., Lee, P. A., and Midgley, A. R., Jr. (1969). *J. Clin. Endocrinol. Metab.* **29,** 1281.

Jailer, J. W., and Knowlton, A. E. (1950). *J. Clin. Invest.* **29,** 1430.

Jepson, J. H. (1968). *Can. Med. Ass. J.* **98,** 844.

Jepson, J. H., and Friesen, H. G. (1968). *Brit. J. Haematol.* **15,** 465.

Jepson, J. H., and Lowenstein, L. (1968a). *Brit. J. Haematol.* **14**, 555.
Jepson, J. H., and Lowenstein, L. (1968b). *Can. J. Physiol. Pharmacol.* **46**, 573.
Jirasek, J. E. (1967). *Endocrinol. Testis, Ciba Found. Symp.* p. 3.
Johannisson, E. (1968). *Acta Endocrinol. (Copenhagen), Suppl.* **130**.
Jones, K. M., Lloyd-Jones, R., Rondel, A., Tait, J. F.. Tait, S. A. S., Bulbrook, R. D., and Greenwood, F. C. (1959). *Acta Endocrinol. (Copenhagen)* **30**, 321.
Josimovich, J. B. (1966). *Endocrinology* **78**, 707.
Josimovich, J. B. (1968a). *Endocrinology* **83**, 530.
Josimovich, J. B. (1968b). *In* "Clinical Endocrinology II" (E. B. Astwood and C. E. Cassidy, eds.), p. 658, Grune & Stratton, New York.
Josimovich, J. B. (1970). Personal communication.
Josimovich, J. B., and Atwood, B. L. (1964). *Amer. J. Obstet. Gynecol.* **88**, 867.
Josimovich, J. B., and Brande, B. L. (1964). *Trans. N. Y. Acad. Sci.* [2] **27**, 16?
Josimovich, J. B., and MacLaren, J. A. (1962). *Endocrinology* **71**, 209.
Josimovich, J. B., and Mintz, D. H. (1968). *Ann. N. Y. Acad. Sci.* **148**, 488.
Josimovich, J. B., Atwood, B. L., and Goss, D. A. (1963). *Encrinology* **73**, 410.
Josimovich, J. B., Kosor, B., and Mintz, D. H. (1969). *Foetal Autonomy, Ciba Found. Symp.* p. 117.
Josimovich, J. B., Kosor, B., Boccella, L., Mintz, D. H., and Hutchinson, D. L. (1970). *Obstet. Gynecol.* **36**, 244.
Jungmann, R. A., and Schweppe, J. S. (1957). *J. Clin. Endocrinol. Metab.* **27**, 1151.
Kalkhoff, R. K., Richardson, B. L., and Beck, P. (1969). *Diabetes* **18**, 153.
Kaplan, N. M. (1961). *J. Clin. Endocrinol. Metab.* **21**, 1139.
Kaplan, S. L., and Grumbach, M. M. (1964). *J. Clin. Endocrinol. Metab.* **24**, 80.
Kaplan, S. L., and Grumbach, M. M. (1965a). *Science* **147**, 751.
Kaplan, S. L., and Grumbach, M. M. (1965b). *J. Clin. Endocrinol. Metab.* **25**, 1370.
Kaplan, S. L., Gurpide, E., Sciarra, J. J., and Grumbach, M. M. (1968). *J. Clin. Endocrinol. Metab.* **28**, 1450.
Karkun, J. N., and Sen, D. P. (1963). *Ann. Biochem. Exp. Med.* **23**, 81.
Katz, H. P., Grumbach, M. M., and Kaplan, S. L. (1969). *J. Clin. Endocrinol. Metab.* **29**, 1414.
Kido, I. (1937). *Zentralbl. Gynaekol.* **61**, 1551.
Klimek, R., and Bieniasz, A. (1969). *Amer. J. Obstet. Gynecol.* **104**, 959.
Klopper, A. (1970). *Amer. J. Obstet. Gynecol.* **107**, 807.
Kock, H., von Kessel, H., Stolte, L., and von Leusden, H. (1966). *J. Clin. Endocrinol. Metab.* **26**, 1128.
Koed, H. J., and Hamburger, C. (1968). *Acta Endocrinol. (Copenhagen)* **59**, 629.
Konsuloff, S. (1934). *Klin. Wochenschr.* **13**, 776.
Kulseng-Hanssen, K. (1951). *Acta Obstet. Gynecol. Scand.* **30**, 420.
Lajos, L. (1960). *Acta Endocrinol. (Copenhagen)*, **51**, *Suppl.*, 681.
Lajos, L., Nagy, D., and Gáti, I. (1959). *Gynaecologia* **148**, 59.
Lauritzen, C., and Lehmann, W. D. (1967). *J. Endocrinol.* **39**, 173.
Lauritzen, C., Shackelton, C. H. L., and Mitchell, F. L. (1969). *Acta Endocrinol. (Copenhagen)* **61**, 83.
Leake, N., and Burt, R. L. (1969). *Obstet. Gynecol.* **34**, 471.
Lee, T. H., and Lee, M. S. (1969). *J. Clin. Endocrinol. Metab.* **29**, 660.
LeMaire, W. J., Conly, P. W., Moffet, A., and Cleveland, W. W. (1970). *Amer. J. Obstet. Gynecol.* **108**, 132.
Levin, L. (1944). "Chemistry and Physiology of Hormones." *Amer. Ass. Advance. Sci.*, Washington, D. C.

Li, C. H., Grumbach, M. M., Kaplan, S. L., Josimovich, J. B., Friesen, H., and Catt, K. J. (1968). *Experientia* **24**, 1288.

Little, B., Smith, O. W., Jessiman, A. G., Selenkow, H. A., Vant't Hoff, W., Eglin, J. M., and Moore, F. D. (1958). *J. Clin. Endocrinol. Metab.* **18**, 425.

Lloyd, C. W., Hughes, E. C., Lobotsky, J., and Rienzo, J. (1951). *J. Clin. Endocrinol.* **11**, 786.

Loraine, J. A., and Bell, E. T. (1966). "Hormone Assays and Their Clinical Application." Second Ed., p. 95. Livingstone, Edinburgh and London.

Loraine, J. A., and Matthew, G. D. (1950). *J. Obstet. Gynaecol. Brit. Emp.* **57**, 542.

Loraine, J. A., and Matthew, G. D. (1953). *J. Obstet. Gynaecol. Brit. Emp.* **60**, 640.

Lunenfeld, B., and Eshkol, A. (1967). *Vitam. Horm.* (*New York*) **25**, 137.

McCarthy, C., and Pennington, G. W. (1964). *Amer. J. Obstet. Gynecol.* **89**, 1074.

McCartney, C. P., Vallach, F. J., and Pottinger, R. E. (1952). *Amer. J. Obstet. Gynecol.* **63**, 847.

McCormick, J. B. (1954). *Obstet. Gynecol.* **3**, 58.

McKenzie, J. M. (1958). *Endocrinology* **63**, 372.

Malaisse, W. J., Fracine, M., Picard, C., and Flement-Durand, J. (1969). *Endocrinology* **84**, 41.

Martin, J. M., and Friesen, H. (1969). *Endocrinology* **84**, 619.

Matthies, D. L., and Diczfalusy, E. (1968). *In* "Program, International Symposium on the Foeto-Placental Unit" (A. Pecile and C. Finzi, eds.), Int. Congr. Ser. No. 170, Abstract, p. 34. Excerpta Med. Found., Amsterdam.

Melby, J. C., Dale, S. L., Wilson, T. E., and Nichols, A. S. (1966). *Clin. Res.* **14**, 283 (Abstr.).

Merimee, T. J., Rabinowitz, D., Riggs, L., Rimoin, D., and McKusick, V. A. (1967). *N. Engl. J. Med.* **276**, 434.

Midgley, A. R., Jr. (1966). *Endocrinology* **79**, 10.

Midgley, A. R., Jr., and Jaffe, R. B. (1968). *J. Clin. Endocrinol. Metab.* **28**, 1712.

Midgley, A. R., Jr., and Pierce, G. B., Jr. (1962). *J. Exp. Med.* **115**, 289.

Mikhail, G., and Allen, W. M. (1967). *Amer. J. Obstet. Gynecol.* **99**, 308.

Mintz, D. H., Stock, R., Finster, J. L., and Taylor, A. L. (1968). *Metab., Clin. Exp.* **17**, 54.

Mishell, D. R., Jr., Wide, L., and Gemzell, C. A. (1963). *J. Clin. Endocrinol. Metab.* **23**, 125.

Mori, K. F. (1969). *Endocrinology* **85**, 330.

Mori, K. F. (1970). *Endocrinology* **86**, 97.

Murakawa, S., and Raben, M. S. (1968). *Endocrinology* **83**, 645.

Nelson, W. W., and Greene, R. R. (1958). *Amer. J. Obstet. Gynecol.* **76**, 66.

Newton, W. H. (1938). *Physiol. Rev.* **18**, 419.

Niemi, M., Ikonen, M., and Hervonen, A. (1967). *Endocrinol. Testis, Ciba Found. Symp.* p. 3.

Northcutt, R. C., and Albert, A. (1970). *J. Clin. Endocrinol. Metab.* **31**, 91.

Odell, W. D., Bates, R. W., Rivlin, R. S., Lipsett, M. B., and Hertz, R. (1963). *J. Clin. Endocrinol. Metab.* **23**, 658.

Odell, W. D., Wilber, J. F., and Utiger, R. D. (1967). *Recent Progr. Horm. Res.* **23**, 47.

Odell, W. D., Abraham, G., Randar Raud, H., Swerdloff, R. S., and Fisher, D. A. (1969a). *Acta Endocrinol.* (*Copenhagen*), *Suppl.* **142**, 54.

Odell, W. D., Reichert, L. E., and Bates, R. W. (1969b). *In* "Protein and Polypeptide Hormones" (M. Margoulies ed.), Int. Congr. Ser. No. 161, p. 124. Excerpta Med. Found., Amsterdam.

Ogier, E. (1956). *Arch. Int. Pharmacodyn. Ther.* **103**, 34.

Palmer, R., Blair, J. A., Eriksson, G., and Diczfalusy, E. (1966). *Acta Endocrinol. (Copenhagen)* **53**, 407.

Palmisano, A. (1948a). *Boll. Soc. Ital. Biol. Sper.* **24**, 1185.

Palmisano, A. (1948b). *Boll. Soc. Ital. Biol. Sper.* **24**, 1293.

Parlow, A. F. (1958). *Fed. Proc., Fed. Amer. Soc. Exp. Biol.* **17**, 402.

Parlow, A. F. (1961). *In* "Human Pituitary Gonadotropins" (A. Albert, ed.), p. 300. Thomas, Springfield, Illinois.

Parlow, A. F., Daane, T. A., and Dignam, W. J. (1970). *J. Clin. Endocrinol. Metab.* **31**, 213.

Petrusz, P. (1969). *Acta Endocrinol. (Copenhagen), Suppl.* **142**, 77.

Plate, W. P. (1952). *Acta Endocrinol. (Copenhagen)* **11**, 119.

Pochin, E. E. (1952). *Clin. Sci.* **11**, 441.

Pommerenke, W. T. (1934). *Amer. J. Obstet. Gynecol.* **27**, 708.

Reisfeld, R. A., Bergenstal, D. M., and Hertz, R. (1959). *Arch. Biochem. Biophys.* **81**, 456.

Reisfeld, R. A., Lewis, U. J., Brink, N. G., and Steelman, S. L. (1963). *Endocrinology* **71**, 559.

Rerup, C., and Melander, A. (1965). *Acta Endocrinol. (Copenhagen)* **50**, 177.

Rice, B. F., Hammerstein, J., and Savard, K. (1964a). *J. Clin. Endocrinol. Metab.* **24**, 606.

Rice, B. F., Hammerstein, J., and Savard, K. (1964b). *Steroids* **4**, 199.

Rice, B. F., Ponthier, R., and Sternberg, W. (1968). *J. Clin. Endocrinol. Metab.* **28**, 1071.

Rizkallah, T., Gurpide, E., and Vande Wiele, R. L. (1969). *J. Clin. Endocrinol. Metab.* **29**, 92.

Robyn, C., Petrusz, P., and Diczfalusy, E. (1969). *Atca Endocrinol. (Copenhagen)* **60**, 137.

Rushworth, A. G. J., Orr, A. H., and Bagshawe, K. D. (1968). *Brit. J. Cancer* **22**, 253.

Sala, N., and Fisch, L. (1965). *Amer. J. Obstet. Gynecol.* **91**, 1069.

Salvatierra, V. (1954). *Arch. Gynaekol.* **184**, 617.

Samaan, N., Yen, S. S. C., Friesen, H., and Pearson, O. H. (1966). *J. Clin. Endocrinol. Metab.* **26**, 1303.

Samaan, N., Yen, S. S. C., Gonzales, D., and Pearson, O. H. (1968). *J. Clin. Endocrinol. Metab.* **28**, 485.

Samaan, N., Bradbury, J. T., and Goplerud, C. (1969). *Amer. J. Obstet. Gynecol.* **104**, 781.

Sandler, M., and Baldock, E. (1963). *J. Obstet. Gynaecol. Brit. Commonw.* **70**, 279.

Savard, K., Marsh, J. M., and Rice, B. F. (1965). *Recent Progr. Horm. Res.* **21**, 285.

Saxena, B. N., Refetoff, S., Emerson, K., Jr., and Selenkow, H. A. (1968a). *Amer. J. Obstet. Gynecol.* **101**, 874.

Saxena, B. N., Goldstein, D. P., Emerson, K., Jr., and Selenkow, H. A. (1968b). *Amer. J. Obstet. Gynecol.* **102**, 115.

Saxena, B. N., Emerson, K., Jr., and Selenkow, H. A. (1969). *N. Engl. J. Med.* **281**, 225.

Schalch, D. S., Boon, R. C., and Lee, L. A. (1967). Secretion of human chorionic gonadotropin (HCG) and human placental lactogen (HPL) during pregnancy: Measurement by radioimmunoassay (Abstract). *In:* Program, 49th Annual Meeting of the Endocrine Society, Bar Harbour, Florida, p. 61.

Schlaff, S., Rosen, S. W., and Roth, J. (1968). *J. Clin. Invest.* **47,** 1722.

Schlumberger, H. D., and Blobel, R. (1969). *Z. Naturforsch. B* **24,** 54.

Schlumberger, H. D., and Blobel, R. (1967). *Med. Welt* **52,** 3157.

Schumacher, G., Uhlig, H., Blobel, R., Mohr, E., and Schlumberger, H. D. (1960). *Naturwissenschaften* **47,** 517.

Schwartz, H. S., and Mantel, N. (1963). *Canc. Res.* **23,** 1724.

Schwers, J., and Fanard, A. (1958). *In* "Le placenta humain" (J. Snoeck, ed.), p. 612. Masson, Paris.

Sciarra, J. J., Kaplan, S. L., and Grumbach, M. M. (1963). *Nature (London)* **199,** 1005.

Segaloff, A., Sternberg, W. H., and Gaskill, C. J. (1951). *J. Clin. Endocrinol.* **11,** 936.

Selenkow, H. A., Saxena, B. N., Dana, C. L., and Emerson, K., Jr. (1969). *In* "The Foeto-Placental Unit" (A. Pecile and C. Finzi, eds.), Int. Congr. Ser. No. 183, p. 340. Excerpta Med. Found., Amsterdam.

Selye, H., Collip, J. B., and Thomson, D. L. (1933). *Proc. Soc. Exp. Biol. Med.* **30,** 589.

Semm, K. (1960). *Geburtsh. Gynaekol.* **195,** Suppl.

Senior, J. B., Fahim, I., Sullivan, F. M., and Robson, J. M. (1963). *Lancet* **2,** 553.

Shabanah, E. H., Toth, A., and Maughan, G. (1964). *Amer. J. Obstet. Gynecol.* **89,** 841.

Shepard, T. H. (1967). *J. Clin. Endocrinol. Metab.* **27,** 945.

Sherwood, L. M. (1967). *Proc. Nat. Acad. Sci. U. S.* **58,** 2307.

Sherwood, L. M. (1969). *In* "Progress in Endocrinology" (C. Gual, ed.), Int. Congr. Ser. No. 184 p. 394. Excerpta Med. Found., Amsterdam.

Shizume, K., and Lerner, A. B. (1954). *J. Clin. Endocrinol. Metab.* **14,** 1491.

Shome, B., Parlow, A. F., Ramirez, V. D., Elrick, H., and Pierce, J. G. (1968a). *Arch. Biochem. Biophys.* **126,** 444.

Shome, B., Brown, D. M., Howard, S. M., and Pierce, J. G. (1968b). *Arch. Biochem. Biophys.* **126,** 456.

Short, R. V. (1969). *Foetal Autonomy, Ciba Found. Symp.* p. 2.

Siegler, A. M., Zeichner, S., Rubenstein, L., Wallace, E. Z., and Carter, A. C. (1959). *Amer. J. Obstet. Gynecol.* **78,** 369.

Sims, E. A. H. (1970). *Amer. J. Obstet. Gynecol.* **107,** 154.

Singer, W., Desjardins, P., and Friesen, H. G. (1970). *Obstet. Gynecol.* **36,** 222.

Skinner, S. L., Lumbers, E. R., and Symonds, E. M. (1968). *Amer. J. Obstet. Gynecol.* **101,** 529.

Smith, G. V., and Smith, O. W. (1934). *Amer. J. Physiol.* **107,** 128.

Smith, G. V., and Smith, O. W. (1939). *Amer. J. Obstet. Gynecol.* **38,** 618.

Smith, G. V., and Smith, O. W. (1948). *Physiol. Rev.* **28,** 1.

Smith, O. W., and Smith, G. V. (1937). *Amer. J. Obstet. Gynecol.* **33,** 365.

Solomon, S., and Friesen, H. G. (1968). *Annu. Rev. Med.* **19,** 399.

Soma, H., Ehrmann, R. L., and Hertig, A. T. (1961). *Obstet. Gynecol.* **18,** 704.

Spellacy, W. N. (1969). *S. Med. J.* **62,** 1054.

Spellacy, W. N. (1967). *Obstet. Gynecol.* **29,** 430.

Spellacy, W. N., and Buhi, W. C. (1969). *Amer. J. Obstet. Gynecol.* **105,** 888.

Spellacy, W. N., and Goetz, F. C. (1963). *N. Engl. J. Med.* **268,** 988.

Spellacy, W. N., Carlson, K. L., and Birk, S. A. (1966). *Amer. J. Obstet. Gynecol.* **96,** 1164.

Spellacy, W. N., Buhi, W. C., and Birk, S. A. (1970a). *Obstet. Gynecol.* **36,** 238.

Spellacy, W. N., Teoh, E. S., and Buhi, W. C. (1970b). *Obstet. Gynecol.* **35,** 685.

Stewart, H. L., Jr. (1951). *Amer. J. Obstet. Gynecol.* **61,** 990.

Stolte, L. A. M., Bakker, J. H. J., Verboom, E., and Dauvillier, P. W. (1952). *Lancet* **2**, 737.

Stolte, L. A. M., Bakker, J. H. J., Verboom, E., and Dauvillier, P. W. (1953). *Ned. Tijdschr. Geneesk.* **97**, 21.

Strott, C. A., and Lipsett, M. B. (1968). *J. Clin. Endocrinol. Metab.* **28**, 1426.

Subrahmanyam, S. (1959). *Indian J. Med. Sci.* **13**, 756.

Sulman, F. G., and Bergmann, F. (1953). *J. Obstet. Gynaecol. Brit. Emp.* **60**, 123.

Suwa, S., and Friesen, H. (1969a). *Endocrinology* **85**, 1028.

Suwa, S., and Friesen, H. (1969b). *Endocrinology* **85**, 1037.

Suzuki, M. (1954). *J. Jap. Obstet. Gynecol.* **1**, 223.

Symonds, E. M., Stanley, M. A., and Skinner, S. L. (1968). *Nature (London)* **217**, 1152.

Tallberg, T., Rouslahti, E., and Ehnholm, C. (1965). *Ann. Med. Exp. Biol. Fenn.* **43**, 67.

Tashima, C. K., Timberger, R., Burdick, R., Leavy, M., and Rawson, R. W. (1965). *J. Clin. Endocrinol. Metab.* **25**, 149.

Telegdy, G., Weeks, J. W., Wiqvist, N., and Diczfalusy, E. (1970). *Acta Endocrinol. (Copenhagen)* **63**, 105.

Teoh, E. S., and Sivasamboo, R. (1968). *J. Obstet. Gynaecol. Brit. Commonw.* **75**, 724.

Thiede, H. A., and Choate, J. W. (1963). *Obstet. Gynecol.* **22**, 433.

Torda, C. (1942). *Proc. Soc. Exp. Biol. Med.* **51**, 398.

Troen, P. (1959). *In* "Recent Progress in the Endocrinology of Reproduction" (C. W. Lloyd, ed.), p. 299. Academic Press, New York.

Troen, P. (1961). *J. Clin. Endocrinol. Metab.* **21**, 895.

Tulsky, A. S., and Koff, A. K. (1957). *Fert. Steril.* **8**, 118.

Turkington, R. W. (1968). *Endocrinology* **82**, 575.

Turkington, R. W. (1970). *Res. Reprod. (IPPF)* **2**, 2.

Turkington, R. W., and Topper, Y. J. (1966). *Endocrinology* **79**, 175.

Turtle, J. R., and Kipnis, D. M. (1967). *Biochim. Biophys. Acta* **144**, 583.

Tyson, J. E., Rabinowitz, D., Merimee, T. J., and Friesen, H. (1969). *Amer. J. Obstet. Gynecol.* **103**, 313.

Ueda, Y., Mochizuki, M., Kishimoto, Y., Washio, T., Mizusawa, S., and Ishigami, O. (1964). *Endocrinol.* **11**, 67.

Varangot, J., Cédard, L., and Yannotti, S. (1965). *Amer. J. Obstet. Gynecol.* **92**, 534.

Varma, K., Selenkow, H. A., and Emerson, K., Jr. (1970). Personal communication.

Varon, H. H. (1959). *Proc. Soc. Exp. Biol. Med.* **100**, 609.

Velardo, J. T. (1959). *Ann. N. Y. Acad. Sci.* **80**, 65.

Villee, D. B., (1969a). *N. Engl. J. Med.* **281**, 473.

Villee, D. B. (1969b). *N. Engl. J. Med.* **281**, 533.

Waltz, H. K., Tullner, W. W., Evans, V. J., Hertz, R., and Earle, W. R. (1954). *J. Nat. Cancer Inst.* **14**, 1173.

Watanabe, M., Meeker, C. I., Gray, M. J., Sims, E. A. H., and Solomon, S. (1963). *J. Clin. Invest.* **42**, 1619.

White, P., and Hunt, H. J. (1943). *J. Clin. Endocrinol. Metab.* **3**, 500.

Wide, L. (1962). *Acta Endocrinol. (Copenhagen), Suppl.* **70**.

Wide, L. (1969). *Lancet* **2**, 863.

Wide, L., and Hobson, B. M. (1964). *Lancet* **2**, 699.

Wide, L., and Hobson, B. (1967). *Acta Endocrinol. (Copenhagen)* **54**, 105.

Wide, L., Johannisson, E., Tillinger, K. G., and Diczfalusy, E. (1968). *Acta Endocrinol. (Copenhagen)* **59**, 579.

Wilde, C. E., Orr, A. H., and Bagshawe, K. D. (1967). *J. Endocrinol.* **37**, 23.

Wilde, C. E., Orr, A. H., and Bagshawe, K. D. (1965). *Nature (London)* **205**, 191.

Wright, A. D., and Joplin, G. F. (1966). *Proc. Roy. Soc. Med.* **59**, 1280.

Yamamoto, M., and Morioka, T. (1956). *Yakugaku Zasshi* **76**, 1038.

Yen, S. S. C., Samaan, N., and Pearson, O. H. (1967). *J. Clin. Endocrinol. Metab.* **27**, 1341.

Yen, S. S. C., Llerena, O., Little, B., and Pearson, O. H. (1968a). *J. Clin. Endocrinol. Metab.* **28**, 1763.

Yen, S. S. C., Pearson, O. H., and Rankin, J. S. (1968b). *Obstet. Gynecol.* **32**, 86.

Yen, S. S. C., Vela, P., and Tsai, C. C. (1970). *J. Clin. Endocrinol. Metab.* **31**, 29.

Yogo, I. (1969). *Endocrinol. Jap.* **16**, 215.

Yoshimi, T., Strott, C. A., Marshall, J. R., and Lipsett, M. B. (1969). *J. Clin. Endocrinol. Metab.* **29**, 225.

Zarrow, M. X., Holmström, E. G., and Salhanick, H. A. (1955). *J. Clin. Endocrinol. Metab.* **15**, 22.

Zondek, B. (1942). *J. Obstet. Gynaecol. Brit. Emp.* **49**, 397.

Zuckerman, J. E., Fallon, V., Tashjian, A. Jr., Levine, L., and Friesen, H. G. (1970). *J. Clin. Endocrinol. Metab.* **30**, 769.

Zuspan, F. P. (1970a). *J. Clin. Endocrinol. Metab.* **30**, 357.

Zuspan, F. P. (1970b). *Amer. J. Obstet. Gynecol.* **107**, 664.

Zuspan, F. P., Barnes, A. C., and Dillhoefer, J. R. (1958). *Amer. J. Obstet. Gynecol.* **76**, 619.

Zuspan, F. P., Nelson, G. H., and Ahlquist, R. P. (1967). *Amer. J. Obstet. Gynecol.* **99**, 709.

The Biosynthesis of Vitamins E and K and Related Compounds

D. R. THRELFALL*

Department of Biochemistry and Agricultural Biochemistry,
University College of Wales, Aberystwyth, Wales (U.K.)

I. INTRODUCTION

The past five years have been active and rewarding ones for those studying the biosynthesis of the vitamins E and K, since in this short time the outlines and many of the details of the pathways involved in their formation have been elucidated. The rapid progress which has been made owes much to the ready availability of a wide range of radioactive isotopes, to the marked improvements in the techniques of lipid fractionation and purification by chromatographic methods, and to parallel studies on the biosynthesis of biogenetically related compounds.

The two groups of vitamins have many biogenetic features in common; however, the obvious difference is that the synthesis of the vitamins K requires the formation of a naphthoquinone ring whereas that of the vitamins E requires the formation of a benzene nucleus. In this article, because of this difference and for the sake of clarity, the biosynthesis of the two groups is dealt with in separate sections, even though this leads to some overlap of subject matter. Each section starts with a brief review of the distribution of the vitamins and their chemically closely

*Present address: Department of Botany, The University, Hull, England.

related compounds and then goes on to consider in detail the biogenetic pathways responsible for their formation.

II. The Vitamins K and Related Compounds

The vitamin K group is defined by the IUPAC-IUB Commission of Biological Chemistry (1967) as being made up of vitamin K_1 (phylloquinone; 2-methyl-3-phytyl-1,4-naphthoquinone) (I) and the vitamins K_2 (menaquinones; 2-methyl-3-all-*trans*-polyprenyl-1,4-naphthoquinones) (II). The definition quite correctly excludes the various modified

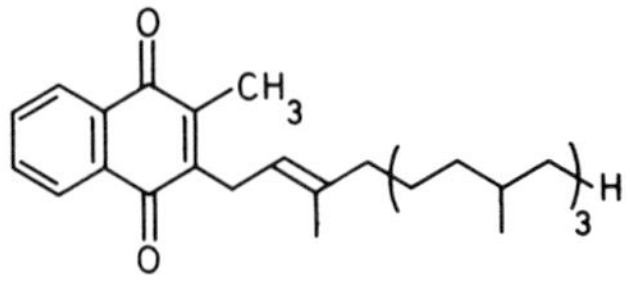

(I)

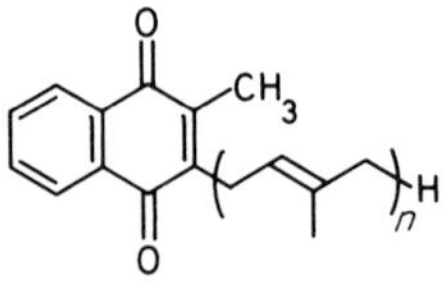

(II)

forms of these vitamins which occur naturally and have yet to be shown to have vitamin activity. These forms, however, must be taken into consideration when the chemistry, distribution, or biosynthesis of the vitamins K is presented. This section, therefore, will deal with the distribution and biosynthesis of (a) phylloquinone, demethylphylloquinone, and hydroxyphylloquinone (the phylloquinone family) in higher plants and algae and (b) menaquinones, demethylmenaquinones, and partly saturated menaquinones (the menaquinone family) in bacteria and some fungi.

A. Distribution in Bacteria and Plants

1. Phylloquinone Family

This is made up of phylloquinone (I), demethylphylloquinone (III), and hydroxyphylloquinone. Phylloquinone is present in the photosynthetic and some nonphotosynthetic tissues of higher plants and in many green, brown, red, and blue-green algae (Egger, 1965; Lichtenthaler, 1968a). In the photosynthetic regions of higher plants it is found in the lamellae and osmiophilic globules of the chloroplast (Lichtenthaler, 1969; Lichtenthaler and Tevini, 1970) ; in nonphotosynthetic tissues it is probably present in other differentiations of plastids known as leucoplasts (roots, rhizomes, chymochromous petals), etioplasts (etiolated tissues), and chromoplasts (ripening fruits, plasmochromous petals) (Lichtenthaler, 1968b). Demethylphylloquinone (III) has so far

(III)

been detected only in spinach chloroplasts (McKenna et al., 1964), and hydroxyphylloquinone (2-methyl-3-monohydroxyphytyl-1,4-naphthoquinone; the position of the hydroxyl group in the side chain is unknown) has been found only in the blue-green alga Anacystis nidulans (C. F. Allen et al., 1967) and the green algae Chlorella pyrenoidosa (Whistance and Threlfall, 1970a) and Euglena gracilis strain Z (Gullis, 1971).

2. Menaquinone Family

This is made up of (a) menaquinones (II), (b) demethylmenaquinones (V), and (c) partly saturated menaquinones.

a. Menaquinones. Menaquinones possessing side chains varying in length from C_5 (II; $n = 1$) to C_{65} (II; $n = 13$) have been isolated from Gram-positive bacteria (Bishop and King, 1962; Bishop et al., 1962; Jacobsen and Dam, 1960; Jeffries et al., 1967; Noll et al., 1960), anaerobic and facultative nonphotosynthetic Gram-negative bacteria (Maroc et al., 1970; Tornabene et al., 1969; Weber et al., 1970; Whistance et al., 1969), and photosynthetic bacteria (Maroc et al., 1968; Osnitskaya et al., 1964; Redfearn and Powls, 1967). Until fairly recently it was assumed that most menaquinone-containing organisms possessed a single homolog; however, the demonstrations that the Gram-positive bacterium Staphylococcus aureus contains menaquinone-1 through -8 (Hammond and White, 1969a), the photosynthetic bacterium Chromatium strain D contains menaquinone-3 through -8 (Whistance and Threlfall, 1970d), sewage sludge contains menaquinone-10 through -13 (Rietz et al., 1970), and human and bovine liver contain menaquinone-7 through -12 (Matschiner and Amelotti, 1968; Rietz et al., 1970) suggests that most organisms contain a series of menaquinones, the major homolog (usually menaquinone-7, -8, or -9) constituting some 85–95% of the total. Two derivatives of menaquinone-7, 1'-oxomenaquinone-7 (chlorobiumquinone) (IV) and 1'-hydroxymenaquinone-7, have been isolated from the photo-

(IV)

synthetic bacteria *Chlorobium thiosulphatophilum* and *Chloropseu-domonas ethylicum* (Powls and Redfearn, 1968; Powls *et al.*, 1968); biogenetic studies have provided some evidence that chlorobiumquinone is a metabolite of menaquinone-7 in *Chlorobium thiosulphatophilum* (Bartlett, 1968). Intracellular distribution studies have shown that menaquinones are concentrated in the protoplast membranes of Gram-positive and facultative Gram-negative bacteria (see Pennock, 1966) and the chromatophores of photosynthetic bacteria (Fuller *et al.*, 1961).

b. *Demethylmenaquinones* (V). Demethylmenaquinones have been iso-

(V)

lated from menaquinone-containing facultative and green photosynthetic Gram-negative bacteria (Bartlett, 1968; Dolin and Baum, 1965; Whistance *et al.*, 1969), two non-menaquinone-containing Gram-positive bacteria (Dolin and Baum, 1965; Lester *et al.*, 1964) and a higher plant (Sandermann and Simatupang, 1962). The side chains range in length from C_5 (V; $n = 1$) in teak wood and from C_{25} (V; $n = 5$) to C_{40} (V; $n = 8$) in bacteria. In the menaquinone-containing bacteria, the side chain is of the same length as that of the principal menaquinone homolog (menaquinone-8). Two derivatives of demethylmenaquinone-7, 4-*O*-

(VI)

(VII)

methyl-2-heptaprenylnaphthoquinol (VI) and 1-O-methyl-2-demethyl-
menachromenol-6 (VII), have been isolated from *Chlorobium thiosulphatophilum* and *Chloropseudomonas ethylicum* (Powls, 1970); the
monoprenyl homolog of 1-O-methyl-2-demethylmenachromenol-6, la-
pachenol, has been isolated from plant tissues (Geissman, 1967). Demethylmenaquinones are localized in the protoplast membranes of
facultative Gram-negative and Gram-positive bacteria (see Pennock,
1966).

 c. Partly Saturated Menaquinones. These menaquinones have a more
limited distribution. Dihydromenaquinone-10, -9 [menaquinone-9(H_2)],
-8, and -7 are found in some members of the *Micrococcaceae* family of
Gram-positive bacteria, in some strains of the fungus *Streptomyces* and
in sewage sludge (Jeffries *et al.*, 1967; Phillips *et al.*, 1969; Rietz *et al.*,
1970); *Streptomyces* sp. contain also tetrahydro-, hexahydro- and
octahydromenaquinone-9, and sewage sludge contains tetrahydro-,
hexahydro-, octahydro-, and decahydromenaquinone-8, -9, and -10
(Phillips *et al.*, 1969; Rietz *et al.*, 1970). It has been shown that the
menaquinone-9(H_2) fraction from *Mycobacterium phlei* is made up of
3'-*trans*-menaquinone-9(II-H_2) (VIII) and small amounts of 3'-*cis*-
menaquinone-9(II-H_2) (IX) (Gale *et al.*, 1963; Dunphy *et al.*, 1968).

(VIII)

(IX)

 In Gram-positive bacteria the partly saturated menaquinones are associated with the protoplast membranes (see Pennock, 1966).

B. BIOSYNTHESIS OF THE NAPHTHOQUINONE NUCLEUS

1. *Involvement of the Shikimic Acid Pathway*

 Before 1964 nothing was known about the biosynthetic origins of the
naphthoquinone nuclei of the menaquinones and phylloquinone. In that

year, however, attention was focused on the shikimic acid pathway of aromatic biosynthesis as a source of the naphthoquinone nucleus by the observation that when the facultative Gram-negative bacterium *Escherichia coli* is grown in the presence of D-[G-^{14}C]shikimic acid radioactivity is incorporated into menaquinone-8 (Cox and Gibson, 1964). Since then it has been shown that radioactivity from D-[G-^{14}C]shikimic acid is incorporated into menaquinones by Gram-positive (*Bacillus megaterium, Bacillus subtilis, Sarcina lutea, Micrococcus lysodeikticus,* and *Staphylococcus aureus*) and facultative Gram-negative bacteria (*Escherichia coli* and *Proteus vulgaris*), demethylmenaquinones by facultative Gram-negative bacteria (*Escherichia coli*), menaquinones (H$_2$) by Gram-positive bacteria (*Mycobacterium phlei*), and phylloquinone by higher plants (*Zea mays*) (Campbell *et al.*, 1967; Cox and Gibson, 1964, 1966; Ellis and Glover, 1968; Guérin *et al.*, 1970; Hammond and White, 1969b; Leistner *et al.*, 1967; Whistance *et al.*, 1966b, 1967). In addition it has been found that multiple aromatic auxotrophs of *Escherichia coli* (83-1 and 156-63) and *Staphylococcus aureus* (SHSLI) that are blocked before shikimic acid do not produce any menaquinone unless the growth medium is supplemented with this acid (Dansette and Azerad, 1970; Sasarman *et al.*, 1969).

The shikimic acid pathway of aromatic biosynthesis is found in bacteria and plants, but not in animals. The pathway has largely been worked out using heterotrophic bacteria (Gibson and Pittard, 1968); however, it appears that most of the details are the same for green plants (see Yoshida, 1969). It consists of a common pathway leading from phosphoenolpyruvate and erythrose 4-phosphate through shikimate to chorismate, after which there is branching to the individual pathways which lead to phenylalanine, tyrosine, tryptophan, 4-aminobenzoate, *p*-hydroxybenzoate, and 2,3-dihydroxybenzoate (Fig. 1). The aspects of the formation of the naphthoquinone nucleus by this pathway which have been investigated are the contribution made by the carbon atoms of shikimic acid, the position of the branch point, the source of the carbon atoms not contributed by shikimic acid, and the nature of the pathway from the branch point to the first naphthalenic intermediate.

2. Contribution Made by Shikimic Acid

Despite the fact that the incorporation of radioactivity from D-[G-^{14}C]shikimic acid into menaquinones has been demonstrated in many baceteria, in three cases only have chemical degradations of the biosynthetic products been performed. Indeed the contribution made by the carbon atoms of D-[G-^{14}C] shikimic acid to the naphthoquinone nucleus was not fully appreciated until 1967. In 1966, Cox and Gibson carried

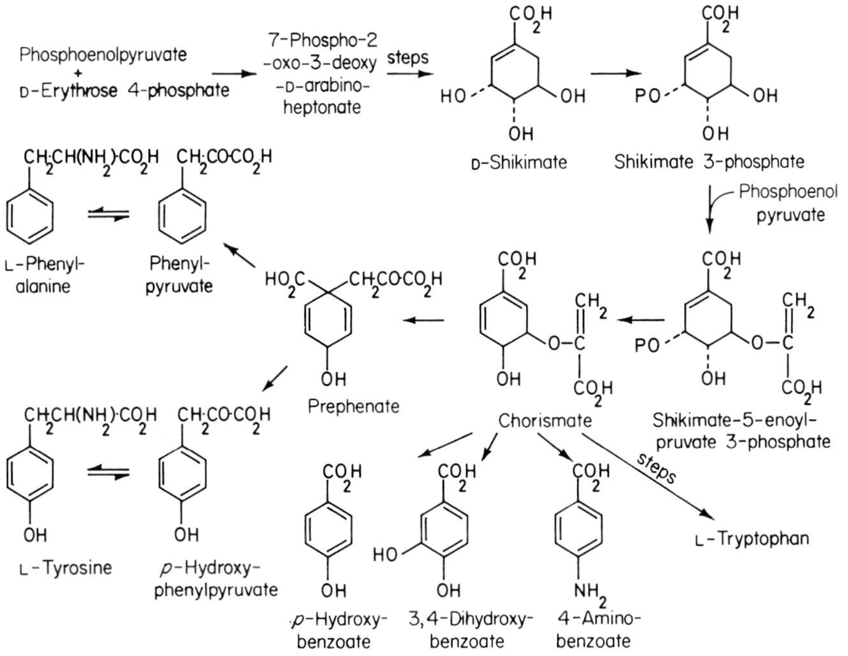

Phosphoenolpyruvate
+
D-Erythrose 4-phosphate

7-Phospho-2
-oxo-3-deoxy
-D-arabino-
heptonate

steps

D-Shikimate   Shikimate 3-phosphate

Phosphoenol pyruvate

L-Phenyl-alanine   Phenyl-pyruvate

Prephenate   Chorismate   Shikimate-5-enoyl-pruvate 3-phosphate

L-Tyrosine   p-Hydroxy-phenylpyruvate

p-Hydroxy-benzoate   3,4-Dihydroxy-benzoate   4-Amino-benzoate

L-Tryptophan

steps

FIG. 1. The shikimic acid pathway of aromatic biosynthesis. In higher plants, 3,4-dihydroxybenzoate and p-hydroxybenzoate are formed from 3-dehydroshikimate (see Yoshida, 1969) and phenylalanine (see Fig. 11), respectively.

out a partial degradation of menaquinone-8 from *Escherichia coli* and concluded that the benzenoid ring (ring A) is formed from shikimic acid. A year later, however, Leistner *et al.* (1967), prompted by their finding that all seven carbon atoms of shikimic acid are used in the biosynthesis of the simple naphthoquinone lawsone (2-hydroxy-1,4-naphthoquinone) by the higher plant *Impatiens balsamina* (Zenk and Leistner, 1967), degraded the menaquinone-7 from *Bacillus megaterium* and found that in addition to the benzenoid ring one of the carbonyl carbon atoms of ring B is formed from shikimic acid. At about the same time Campbell *et al.* (1967) obtained similar results for the menaquinone-9(II-H$_2$) from *Mycobacterium phlei*. Both groups of workers concluded that the carbon skeleton of shikimic acid is incorporated as a C$_6$–C$_1$ unit, the alicyclic ring giving rise to the benzenoid ring and the carboxyl carbon atom either giving rise to one of the carbonyl carbon atoms or contributing equally to both carbonyl carbon atoms (Fig. 2).

Recently, Leduc *et al.* (1970) have determined the pattern of incorporation of radioactivity from DL-[1,6-^{14}C]shikimic acid and D-[3-^{3}H]-

shikimic acid into the benzenoid ring of menaquinone-9 (II-H_2) by *Mycobacterium phlei* (in this article shikimic acid is numbered through the double bond). They found that the ethylenic carbon atoms (C-1 and -2) give rise to the carbon atoms forming the bridge (C-9 and -10) between the fused rings and that C-3 either gives rise to C-5 or C-8 or contributes equally to C-5 and -8 (Fig. 2). The uncertainty about the actual contributions made by the various carbon atoms is due to the symmetrical nature of one of the chemical degradation products. Some light on this aspect has come from studies on the incorporation of D-[G-^{14}C]shikimic acid and DL-[1,6-^{14}C]shikimic acid into juglone (5-hydroxy-1,4-naphthoquinone), a plant quinone whose 5-hydroxy group confers assymetry on its chemical degradation products. The results of these studies showed that C-1 and -2 of shikimic acid give rise to C-9 and -10, and that C-7 and -6 contribute equally to C-1 and -4 and C-3 and -6, respectively (Leistner and Zenk, 1968a). These findings show that (a) the intermediates involved in the early stages of naphthoquinone biosynthesis are of such a nature that the assymetry of the alicyclic ring of shikimic acid is preserved, i.e., C-2 and -6, and C-3 and -5 do not become equivalent, and (b) a symmetrical 1,4-dihydroxy intermediate (naphthoquinol?) is involved in the biosynthesis of juglone and presumably menaquinones and phylloquinone also.

3. The Branch Point of Naphthoquinone Biosynthesis

The branch point on the shikimic acid pathway for menaquinone biosynthesis is either at chorismate or, more unlikely, at prephenate. It is placed at chorismate or beyond by the facts that *Escherichia coli* 159-4, a multiple aromatic auxotroph blocked between shikimate and shikimate

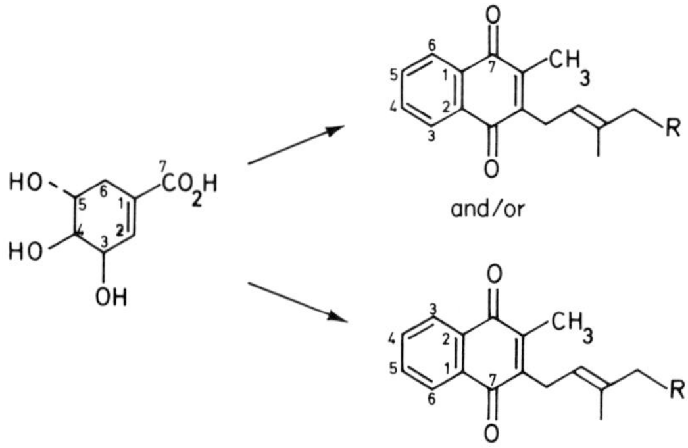

Fig. 2. Contribution made by the carbon atoms of shikimic acid to the naphthoquinone ring of menaquinone.

5-phosphate, and *Klebsiella aerogenes* (*Aerobacter aerogenes*) 170-44, a multiple aromatic auxotroph blocked between 5-enoylpyruvylshikimate 3-phosphate and chorismate, are unable to synthesize menaquinones (Cox and Gibson, 1966; Dansette and Azerad, 1970). It is restricted to chorismate or prephenate both on theoretical grounds and on the basis of negative results obtained in radioactive tracer experiments and isotope competition experiments. At the outset it is possible to eliminate (a) the intermediates on the prephenate to tyrosine and prephenate to phenyl-alanine pathways, because they do not retain C-7 of shikimate, (b) *p*-hydroxybenzoate, because in its formation C-2 and -6 and C-3 and -5 of shikimate become equivalent and this does not occur in menaquinone biosynthesis (Section II,B,2), and (c) 4-aminobenzoate, because the multiple aromatic auxotrophs *Escherichia coli* 159-4 and *Klebsiella aerogenes* 170-44, which require this compound for growth, do not produce mena-quinones (Cox and Gibson, 1966; Dansette and Azerad, 1970). Dihy-droxybenzoate and, although for the reasons given above they cannot be intermediates, *p*-hydroxybenzoate, *p*-hydroxyphenylpyruvate, and phenyl-pyruvate have been eliminated by radioactive tracer and isotope com-petition experiments (Campbell *et al.*, 1967; Cox and Gibson, 1964, 1966; Guérin *et al.*, 1970; Leistner *et al.*, 1967). Early in the course of these investigations it was found that 3,4-dihydroxybenzaldehyde will reduce the incorporation of radioactivity from D-[G-14C]shikimic acid into menaquinone-8 by *Escherichia coli,* which suggested that it is an inter-mediate (Cox and Gibson, 1964, 1966). However, although the isotope competition effect has been confirmed (Leistner *et al.*, 1967), radioactivity from 14C and 3H species of 3,4-dihydroxybenzaldehyde is not incorporated into menaquinones by *Klebsiella aerogenes, Bacillus megaterium, Esch-erichia coli, Mycobacterium phlei,* and *Proteus vulgaris* (Campbell *et al.*, 1967; Guérin *et al.*, 1970; Leistner *et al.*, 1967). The tryptophan pathway has not been examined as a source of intermediates; however, it is un-likely that any of the compounds on this pathway are involved.

In higher plants the branch point for phylloquinone biosynthesis is probably at the same position. The only evidence in support of this is that radioactivity from *p*-hydroxy[U-14C]phenylpyruvic acid, [U-14C]-phenylpyruvic acid, *p*-hydroxy[U-14C]benzoic acid, 3,4-dihydroxy-[U-14C]benzoic acid, L-[U-14C]tyrosine, and L-[U-14C]phenylalanine is not incorporated into phylloquinone by French bean shoots (*Phaseolus vulgaris*), maize shoots (*Zea mays*), and ivy leaves (*Hedera helix*) (Whistance and Threlfall, 1967, 1968b, 1970a; Whistance *et al.*, 1966b, 1967). Leistner and Zenk (1968a) reported that although radioactivity from [G-14C]chorismic acid is incorporated into phenylalanine and tyrosine by *Juglans regia*, it is not incorporated into the shikimic acid-derived naphthoquinone juglone: however, before this result is accepted as evidence against the involvement of this acid in the biosynthesis of plant naphthoquinones, the fact must be taken into account that chorismic acid and its salts are unstable and decompose under physiological conditions to give a mixture of *p*-hydroxybenzoate and prephenate (F. Gibson, 1964; M. I. Gibson and Gibson, 1964).

4. The Nature of the Pathway from the Branch Point to the First Naphthalenic Intermediate

The nature of the pathway from the branch point to the first naphthalenic compound is only now beginning to emerge. Most investigators have chosen to attack this problem by attempting to determine the source of the three-carbon unit which together with shikimic acid forms the naphthoquinone nucleus.

The first reports came from Cox and Gibson (1966) and Campbell *et al.* (1967), who obtained some incorporation of radioactivity from [1,2-^{14}C]acetic acid into the quinone rings of menaquinone-8 in *Escherichia coli* and menaquinone-9(II-H$_2$) in *Mycobacterium phlei*. This was

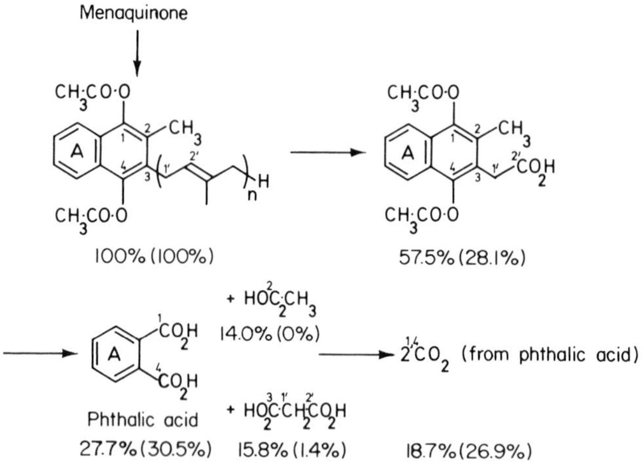

Fig. 3. Chemical degradation of menaquinone-8 labeled from either L-[U-^{14}C]glutamic acid or DL-[2-^{14}C]glutamic acid (after Robins *et al.*, 1970). The radioactivity from either L-[U-^{14}C]glutamic acid (unparenthesized figures) or DL-[2-^{14}C]glutamic acid (parenthesized figures) that was present in the various degradation products is given as a percentage of the total radioactivity incorporated into the menaquinone molecule.

followed by the report of Leistner and Zenk (1968a) that in *Juglans regia* [2-^{14}C]acetic acid or malonic acid labels C-2 and/or C-3 of juglone, but that the malonic acid carboxyl group is not incorporated; [2,3-^{14}C]fumaric acid and succinic acid were also found to be precursors. The possibility that the C_3-unit is derived from the enoylpyruvyl side chain of chorismate itself was raised when Hammond and White (1969b) found that [2-^{14}C]glycerol contributed some radioactivity to the menaquinones of *Staphylococcus aureus;* however, this was discounted when it was shown that in *Escherichia coli* and *Mycobacterium phlei* neither [1,3-^{14}C]glycerol nor [1-^{14}C]pyruvic acid are incorporated into the menaquinone fraction (Robins *et al.*, 1970).

The problem was resolved finally when it was shown that radioactivity from DL-[2-^{14}C]glutamic acid is incorporated into C-1 and/or C-4 of juglone by *Juglans regia* (Campbell, 1969) and menaquinone-8 by *Escherichia coli* and from L-[U-^{14}C]glutamic acid is incorporated into C-1 (and/or C-4), -2, and -3 of menaquinone-8 by *Escherichia coli* and menaquinone-9(II-H$_2$) by *Mycobacterium phlei* (Robins *et al.*, 1970). In these experiments the interpretation of the results obtained for the degradation of the menaquinones is complicated by the fact that exten-

F$_{IG}$. 4. Proposed pathway for the biosynthesis of the naphthoquinone nucleus of menaquinones by bacteria and of lawsone by *Impatiens balsamina*. After Campbell (1969) and Robins *et al.* (1970).

sive metabolism of the [^{14}C]glutamic acid occurs and only some 30–60% of the radioactivity incorporated into the molecules is present in the relevant atoms (Fig. 3). Nevertheless, they are consistent with the view that the C_3-unit can be formed from C-2, -3, and -4 of glutamate, and this led Campbell (1969) and Robins et al. (1970) to put forward a pathway for the formation of the naphthoquinone nucleus which has as its first step the condensation of shikimate with a succinylsemialdehyde thiamine pyrophosphate anion (Fig. 4). Unfortunately, the pathway suggested has the branch point at shikimate, a proposal which is not in keeping with the experimental evidence (Section II,B,3). This discrepancy, however, was resolved by Dansette and Azerad (1970), who proposed that the first step is the condensation with concomitant dehydration of chorismate with a C_4 derivative of glutamate, which might be the succinyl-semialdehyde thiamine pyrophosphate anion of Robins et al. (1970), followed by a simple elimination reaction to form O-succinylbenzoate (Fig. 5). They also made the point that in terms of Michael

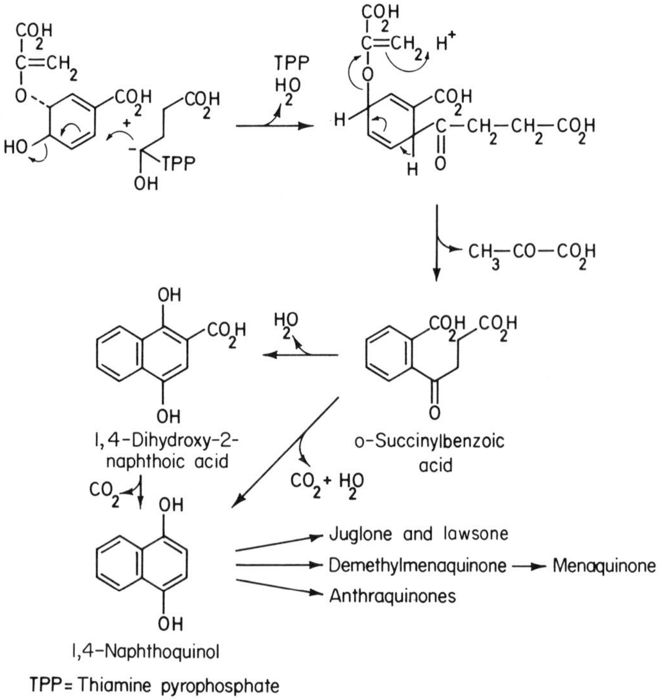

FIG. 5. Proposed pathway for the biosynthesis of the menaquinones by bacteria and naphthoquinones and anthraquinones by higher plants. After Dansette and Azerad (1970).

addition on a carbonyl-activated double bond an alternative and more attractive possibility is the attack of the same carbanion on isochorismic acid. In support of their proposals Dansette and Azerad (1970) showed that when *Escherichia coli* 83-1 and 156-53, multiple aromatic auxotrophs blocked in the early reactions of aromatic biosynthesis, are cultured on an aromatic supplement and O-succinylbenzoic acid they formed the same amounts of menaquinone-8 as when grown in the presence of shikimic acid. With *Escherichia coli* 159-4, which is blocked after shikimate, and *Klebsiella aerogenes* 170-44, which is blocked between 5-enoylpyruvyl shikimate-3-phosphate and chorismate, only O-succinylbenzoic acid is effective. Finally, they synthesized O-succinyl[$carboxy$-^{14}C]benzoic acid and showed that the radioactivity is incorporated into C-1 and/or C-4 of menaquinone-9(II-H_2) by *Mycobacterium phlei*, of demethylmenaquinone-8 and menaquinone-8 by *Klebsiella aerogenes* and *Escherichia coli*, of lawsone by *Impatiens balsamina*, of juglone by *Juglans regia*, and the anthraquinone pseudopurpurine by *Rubia peregrina*.

Dansette and Azerad (1970) proposed that O-succinylbenzoate is cyclized to form 1,4-dihydroxy-2-naphthoate, the first naphthalenic compound on the pathway, and this is then decarboxylated to give 1,4-naphthoquinol (Fig. 5). The unstable 1,4-dihydroxy-2-naphthoic acid has been prepared; however, in an isotope competition experiment it did not reduce the incorporation of O-succinyl[$carboxy$-^{14}C]benzoic acid into lawsone by young shoots of *Impatiens balsamina* (Dansette and Azerad, 1970). It has been reported that radioactivity from 1,4-[1-^{14}C]- and 1,4-[1,4,5,8-^{14}C]naphthoquinone is incorporated into menaquinone-8 by the mutant *Klebsiella aerogenes* 170-44 (Guérin *et al.*, 1970), 1,4-[5,8,?-^3H]naphthoquinone is incorporated into menaquinone-9 by the anaerobic bacterium *Bacteroides melaninogenicus* (*Fusiformis nigrescens*) (Martius and Leuzinger, 1964) and 1,4-[2,3,9,10-^{14}C]naphthoquinone is incorporated into juglone by *Juglans regia* and the anthraquinone alizarin by *Rubia tinctorum* (Leistner and Zenk, 1968a,b). It is of note that in these experiments 1,4-naphthoquinone rather than the postulated intermediate 1,4-naphthoquinol was administered.

Further support for the pathway of Dansette and Azerad (1970) is the demonstration that ^{18}O from [^{18}O]H_2O but not from $^{18}O_2$ is incorporated into menaquinone-9(II-H_2) by *Mycobacterium phlei* (Snyder and Rapoport, 1970). A finding which provides very good evidence that both oxygen atoms are derived from the precursors which go to form the carbon skeleton of the naphthoquinone nucleus and that aromatic hydroxylation is virtually excluded.

In the early stages of the investigations concerned with the nature of

the naphthalenic compounds involved in the biosynthesis of naphthoquinones, Sanderman and Simatupang (1967), on comparative phytochemical grounds, had proposed that α-naphthol might be a precursor of
some of the naphthalenic compounds found in nature. In support of this
proposal Leistner et al. (1967) showed that radioactivity from α-[1-^{14}C]-
naphthol is incorporated into C-1 and/or C-4 of menaquinone-7 by
Bacillus megaterium. Since then it has been reported that radioactivity
from α-[1-^{14}C]naphthol is incorporated into menaquinones by the Gram-
positive bacterium Staphylococcus aureus and the Gram-negative bacterium Klebsiella aerogenes 170-44 (Guérin et al., 1970; Hammond and
White, 1969b; Hurd, 1970), but not by the Gram-positive bacteria
Bacillus megaterium, Bacillus subtilis, Micrococcus lysodeikticus, Micrococcus phlei, and the Gram-negative bacteria Escherichia coli, Proteus
mirabilis, and Proteus vulgaris and phylloquinone by maize shoots
(Brown et al., 1968; Guérin et al., 1970; Ellis and Glover, 1968; R. A.
Hall, 1970; Hurd, 1970). The simplest way of explaining these anomalous
results and of rationalizing the part played by α-naphthol in the biosynthesis of menaquinones is to propose that it is an aberrant precursor and
that those organisms which can utilize it possess the necessary enzyme
to convert it into 1,4-naphthoquinol.

C. Source of the 2-Methyl Group

1. The Methyl Donor

The source of the 2-methyl group is the S-methyl group of L-methionine. Thus, it has been shown that radioactivity from L-[Me-^{14}C]-
methionine is incorporated into the 2-methyl groups of menaquinone-7
and chlorobiumquinone by the photosynthetic bacterium Chlorobium
thiosulphatophilum (Bartlett, 1968), menaquinone-8 by the photosynthetic bacterium Chromatium strain D and the facultative Gram-negative
bacterium Escherichia coli (Whistance and Threlfall, 1970d), mena-
quinone-9 by the anaerobic Gram-negative bacterium Bacteroides
melaninogenicus (Martius and Leuzinger, 1964), menaquinone-9 (II-H_2)
by the Gram-positive bacterium Mycobacterium phlei (Guérin et al.,
1965), and phylloquinone by the alga Euglena gracilis, maize shoots and
ivy leaves (Threlfall et al., 1968; Whistance and Threlfall, 1968b, 1970d).

2. The Mechanism of Methylation

Studies with DL-[Me-$^2H_3$]methionine and L-[Me-^{14}C, ^{3}H]methionine
have established that the 2-methyl groups of menaquinone-8 in Escherichia coli, menaquinone-9 in Mycobacterium smegatis and phylloquinone
in maize shoots are formed by transmethylation (Jackman et al., 1967;

Jauréguiberry *et al.*, 1966; Threlfall *et al.*, 1967a, 1968). Azerad *et al.* (1967) found that in cell free extracts of *Mycobacterium phlei* the electrophile *S*-adenosyl-L-methionine is the immediate donor of the 2-methyl group of menaquinone-9(II-H$_2$). These findings indicate that the transmethylation reaction will proceed as shown in Fig. 6. It would appear that the nucleophile for the reaction, depending on the organism examined, can be either naphthoquinol (Section II,E,1) or demethyl-menaquinol (Section II,C,3).

3. Properties of the Mycobacterium phlei Methyltransferase

The properties of the methyltransferase involved in the formation of menaquinone-9(II-H$_2$) by *Mycobacterium phlei* have been extensively studied. Azerad *et al.* (1967) provided evidence that the natural substrate for the enzyme is demethylmenaquinone-9, when they demonstrated that the 10,000 g supernatant fraction from cells ruptured with ultrasound is able to form [Me-^{14}C]menaquinone-9 from demethylmenaquinone-9 and *S*-adenosyl-L-[Me-^{14}C]methionine and then to reduce it to [Me-^{14}C]menaquinone-9(II-H$_2$) when NADPH or NADH is added. Further studies with dialyzed cell free preparations have shown that the acceptor molecule must have an unmodified naphthoquinone ring and a *trans*-$\beta\gamma$-unsaturated side chain of at least two isoprene units in length (Samuel and Azerad, 1969). The preparation is active for demethyl-menaquinone-2 through to demethylmenaquinone-9, the activity reaching a maximum for demethylmenaquinone-3 and -4 and then decreasing with increasing chain length. It is of note that naphthoquinone could not be tested as an acceptor molecule, because it was found to be impossible to recover added menadione (due to its high affinity for protein sulfhydryl groups) from the incubation mixtures. However, the dependence of transmethylase activity on the presence of a polyprenyl side chain indicates that it would not be methylated in this system. The finding that the maximal rate of activity is obtained with a side chain considerably

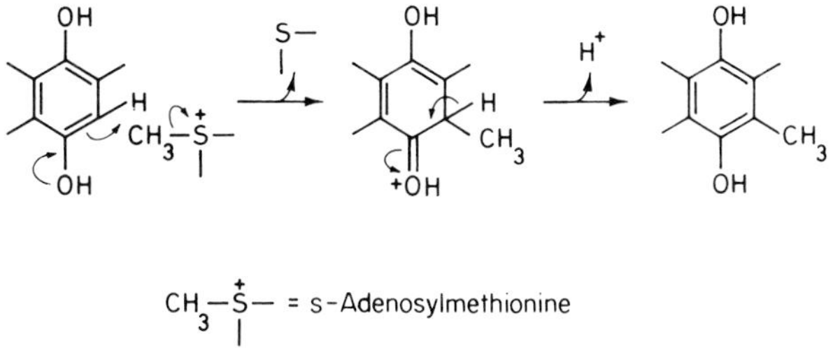

$$CH_3-\overset{+}{\underset{|}{S}}- = \text{s-Adenosylmethionine}$$

FIG. 6. A mechanism for the transmethylation reactions involved in the biosynthesis of isoprenoid quinones and chromanols.

shorter than that of the proposed natural substrate (demethylmena-quinone-9) indicates that *in vivo* the rate of synthesis of demethylmena-quinone-9 must be greater than the rates of synthesis of its homologs. An alternative explanation is that in these experiments the efficiency of the technique used to solubilize the demethylmenaquinones was greater for the less hydrophobic short-chain homologs.

Catala *et al.* (1970) have recently reported that the S-adenosyl-L-methionine:demethylmenaquinone transferase is associated with the membrane, has a pH optima of 8, and is strongly inhibited by p-hydroxy-mercuribenzoate. Demethylmenaquinone provides no protection against the inhibitor and S-adenosyl-L-methionine affords only partial protection.

For all of the enzyme studies described above, demethylmenaquinones were used as acceptor molecules, despite the fact that on mechanistic grounds the acceptor molecules should be quinols (Section II,C,2). In an attempt to rationalize this apparent anomaly, Lederer (1969) pro-posed that demethylmenaquinone first reacts with the sulfhydryl group of the methyltransferase to produce a 2-thioether of demethylmena-quinol which is amenable to attack by the electrophile S-adenosyl-L-methionine; after which the enzyme is eliminated by a reversal of the thiolation reaction (Fig. 7). Evidence against this type of mechanism is provided by the observation that preincubation of a methyltransferase

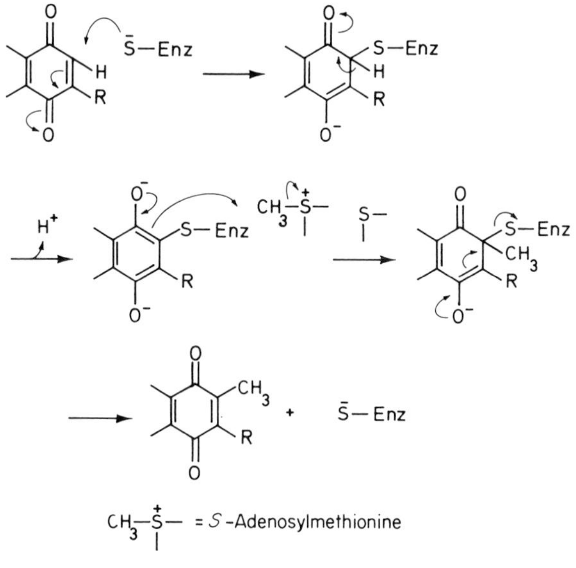

FIG. 7. Proposed mechanism for the C-methylation of demethylmenaquinone by cell-free extracts of *Mycobacterium phlei*. After Lederer (1969).

preparation with demethylmenaquinone does not prevent its inhibition by p-hydroxymercuribenzoate (Catala *et al.*, 1970). A more attractive explanation, based on the mechanism of the reaction between the sulfhydryl group of glutathione and menadione (Nickerson *et al.*, 1963), is that in the incubation systems used two molecules of demethylmenaquinone and one molecule of a sulfhydryl protein (not necessarily the methyltransferase) or, in those incubations in which it was present, mercaptoethanol reacted to produce one molecule of a 2-thioether of demethylmenaquinone and one molecule of demethylmenaquinol; the latter then acted as the acceptor molecule for the methyltransferase. In the undialyzed methyl transferase preparations demethylquinone was possibly reduced to the quinol by the action of an appropriate reductase.

D. FORMATION OF THE 3-POLYPRENYL GROUP

1. *Source of the 3-Polyprenyl Group*

The details of the formation of the 3-all-*trans*-polyprenyl groups of the menaquinones and demethylmenaquinones, the 3-all-*trans*-polyprenyl (H_X) group of the partly saturated menaquinones, the 3-phytyl group of phylloquinone and the modified forms of these groups found in 3'-*cis*-menaquinone(II-H_2), chlorobiumquinone, hydroxymenaquinone-7, and hydroxyphylloquinone are still far from clear. It is believed that they are synthesized independently of the nuclei as all-*trans*-polyprenylphosphates, the allylic groups of which are then transferred to either naphthoquinol or menadiol (Section II,E,1) in an electrophilic aromatic.substitution reaction (Fig. 8). The various modifications to the polyprenyl units probably take place after they have been coupled to the nuclei. An alternative method of synthesis is the isopentylation of the nucleus fol-

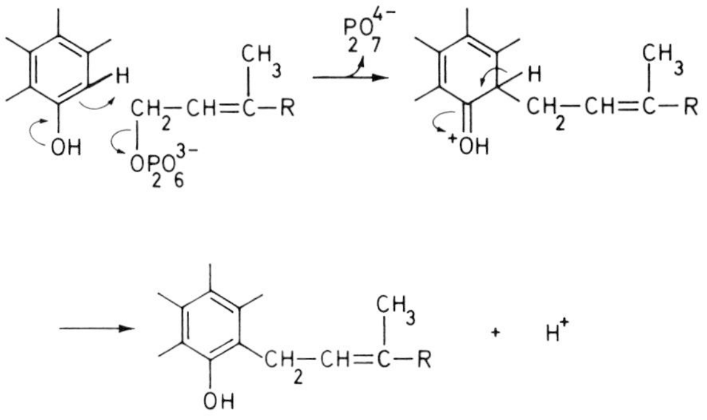

FIG. 8. A mechanism for the polyprenylation reactions involved in the biosynthesis of isoprenoid quinones and chromanols.

lowed by stepwise addition of isopentyl groups; however, apart from the report that chain elongation of α-tocopherolquinone to form tocoquinone-10 can take place in animals (Martius, 1962; Martius and Furer, 1962), there is no evidence to support this type of pathway (Krishnamurthy and Bieri, 1963; Mellors and Barnes, 1966; Plack and Bieri, 1964; Seward and Corwin, 1963).

2. Incorporation of Mevalonic Acid

It has been shown that radioactivity from DL-[2-^{14}C]mevalonic acid, the specific distal precursor of the basic isoprene unit of terpenoid compounds, is incorporated into the 3-phytyl groups of phylloquinone by tobacco leaves (*Nicotiana tabacum*) (Griffiths *et al.*, 1968) and young maize shoots (Dada *et al.*, 1968; Threlfall *et al.*, 1967b). The evidence for the involvement of this acid in the formation of the 3-polyprenyl groups of menaquinones is still far from satisfactory. Hammond and White (1969b) obtained a small incorporation of radioactivity from DL-[2-^{14}C]mevalonic acid and DL-[5-^{3}H]mevalonic acid into the 3-octaprenyl group of menaquinone-8 in *Staphylococcus aureus* and Sarikabuhti (1968) has reported that cell free preparations of *Mycobacterium phlei* will incorporate small amounts of radioactivity from DL-[2-^{14}C]mevalonic acid into menaquinone-9 (II-H$_2$). All other attempts to incorporate mevalonic acid into bacterial menaquinones (and ubiquinones) have so far failed (Raman *et al.*, 1965; Ramasarma and Ramakrishnan, 1961; Whistance and Threlfall, 1970d). This failure is usually attributed to the inability of the acid to enter the cell and reach the site of polyprenylpyrophosphate synthesis, rather than to its noninvolvement in menaquinone biosynthesis.

3. The Formation of Polyprenylpyrophosphates

The pathway by which mevalonate gives rise to the γ,γ-dimethyl-allyl- through to all-*trans*-tridecaprenylpyrophosphates required for the biosynthesis of monoprenyl through to tridecaprenylnaphthoquinones is probably an extended version of the well-authenticated pathway for the formation of all-*trans*-farnesylpyrophosphate (see Popják, 1970), required for the biosynthesis of sterols (see Clayton, 1965), the all-*trans*-farnesyl-poly-*cis* family of prenols (see Hemming, 1970), etc., and all-*trans*-geranylgeranylpyrophosphate (see Porter, 1969), required for the biosynthesis of carotenoids (see Porter, 1969), all-*trans*-polyprenols, the all-*trans*-geranyl-poly-*cis* family of prenols (see Hemming, 1970), etc. (Fig. 9). The key compound is isopentenylpyrophosphate, formed from mevalonate via mevalonatepyrophosphate, since its stepwise condensation in the appropriate stereospecific manner with allylic

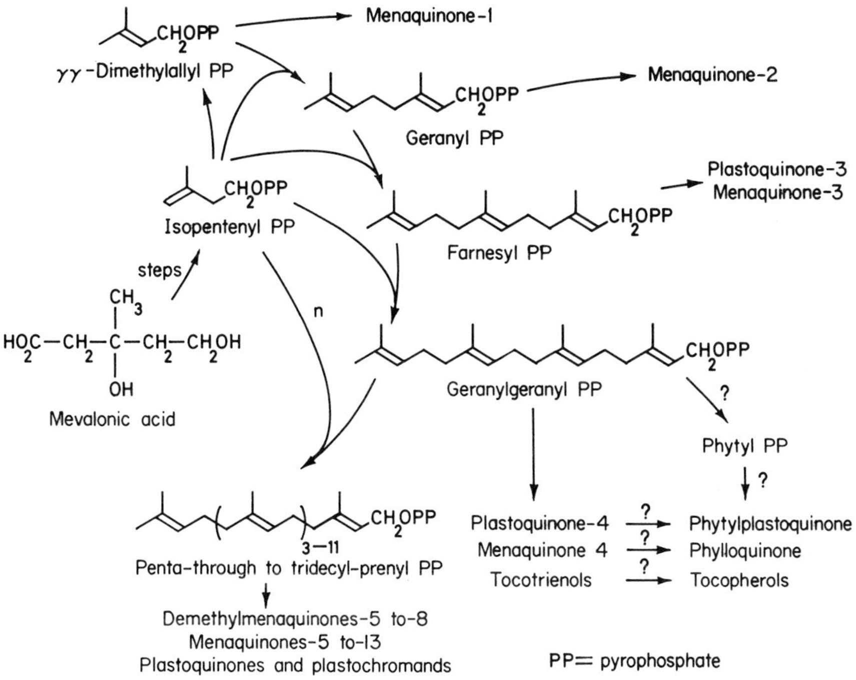

FIG. 9. Formation of all-*trans*-polyprenylpyrophosphates required for the biosynthesis of isoprenoid quinones and chromanols.

pyrophosphates leads to the formation of the all-*trans* (Fig. 9), all-*trans*-farnesyl-poly-*cis*, and all-*trans*-geranyl-poly-*cis* series of alcohol pyrophosphates.

The stereochemistry of the formation of the double bonds can be followed using $(3RS)$-$[2$-$^{14}C,(4R)$-4-$^3H_1]$- and $(3RS)$-$[2$-$^{14}C,(4S)$-4-$^3H_1]$mevalonic acids. Thus in the formation of a *trans* configuration the *pro*-R hydrogen at C-2 of isopentenylpyrophosphate (which corresponds to the *pro*-S hydrogen at C-4 of mevalonic acid) is eliminated and the *pro*-S hydrogen is retained; in the formation of a *cis* configuration the reverse takes place (see Popják, 1970) (Fig. 10). Dada *et al.* (1968) showed that only from $(3RS)$-$[2$-$^{14}C,(4R)$-4-$^3H_1]$mevalonic acid is ^3H incorporated into phylloquinone in maize shoots, which establishes that all four isoprene units of the 3-phytyl group are biogenetically *trans*. A result that is consistent with the view that the phytyl group is formed by reduction of an all-*trans*-geranylgeranyl group.

A limited amount of work has been done on the nature and intra-cellular distribution of synthetases which might be concerned with the

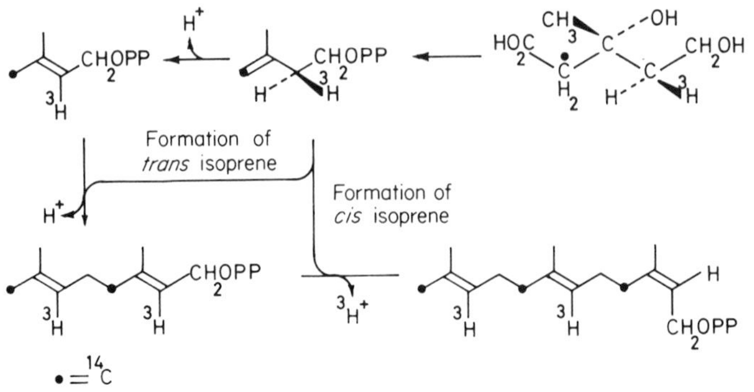

Fig. 10. Incorporation of $[2\text{-}^{14}C,(4R)\text{-}4\text{-}^{3}H_1]$mevalonic acid into *cis* and *trans* isoprene residues. In the case of $[2\text{-}^{14}C,(4S)\text{-}4\text{-}^{3}H_1]$mevalonic acid tritium is lost in the formation of a *trans* residue and retained in the formation of a *cis* residue.

formation of the allylic pyrophosphates used for the synthesis of menaquinones and phylloquinone.

Kandutsch *et al.* (1964) and C. M. Allen *et al.* (1967) have isolated two synthetases from *Micrococcus lysodeikticus*, the first of which will synthesize geranylgeranylpyrophosphate from isopentenylpyrophosphate and γ,γ-dimethylallylpyrophosphate, and the second of which will synthesize from penta- through to decaprenylpyrophosphate (with septa- and octa- predominating) from farnesylpyrophosphate and isopentenylpyrophosphate. Obviously the concerted action of these two synthesases could be responsible for the formation of the nonaprenylpyrophosphate required for the synthesis of menaquinone-9(II-H$_2$). Christenson *et al.* (1969) reported the isolation from *Salmonella newingtonii* of a particulate synthetase which forms the undecaprenylpyrophosphate used in the synthesis of antigenic lipopolysaccharide and a soluble synthetase which forms polyprenols with chain lengths shorter than C$_{55}$ and could produce the menaquinone side chain. The criticism which must be leveled against these proposals is that the stereochemical properties of the products of the synthetases are unknown, and it may be that they are producing *cis-trans*-polyprenylpyrophosphates, not the required all-*trans*-polyprenylpyrophosphates.

In higher plants it has been shown that geranylgeranylpyrophosphate, the allylic pyrophosphate required for phylloquinone synthesis, can be made from mevalonic acid by endosperm of *Echinocystis macrocarpa* (Oster and West, 1968), pea homogenates (Graebe, 1967; Pollard *et al.*, 1966), and tomato plastids (Suzue and Porter, quoted in Porter, 1969) and from isopentenylpyrophosphate and farnesylpyrophosphate by enzymes isolated from tomato fruit plastids (Jungalwala and Porter, 1967) and carrot roots (Nandi and Porter, 1964).

4. Evidence for the 3-Polyprenylation Reaction

Indirect evidence in support of the view that the polyprenyl group is added as a preformed unit (Section II,D,1) comes from the fact that polyprenylsynthetases capable of synthesizing polyprenylpyrophosphates of the required lengths are found in nature (Section II,D,3). Direct evidence comes from the fact that rat liver mitochondria and chicken and rat liver and heart cell cultures are capable of synthesizing menaquinone-3, -4, and -9 from menadione and farnesyl-, geranylgeranyl-, and nonaprenyl(solanesyl)pyrophosphates, respectively (Schiefer and Martius, 1960; Stoffel and Martius, 1960).

Further support comes from the demonstration that chromatophores from the photosynthetic bacterium *Rhodospirillum rubrum* and mitochondria from rat kidney, brain, and liver do not synthesize 4-carboxy-2-polyprenylphenol (X), the first polyprenylated intermediate

(X)

in the biosynthesis of ubiquinone, from *p*-hydroxybenzoic acid and isopentenylpyrophosphate unless they are supplemented with polyprenylpyrophosphate synthetase from *Micrococcus lysodeikticus* (Raman *et al.*, 1969; Winrow and Rudney, 1969). These findings demonstrate quite clearly that 4-carboxy-2-polyprenylphenols cannot be synthesized by 2-isopentylation of *p*-hydroxybenzoic acid followed by the stepwise addition of isopentyl groups, but that a preformed side chain is required.

5. Hydrogenation of the Polyprenyl Group

An interesting aspect of the biosynthesis of menaquinones(H_X) and phylloquinone is how and at what stage the side chains are hydrogenated. Azerad *et al.* (1967) have provided some evidence that the menaquinone-9 (II-H_2) in *Mycobacterium phlei* is formed from menaquinone-9 by the action of an NADPH or NADH-dependent reductase (Section II,C,3). In the case of phylloquinone, it is not known whether the geranylgeranyl unit is saturated before or after its addition to the nucleus. Although, as in the case of the hydrogenation reactions involved in the biosynthesis of tocopherols and tocotrienols (Wellburn, 1968, 1970), it is to be expected that an NADPH-dependent reductase is involved.

E. PATHWAYS FROM NAPHTHOQUINOL

1. The Overall Picture

It is now almost certain that 1,4-naphthoquinol is the first naphthalenic compound on the pathway leading from chorismate to the menaquinone and phylloquinone families of compounds and to the simple shikimic acid-derived naphthoquinones and anthraquinones (Section II,B,4). The possible number of pathways leading from naphthoquinol to menaquinones and phylloquinones is limited. Indeed, in the case of demethylmenaquinones the pathway can only be the one given in Eq. (1). In the case of bacterial menaquinones the picture that is beginning to emerge is that menadiol is an intermediate in the biosynthesis of menaquinones by Gram-negative and Gram-positive bacteria [Eq. (2)] and that demethylmenaquinols are intermediates in the biosynthesis of dihydromenaquinones by Gram-positive bacteria [Eq. (3)]. The nature of the terminal steps in the biosynthesis of phylloquinone are still far from clear.

1,4-Naphthoquinol → demethylmenaquinol → demethylmenaquinone   (1)

$$\overset{?}{}$$

1,4-Naphthoquinol → menadiol → menaquinol → menaquinone →
                                              dihydromenaquinone (2)

1,4-Naphthoquinol → demethylmenaquinol → menaquinol → menaquinone →
                                              dihydromenaquinone (3)

It is worth commenting on the fact that although the pathways outlined in Eqs. (2) and (3), for mechanistic reasons (Sections II,C, and II,B), have quinols as substrates for the 2-methylation and 3-prenylation reactions, all the researchers in this field persist in working with quinones.

2. In Gram-Negative Bacteria

The evidence that in Gram-negative bacteria the pathway from 1,4-naphthoquinol to menaquinone is as represented in Eq. (2) has come from a variety of sources. Thus, it has been shown that radioactivity from [Me-^{3}H]menadione and [Me-^{14}C]menadione is incorporated into menaquinones by *Bacteroides melaninogenicus* (Martius and Leuzinger, 1964), and the mutant *Klebsiella aerogenes* 170-44 (Guérin *et al.*, 1970) and that 1,4[1,4-^{3}H]naphthoquinone is converted into menadione before incorporation into menaquinone-9 by *Bacteroides melaninogenicus* (Martius and Leuzinger, 1964).

Against these observations must be set the facts that radioactivity from [*Me*-^{14}C]menadione is not incorporated into menaquinone-8 by *Escherichia coli* (Hurd, 1970) and that the dilution values for the incorporation of 1,4-[1-^{14}C]naphthoquinone, 1,4-[1,4,5,8-^{14}C]naphthoquinone and [*Me*-^{14}C]menadione into menaquinone-8 by the mutant *Klebsiella aerogenes* 170-44 suggest that in this organism menadione is not a true intermediate (Guérin *et al.*, 1970).

The last series of observations would seem to indicate that in *Escherichia coli* and *Klebsiella aerogenes* the pathway for the formation of menaquinone will be the same as the one outlined in Eq. (3). However, it has been found that the specific activities of demethylmenaquinones synthesized from [1-^{14}C]acetate in *Chlorobium thiosulphatophilum* and from DL-[1,6-^{14}C]shikimic acid in *Escherichia coli* are considerably lower than those of the corresponding menaquinones (Bartlett, 1968; Ellis and Glover, 1968), which suggests that demethylmenaquinols cannot be involved in menaquinone biosynthesis in Gram-negative bacteria.

3. *In Gram-Positive Bacteria*

In support of the proposal that menaquinones are produced by the pathway outlined in Eq. (2), it has been reported that radioactivity from [*Me*-^{14}C]menadione is incorporated into menaquinone-7 by *Bacillus megaterium* and menaquinone-8 by *Staphylococcus aureus* (Hammond and White, 1969b; Hurd, 1970), and that mutants of *Staphylococcus aureus* (SHLS2, 3 and 4) which are blocked after shikimate will produce menaquinones when the growth medium is supplemented with menadione (Sasarman *et al.*, 1969).

The evidence that in Gram-positive bacteria dihydromenaquinones are formed by the pathway outlined in Eq. (3) is based solely on the observations that cell-free preparations of *Mycobacterium phlei* are able to methylate added demethylmenaquinone-9 to form menaquinone-9, which is then reduced to menaquinone-9(II-H$_2$) when NADPH or NADH is added (Azerad *et al.*, 1967). It must be pointed out, however, that because of its reactive nature 1,4-naphthoquinone has never been tested in this system as a substrate for the transmethylase, and there is just an outside possibility that it (or more likely its quinol) is the true substrate. In which case the formation of dihydromenaquinones would proceed along the lines outlined in Eq. (2). Against this, however, must be set the observation that radioactivity from [*Me*-^{14}C]menadione is not incorporated into menaquinone-9(II-H$_2$) by *Mycobacterium phlei* (Hurd, 1970).

4. *In Plants*

Nothing is known about the final steps in the biosynthesis of phylloquinone, although it has been shown that radioactivity from $[Me\text{-}^{14}C]$-menadione is not incorporated into it by young maize shoots (R. A. Hall, 1970). The occurrence of demethylphylloquinone in spinach chloroplasts (McKenna et al., 1964) provides some evidence that phytylation precedes methylation. The stage at which the side chain is saturated is also not apparent (Section II,D,5).

F. INTRACELLULAR SITES OF SYNTHESIS

There is little information concerning the sites of synthesis of menaquinones. It is to be expected that in the Gram-positive and nonphotosynthetic Gram-negative bacteria the 1,4-naphthoquinol and menadiol nuclei will be synthesized in the soluble fraction of the cell. They will then pass to the membrane to be polyprenylated with the allylic group of a polyprenylpyrophosphate which has been synthesized either in the cytoplasm or in the cell membrane, methylated (if required), hydrogenated (if required), and sited in a membrane bound electron transport system. In the photosynthetic bacteria it is not unreasonable to suppose that the synthesis of menaquinones will take place entirely within the confines of the chromatophore.

In the case of higher plants there is a considerable body of evidence to suggest that in photosynthetic tissues the overall biosynthesis of phylloquinone takes place within the chloroplast (Section III,F).

III. THE VITAMINS E AND RELATED COMPOUNDS

The vitamin E group is made up of α-, β-, γ-, and δ-tocopherol (XI) and four corresponding unsaturated derivatives, α-, β-, γ-, and δ-tocotrienol (XII). The elucidation of the biosynthesis of these compounds

R₁	R₂	
H	H	δ−Tocopherol
CH₃	H	β−Tocopherol
H	CH₃	γ−Tocopherol
CH₃	CH₃	α−Tocopherol

R₁	R₂	
H	H	δ−Tocotrienol
CH₃	H	β−Tocotrienol
H	CH₃	γ−Tocotrienol
CH₃	CH₃	α−Tocotrienol

(XI)   (XII)

and their γ-hydroxyquinone derivatives, the tocopherolquinones and tocotrienolquinones, has gone hand in hand with studies on the biosynthesis of the chemically and biogenetically closely related plastoquinones and plastochromanols. The tocochromanols, tocoquinones, plastoquinones, and plastochromanols, in addition to their strong chemical and biogenetic links, have in common the fact that their biosynthesis is confined to higher plants, algae, and some fungi.

A. Distribution in Plants

1. Tocopherols, Tocotrienols, Tocopherolquinones, and Tocotrienolquinones (Tocochromanols and Tocoquinones)

Tocopherols (XI) are found in higher plants, in algae, and in some nonphotosynthetic plants, such as yeasts and mushrooms (see Green, 1970). The most widespread tocopherol is α-tocopherol, and this is to be found in the photosynthetic and nonphotosynthetic tissues of higher plants and in many green, brown, red, and blue-green algae (see Green, 1970; Lichtenthaler, 1968a). In the photosynthetic regions of higher plants, it is concentrated mainly in the lamellae and osmiophilic globules (when present) of the chloroplast (Bucke 1968; Lichtenthaler, 1969; Lichtenthaler and Tevini, 1970); in nonphotosynthetic tissues (excluding seed oils) it is probably associated in the main with various differentiations of plastids (Lichtenthaler, 1968b). There is evidence that in spinach (*Spinacea oleracea*) and lilac (*Syringa vulgaris*) leaves, maize shoots (*Zea mays*) and the alga *Euglena gracilis* some of it is associated with the mitochondria (Baszynski *et al.*, 1969; Dilley and Crane, 1963; Griffiths *et al.*, 1967). The non α-tocopherols, with the possible exception of γ-tocopherol, are not nearly as widespread (see Green, 1970). The leaves of higher plants often contain γ-tocopherol (Whistance and Threlfall, 1970d): in ivy (*Hedera helix*) and holly (*Taxus baccata*) it co-occurs with δ-tocopherol (Booth, 1963). It is also present in *Euglena gracilis* (Whistance and Threlfall, 1968b), but in the blue-green alga *Anabaena variabilis* it is replaced by β-tocopherol (Powls and Redfearn, 1967). The intracellular distribution of these tocopherols has not been clearly defined. Booth (1963), reported that in ivy and holly leaves, γ-, and δ-tocopherol are located outside the chloroplast, whereas Dada (1968) found that at least half of the γ-tocopherol is present in chloroplasts from ivy leaves. In nonphotosynthetic tissues the non α-tocopherols are more abundant, particularly in natural oils and fruits (see Green, 1970).

The tocopherolquinones (XIII) are the γ-hydroxyquinone derivatives of the tocopherols, from which they can easily be formed by oxidation with ferric chloride or gold chloride. α-Tocopherolquinone has been iso-

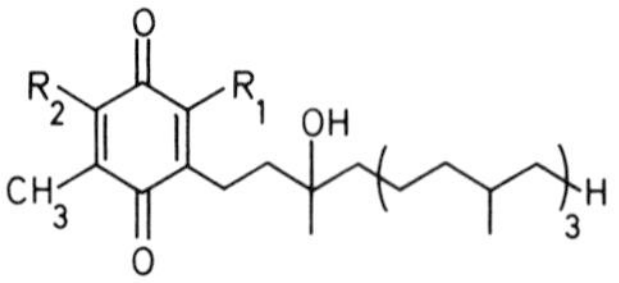

R_1	R_2	
H	H	δ−Tocopherolquinone
CH_3	H	β−Tocopherolquinone
H	CH_3	γ−Tocopherolquinone
CH_3	CH_3	α−Tocopherolquinone

(XIII)

lated from the photosynthetic and nonphotosynthetic regions of higher plants and from many algae (Lichtenthaler, 1968a); however, so far, β-, γ-, and δ-tocopherolquinone have been isolated only from the leaves of a few higher plants (Barr and Arntzen, 1969; Henninger et al., 1963). In higher plants they are concentrated in the lamellae and osmiophilic globules of the chloroplast of green tissue and the leucoplasts, chromoplasts, and etioplasts of nonphotosynthetic tissue (Dilley and Crane, 1963; Barr and Arntzen, 1969; Lichtenthaler, 1968b, 1969; Lichtenthaler and Trevini, 1970).

Tocotrienols (XII) are of limited distribution, and are to be found mainly in seed germ oils (Green, 1958; Pennock et al., 1964). Appreciable amounts of α-, β-, γ- and δ-tocotrienol together with esterified α-, γ- and δ-tocotrienol and α-tocotrienolquinone (XIV), the only tocotrienol-

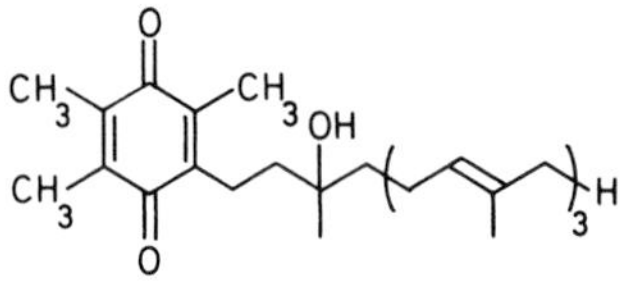

(XIV)

quinone known to occur naturally, are present in the latex of *Hevea brasiliensis* (Dunphy et al., 1965; Whittle et al., 1967).

2. Plastoquinones and Plastochromanols

Plastoquinones are found only in higher plants and algae. The most widely distributed plastoquinones are plastoquinone-9 (XV, $n = 9$), the plastoquinones-B (XVI) and the plastoquinones-C (XVII), and these are to be found in all higher plant and algal species examined (see Barr

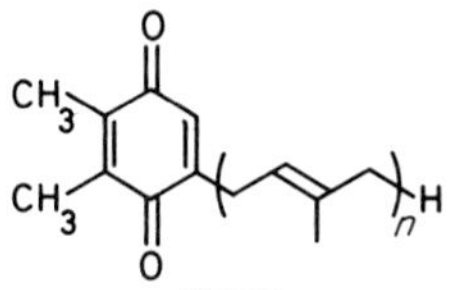

(XV)

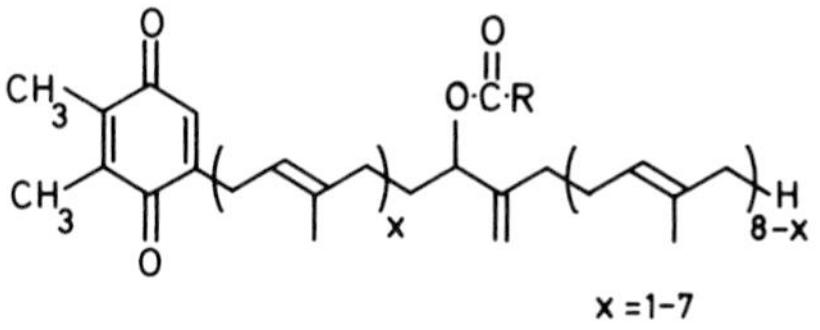

$$CH_3$$

x = 1-7

(XVI)

OH

OH

x = 1-7

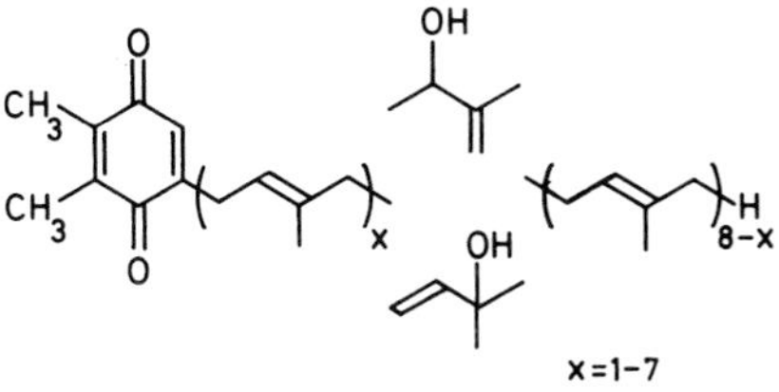

(XVII)

and Crane, 1967; Lichtenthaler, 1968a; Pennock, 1966; Sun *et al.*, 1968). Plastoquinones-Z (monohydroxylated plastoquinones-B) are not nearly so widespread, being confined in the main to higher plants (Wallwork and Pennock, 1968). The only homologs of the above compounds to be isolated are: plastoquinone-8 (XV, $n = 8$) from horse chestnut leaves (*Aesculus hippocastanum*), maize shoots and *Euglena gracilis* (Whistance and Threlfall, 1970c); plastoquinone-4 (XV, $n = 4$) from horse chestnut leaves (Eck and Trebst, 1963); plastoquinone-3 (XV, $n = 3$) from spinach chloroplasts (Misiti *et al.*, 1965); and phytylplastoquinone (XVIII), from strains of *Euglena gracilis* and *Tribonema* (Whistance and Threlfall, 1970b). An interesting metabolite of phytylplastoquinone, phytylplastohydroquinone monomethyl ether (XIX) has been isolated from *Euglena gracilis* (Whistance and Threlfall, 1970b). The intertissue, intracellular, and intraorganelle distribution of the plastoquinones is

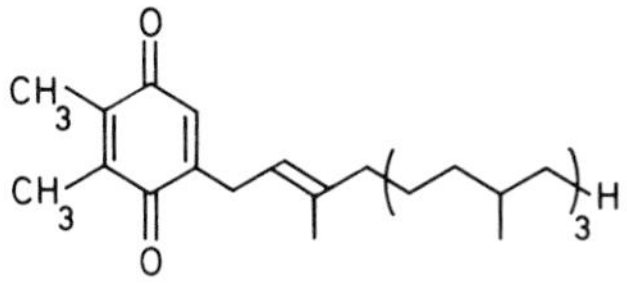

(XVIII)

(XIX)

similar to that of phylloquinone and the tocopherolquinones (Sections II,A,1 and III,A,1) (see Barr *et al.*, 1967; Lichtenthaler, 1968a,b, 1969; Lichtenthaler and Trevini, 1970; Pennock, 1966; Threlfall and Goodwin, 1967).

Cyclic derivatives of plastoquinone-9 and the plastoquinones-B, -C and -Z known as plastochromanols have been isolated from the leaves of higher plants. Plastochromanol-8 (the chromanol of plastoquinone-9) (XX) has been isolated from many plant species; and in Japanese knot-

(XX)

weed (*Polygonum cupsidatum*) it has been shown to be localized in the chloroplasts (Dunphy *et al.*, 1966). Plastochromanols-B, -C, and -Z have so far only been reported to occur in privet leaves (*Lingustrum vulgare*) and Japanese knotweed (Dunphy *et al.*, 1969; Peake *et al.*, 1970b). The chromanol forms of plastoquinone-4 and phytylplastoquinone, γ-toco-trienol and γ-tocopherol, respectively, have been dealt with already (Section III,B,1).

B. BIOSYNTHESIS OF THE AROMATIC AND BENZOQUINONE NUCLEI

It is now clear that the aromatic nuclei of tocochromanols and plasto-chromanols and the *p*-benzoquinone nuclei of tocoquinones and plasto-quinones are formed by the same, though not necessarily common, path-way. The details of this pathway have come mainly from studies on the incorporation of radioactivity from various uniformly and specifically labeled aromatic compounds into phylloquinone, plastoquinone-9, α- and γ-tocopherol, α-tocopherolquinone, ubiquinone-9, β-carotene, and 4-demethylsterols by excised 7-day-old etiolated (dark grown) maize shoots kept under constant illumination for periods of up to 24 hours. This system was used because (a) young seedlings are metabolically very active and (b) it was hoped that the marked incremental synthesis of phylloquinone, plastoquinone-9, and α-tocopherolquinone which takes place on illumination of etiolated maize shoots (Griffiths *et al.*, 1964, 1967) would lead to an enhanced incorporation of radioactivity into these compounds.

1. *Involvement of the Shikimic Acid Pathway*

The first information on the biosynthetic origins of the aromatic and *p*-benzoquinone nuclei of the compounds under consideration came from investigations designed to elucidate the nature of the pathway involved in the formation of the *p*-benzoquinone nucleus of ubiquinone (XXI). It

(XXI)

had been reported that radioactivity from *p*-hydroxy[U-^{14}C]benzoic acid is incorporated into ubiquinone-9 (XXI, $n = 9$), but not into plastoquinone-9 or tocopherols, by maize shoots (Threlfall and Griffiths, 1967) and by *Euglena gracilis* (Powls and Hemming, 1966). In higher plants *p*-hydroxybenzoic acid can be formed from shikimic acid by pathways involving the aromatic amino acids phenylalanine and tyrosine (Neish, 1964) (Fig. 11), and it was while the importance of these pathways in the biosynthesis of ubiquinone-9 by maize shoots was being investigated that it was found that radioactivity from DL-[G-^{14}C]-shikimic acid, L-[U-^{14}C]phenylalanine and L-[U-^{14}C]tyrosine (but not *p*-hydroxy[U-^{14}C]benzoic acid) is incorporated into plastoquinone-9, α- and γ-tocopherol, and α-tocopherolquinone (Whistance *et al.*, 1966b, 1967). Partial chemical degradations of the [^{14}C]plastoquinones-9 and comparisons of the specific radioactivities of the α- and γ-tocopherols and α-tocopherolquinones with those of the β-carotenes and 4-demethylsterols established that the radioactivity had been incorporated into the quinone nuclei of the *p*-benzoquinones and the aromatic nuclei of the chromanols. (The specific radioactivities of β-carotene and 4-demethylsterols provide a measure of the degree of breakdown of the radiosubstrates to give metabolites which can be utilized in the formation of polyprenyl groups and methionine-derived methyl groups.) These results were interpreted as showing that in higher plants the aromatic nuclei of the tocochromanols (and plastochromanols) and the *p*-benzoquinone nuclei of the tocopherolquinones and plastoquinones are formed from the tyrosine branch of the shikimic acid pathway of aromatic biosynthesis (Fig. 11).

In higher plants the compound on the tyrosine pathway which is required for the biosynthesis of tocochromanols, plastochromanols, tocoquinones, and plastoquinones is p-hydroxyphenylpyruvate (Fig. 11). The evidence for this is based on (a) isotope competition experiments (Whistance and Threlfall, 1968b) and (b) the demonstration that p-hydroxy-[U-^{14}C]phenylpyruvic acid is a better precursor than L-[U-^{14}C]tyrosine of the aromatic rings of α- and γ-tocopherol and the p-benzoquinone rings of plastoquinone-9 and α-tocopherolquinone in maize shoots (Whistance et al., 1967; Whistance and Threlfall, 1970a).

In algae the involvement of the shikimic acid pathway in the biosynthesis of plastoquinones, tocopherols (tocotrienols are not found in algae), and tocopherolquinones has still to be demonstrated. However, from what little is known about the formation of aromatic and p-benzoquinone nuclei by algae (Section III,B,3), it would appear that as in

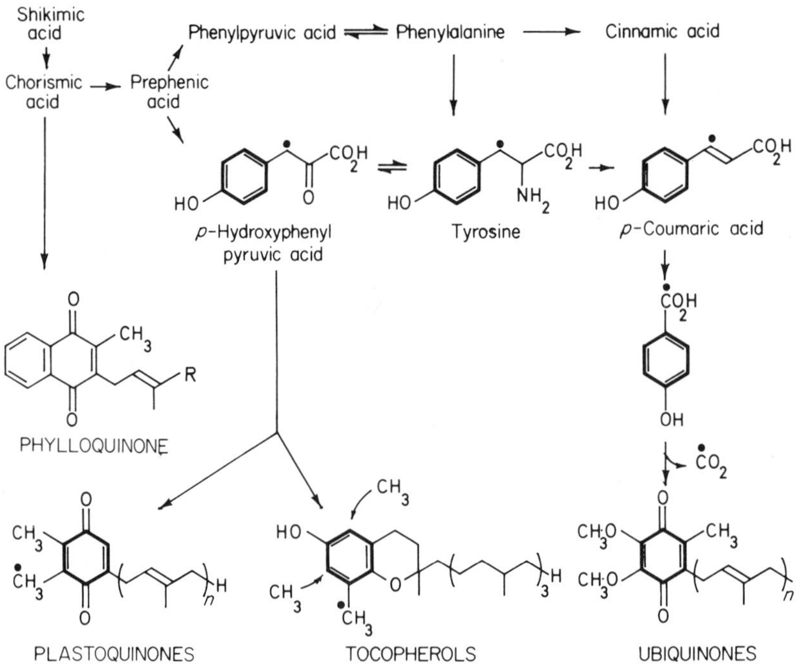

FIG. 11. Involvement of the shikimic acid pathway of aromatic biosynthesis in the biosynthesis of isoprenoid quinones and chromanols by higher plants. After Whistance and Threlfall (1967).

higher plants it will be required for the production of p-hydroxyphenyl-pyruvate.

2. Manner of Incorporation of Shikimic Acid

Whistance and Threlfall (1971) investigated the patterns of incorporation of radioactivity from DL-[1,6-^{14}C]shikimic acid into quinones and chromanols by maize shoots. The results of their investigation showed that C-1, C-2 and -6, C-3 and -5, and C-4 of shikimic acid give rise to C-4, C-3 and -5, C-2 and -6, and C-1 in plastoquinone-9 (2,3-dimethyl-5-solanesyl-1,4-benzoquinone) and C-1, C-2 and -6, C-3 and -5, and C-4 in α-tocopherolquinone (2,3,5-trimethyl-6-monohydroxy-phytyl-1,4-benzoquinone), and C-9, C-8 and -10, C-5 and -7, and C-6 in α- and γ-tocopherol [see (XI) for tocopherol numbering]. These findings show that on the pathway for the biosynthesis of these compounds there is (a) at least one intermediate (p-hydroxyphenylpyruvate) with an aromatic ring which is symmetrical with respect to C-2 and -6 and C-3 and -5 and (b) no symmetrical 1,4-dihydroxy intermediate, i.e., the 4-hydroxyl group of p-hydroxyphenylpyruvate gives rise to the carbonyl group of the p-benzoquinones which is *meta* to the polyprenyl group and to the hydroxyl group of the chromanols (Fig. 11).

3. The Early Steps on the Pathway from p-Hydroxyphenylpyruvate

The rapid elucidation of the first intermediate on the pathway from p-hydroxyphenylpyruvate was due to a somewhat fortuitous sequence of events. Thus, Threlfall et al. (1967a, 1968), following their studies on the incorporation of shikimic acid and the aromatic amino acids into plastoquinone-9, tocopherols, and α-tocopherolquinone by maize shoots, chose to investigate the incorporation of L-[Me-^{14}C,^{3}H]methionine into these compounds and found that in each case one of the nuclear C-methyl groups is not derived from the S-methyl group of L-methionine. The most likely source of this methyl group appeared to be the β-carbon atom of one of the C_6–C_3 compounds on the tyrosine branch of the shikimic acid pathway. This was soon confirmed by partial chemical degradation of radioactive plastoquinone-9, α- and γ-tocopherol, and α-tocopherol-quinone isolated from maize shoots which had been incubated with either DL-[β-^{14}C]tyrosine or DL-[β-^{14}C]phenylalanine (Whistance and Threl-fall, 1967, 1968b). Further experiments with DL-[$ring$-^{14}C]phenylalanine, DL-[α-^{14}C]tyrosine and L-[U-^{14}C]tyrosine established beyond doubt that the aromatic ring carbon atoms and β-carbon atoms of tyrosine (and phenylalanine) are incorporated as a C_6–C_1 unit into plastoquinone-9, α- and γ-tocopherol, and α-tocopherolquinone (Whistance and Threlfall,

1968b) (Fig. 11). Similar findings were obtained for the incorporation of L-[U-^{14}C]tyrosine and DL-[β-^{14}C]tyrosine into plastoquinone-9, tocopherols, and α-tocopherolquinone by ivy leaves (*Hedera helix*) and French bean shoots (*Phaseolus vulgaris*) (Whistance and Threlfall, 1968b). In the experiments with ivy leaves (a tissue which contains appreciable amounts of δ-tocopherol), it was shown that the 8-methyl group of δ-tocopherol is labeled from DL-[β-^{14}C]tyrosine, but not from L-[Me-^{14}C]methionine. In other experiments with *Euglena gracilis*, however, the contribution made by the various carbon atoms of tyrosine to the nuclei of the quinones and chromanols could not be determined because so much radioactivity was incorporated into the polyprenyl groups.

To explain the incorporation of the β-carbon atom of tyrosine (and phenylalanine) into plastoquinone-9, tocopherols, and α-tocopherolquinone, it was postulated that one of the biosynthetic steps in their formation is an intramolecular rearrangement of p-hydroxyphenylpyruvate (the true intermediate, see Section III,B,1) (Whistance and Threlfall, 1967). This postulate, when considered in conjunction with the knowledge that shikimic acid is a distal precursor of the nuclei of plastoquinone-9, tocopherols, and α-tocopherolquinone (Section III,B,1) and with reports of the occurrence in plants of homogentisic acid (Bertel, 1903), homogentisic acid glucoside (Matsumura and Shibata, 1964), and homoarbutin (Inoue et al., 1958), led to the proposal that tocochromanols, plastochromanols, tocoquinones, and plastoquinones might be synthesized by the pathway shown in Fig. 12. The alternative possibility that the C_6-C_1 unit could be formed from the C_6-C_3 acrylic acids (p-coumaric acid and cinnamic acid) produced by nonoxidative deamination of tyrosine and phenylalanine was discounted on the grounds that radioactivity from [β-^{14}C]cinnamic acid is not incorporated into these compounds by maize shoots (Whistance and Threlfall, 1967).

The involvement of homogentisate in the biosynthesis of plastoquinone-9, α- and γ-tocopherol, and α-tocopherolquinone by maize shoots was established in the first place by isotope competition experiments (Whistance and Threlfall, 1968b) and then later confirmed by tracer experiments using [U-^{14}C]homogentisic acid and [α-^{14}C]homogentisic acid (Whistance and Threlfall, 1968a, 1970a). In the latter experiments it was established that the aromatic carbon atoms and α-carbon atom of homogentisic acid are incorporated in the expected manner i.e., as a C_6–C_1 unit (Fig. 12). It was also shown in these studies that radioactivity from [U-^{14}C]homogentisic acid is incorporated in the expected manner into plastoquinones, tocopherols, and tocopherolquinones present in lettuce leaves (*Lactuca sativa*) (plastoquinone-9, α- and γ-tocopherol, and

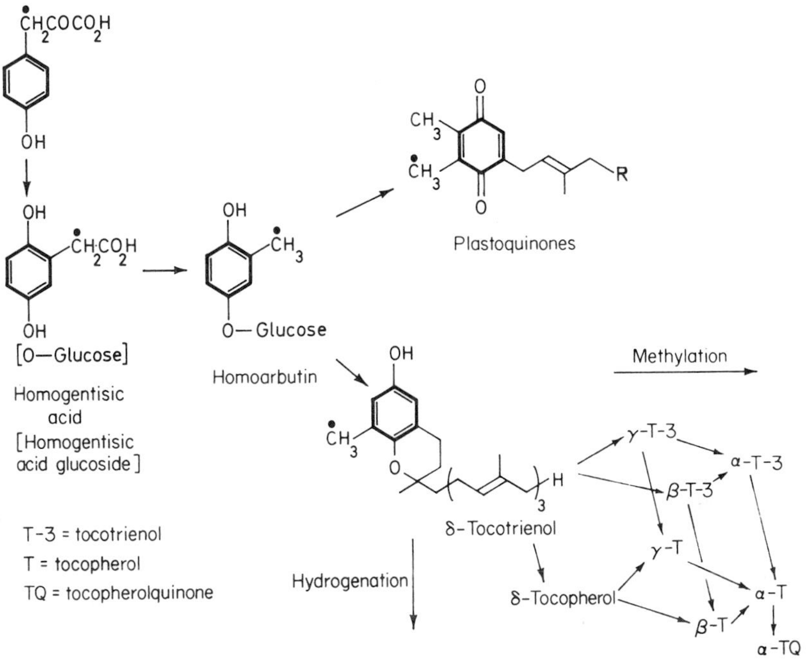

Fig. 12. Proposed pathways for the biosynthesis of plastoquinones, tocochromanols, and tocopherolquinones from p-hydroxyphenylpyruvate. After Whistance and Threlfall (1967).

α-tocopherolquinone), red-veined dock leaves (*Rumex sanguineus*) (plastoquinone-9 and α- and γ-tocopherol), the green algae *Euglena gracilis* (plastoquinone-9 and -8, phytylplastoquinone, and α-tocopherol) and *Chlorella pyrenoidosa* (plastoquinone-9 and α-tocopherol), and the blue-green alga *Anacystis nidulans* (plastoquinone-9) (Whistance and Threlfall, 1970a). More recently it has been reported that radioactivity from [U-^{14}C]homogentisic acid and p-hydroxy[U-^{14}C]phenylpyruvic acid is incorporated into α-, γ-, and δ-tocopherol by rubber plant leaves (*Hevea brasiliensis*) and α-, γ-, and δ-tocotrienol and α-tocopherol by *Hevea* latex (Peake *et al.*, 1970a).

It is almost certain that in higher plants homogentisate is formed from p-hydroxyphenylpyruvate. The evidence for this is that (a) homogentisic acid markedly reduces the incorporation of radioactivity from p-hydroxy[U-^{14}C]phenylpyruvic acid into plastoquinone-9, tocopherols, and α-tocopherolquinone by maize shoots (Whistance and Threlfall, 1970a) and (b) radioactivity from [α-^{14}C]- and [U-^{14}C]homogentisic acid is incorporated far more effectively than from p-hydroxy[β-^{14}C]-

and p-hydroxy[U-^{14}C]phenylpyruvic acid into plastoquinone-9, tocopherols, and α-tocopherolquinone by maize shoots (Whistance and Threlfall, 1970a). The possibility that some homogentisate is formed by o- and m-hydroxylation of phenylacetate, is ruled out by the demonstration that radioactivity from [U-^{14}C]phenylacetate is not incorporated into quinones and chromanols by maize shoots (Whistance and Threlfall, 1970a). The mechanism of the conversion of p-hydroxyphenylpyruvate to homogentisate has still to be elucidated. Although in view of the finding that radioactivity from p-hydroxy[U-^{14}C]phenylacetic acid is not incorporated into plastoquinone-9, tocopherols, and α-tocopherolquinone by maize shoots (Whistance and Threlfall, 1970a), it would seem highly probable that, as proposed by Whistance and Threlfall (1967, 1968b), it will be a concerted reaction involving the utilization of 1 mole of O_2, hydroxylation of the aromatic ring, shift of the side chain, and the formation of CO_2, i.e., similar to the reaction in animals (see Meister, 1965). Support for the side chain shift is provided by the observation that radioactivity from DL-[1,6-^{14}C]shikimic acid is incorporated in the predicted manner into the p-benzoquinone nuclei of plastoquinone-9 and α-tocopherolquinone and the aromatic nuclei of α- and γ-tocopherol by maize shoots (Whistance and Threlfall, 1971). This study also provided conclusive evidence that in these compounds the α-carbon atom of homogentisate gives rise to the methyl groups which are *meta* to the polyprenyl groups, a belief which has been held since the demonstration that the 8-methyl group of δ-tocopherol in ivy can arise from the β-carbon atom of tyrosine (Whistance and Threlfall, 1967) and that the 8-methyl group of δ-tocotrienol in *Hevea* latex is not derived from the S-methyl group of L-methionine (Whittle et al., 1967).

The details of the pathways leading from homogentisate to the tocochromanols, tocoquinones, plastochromanols, and plastoquinones have still to be elucidated. Whistance and Threlfall (1967), on comparative phytochemical grounds, proposed that homogentisate (possibly as its glucoside) is converted into homoarbutin (2-methylquinol-4-β-D-glucoside) (Fig. 12): however, isotope competition experiments have provided evidence that homarbutin and such plausible intermediates as the C_6-C_1 compounds gentisic acid (XXII), gentisaldehyde (XXIII), and gentisylalcohol (XXIV) and their glucosides are not involved (Whistance and Threlfall, 1968b, 1970a, 1970d). Furthermore, it has been shown that radioactivity from [Me-^{14}C]toluquinol (the aglycone of homoarbutin) is not incorporated into plastoquinone-9, tocopherols, and α-tocopherolquinone by maize shoots (Whistance and Threlfall, 1968b). The interpretation which must be placed on these results is that there are no simple C_6-C_1 compounds or glucosides of C_6-C_1 compounds involved in

OH   OH   OH

(structures showing benzene rings with $-CO_2H$, $-CHO$, and $-CH_2OH$ substituents and OH groups)

(XXII)   (XXIII)   (XXIV)

the formation of tocochromanols, tocoquinones, plastochromanols, and plastoquinones.

C. Sources of the Nuclear C-Methyl Groups

1. The Sources of the Methyl Groups

The α-carbon atom of homogentisate is the source of the 8-methyl groups of δ-tocochromanols, the methyl groups of δ-tocoquinones and one of the nuclear methyl groups of each member of the following groups of compounds: plastoquinones, α-, β-, and γ-tocochromanols and α-, β- and γ-tocoquinones (Section III,B,3). In maize shoots the α-carbon has been shown to form the 3-methyl group of plastoquinone-9, the 2-methyl group of α-tocopherolquinone, and the 8-methyl groups of α- and γ-tocopherol (Section III,B,3). Although the pattern of its incorporation into other plastoquinones, tocochromanols, and tocoquinones has still to be determined, it is to be expected that in these also it will give rise to the 3-methyl groups of the dimethyl p-benzoquinones, the 2-methyl groups of the trimethyl p-benzoquinones and the 8-methyl groups of the chromanols.

The S-methyl group of L-methionine gives rise to the remaining methyl groups. It has been shown that radioactivity from L-[Me-^{14}C]methionine is incorporated into the nuclear methyl groups of plastoquinone-9, plasto-quinone-8 (shown for *Euglena gracilis*), phytylplastoquinone (shown for *Euglena gracilis*), α- and γ-tocopherol and α-tocopherolquinone by maize shoots (Threlfall *et al.*, 1968), ivy leaves (Whistance and Threl-fall, 1968b) and *Euglena gracilis* (Gullis, 1971; Whistance and Threlfall, 1970d), and into α-, β-, and γ-tocochromanols and α-tocotrienolquinone (shown for *Hevea* latex) by *Hevea* latex (Whittle *et al.*, 1967) and latex-containing leaves of decorative rubber (Wellburn, 1970).

2. The Mechanism of C-Methylation

An experiment with L-[Me-^{14}C,^{3}H]methionine has shown that the 2-methyl group of plastoquinone-9, the 7-methyl group of γ-tocopherol, the 7- and 8-methyl groups of α-tocopherol, and the 3- and 5-methyl groups of α-tocopherolquinone in maize shoots are formed by transmethylation (Threlfall *et al.*, 1968). It is to be expected that the mechanism of methylation will be the same as the one proposed for the 2-methylation of the naphthoquinol nucleus in vitamin K biosynthesis (Section II,C,2). Some support for the involvement of the electrophile *S*-adenosyl-L-methionine in this reaction is provided by the report that an increased synthesis of α-tocopherol can be obtained by supplementing 2-day-old pea seedlings with methionine in the presence of ATP (Bazynski, 1961).

3. *β-, γ-, and δ-Tocochromanols as Substrates for the Methyltransferases Involved in α-Tocopherol Biosynthesis*

There is some evidence that β-, γ-, and δ-tocochromanols are the substrates for the methyltransferases involved in the biosynthesis of α-tocopherol.

In the first investigations the changes in the amounts and composition of the tocopherols and tocotrienols which take place during seed germination were followed. The results obtained suggested that, depending on the seeds examined, α-tocopherol is formed by methylation and, if required, hydrogenation of stored β- and γ-tocochromanols (barley), β-tocochromanols (wheat), γ-tocochromanols (maize), or γ- and δ-tocopherol (pea) (Bazynski, 1961; Green, 1958). However, in a recent study using wheat seeds, G. S. Hall and Laidman (1968), on the basis of balance experiments and the observation that injected β-tocotrienol did not influence the rate of α-tocopherol synthesis, concluded that the methylation of β- and γ-tocochromanols are not important reactions in the biosynthesis of α-tocopherol during seed germination.

Studies in which the incorporation of radioactivity from L-[*Me*-^{14}C] methionine, [U-^{14}C]homogentisic acid, and *p*-hydroxy[U-^{14}C]phenylpyruvic acid into the tocochromanols by *Hevea* latex was examined have provided some evidence that in this exudate δ- and γ-tocotrienol are the substrates for the transmethylases involved in the biosynthesis of α-tocopherol; i.e., the biosynthetic sequence is

δ-Tocotrienol → γ-tocotrienol → α-tocotrienol → α-tocopherol

(Peake *et al.*, 1970a; Whittle *et al.*, 1967).

Further support for these proposals is provided by the observations that (a) the administration of δ-tocotrienol to latex-containing leaves of decorative rubber (*Ficus elastica*) leads to an appearance of α-, β-, and γ-tocotrienol (the levels of α-, β-, γ-, and δ-tocopherol are unaffected)

and (b) radioactivity from L[*Me*-^{14}C]methionine is only incorporated into α-, β- and γ-tocotrienols and tocopherols in the presence of exogenous δ-tocotrienol (Wellburn, 1970).

Radiochemical incorporation studies have suggested that γ-tocopherol is a precursor of α-tocopherol in maize shoots, French bean shoots, ivy leaves, red-veined dock leaves, and rubber leaves (Dada *et al.*, 1968; Peake *et al.*, 1970a; Threlfall *et al.*, 1968; Whistance and Threlfall, 1968b, 1970a), but that δ-tocopherol is not a precursor of γ-tocopherol in ivy leaves or rubber leaves (Peake *et al.*, 1970a; Whistance and Threlfall, 1968b). These results, however, must be treated with caution until the exact intracellular distribution of δ- and γ-tocopherol and, possibly even α-tocopherol, is known with certainty (Section III,A,1), since it is possible that within the photosynthetic plant cell there is more than one tocopherol-synthesizing site (Section III,F).

D. FORMATION OF THE POLYPRENYL GROUPS

The biosynthesis of the polyprenyl groups of plastoquinones, tocopherolquinones, and tocotrienolquinones and the polyprenyl portions (C-2, -3, and -4 of the chroman ring and the 2-alkyl substituent) of plastochromanols, tocopherols, and tocotrienols is believed to be similar in many respects to that of the 2-polyprenyl groups of menaquinones and phylloquinones (Section II,D).

It has been shown that DL-[2-^{14}C]mevalonic acid is a precursor of the polyprenyl portions of plastoquinone-9, plastoquinones-C, α-tocopherol, γ-tocopherol, and α-tocopherolquinone in maize shoots, barley shoots, and tobacco leaves (Dada *et al.*, 1968; Griffiths *et al.*, 1968; Threlfall *et al.*, 1967b): however, its involvement in the biosynthesis of plastoquinone-8, -4, and -3, plastoquinones-B and -Z, plastochromanols, β- and δ-tocopherol, β-, γ-, and δ-tocopherolquinones, tocotrienols, and α-tocotrienolquinone has still to be demonstrated. In algae all attempts to show the incorporation of this compound into isoprenoid quinones and chromanols have so far failed (Threlfall and Goodwin, 1967). As in the case of bacterial menaquinones, this failure is attributed to the inability of the acid to reach the centers of terpenoid biosynthesis (Section II,D,2).

Indirect evidence that the polyprenyl groups are synthesized independently of the nuclei as all-*trans*-polyprenylpyrophosphates has been obtained from the facts that solanesol (all-*trans*-nonaprenol) is found with plastoquinone-9 in tobacco chloroplasts (Stevenson *et al.*, 1963) and that all-*trans*-geranylgeranylpyrophosphate can be formed by preparations from tocopherol- and tocopherolquinone-containing higher plant tissues and intracellular organelles (Section II,D,3).

The stereochemistry of the biosynthesis of the polyprenyl portions of plastoquinone-9, α-tocopherol, γ-tocopherol, and α-tocopherolquinone by maize shoots has been investigated using (3RS)-[2-^{14}C,(4R)-4-^{3}H$_1$]-mevalonic acid and (3RS)-[2-^{14}C,(4S)-4-^{3}H$_1$]mevalonic acid (Dada et al., 1968). The results obtained showed that each isoprene unit of the polyprenyl portions of these compounds is biogenetically trans. A finding which provides good evidence that the octahydrotetraprenyl groups of tocopherols and tocopherolquinones are formed from all-trans-geranylgeranylpyrophosphate.

The mechanism of the hydrogenation of the tetraprenyl group has been examined by Wellburn (1968, 1970), who found that radioactivity from 4R[4-^{3}H$_1$]NADPH (but not 4S[4-^{3}H$_1$]NADPH) is incorporated into α-tocopherol by seedlings of French bean and oat (Avena sativa) and into α-, β-, γ-, and δ-tocopherol by latex-containing leaves of the

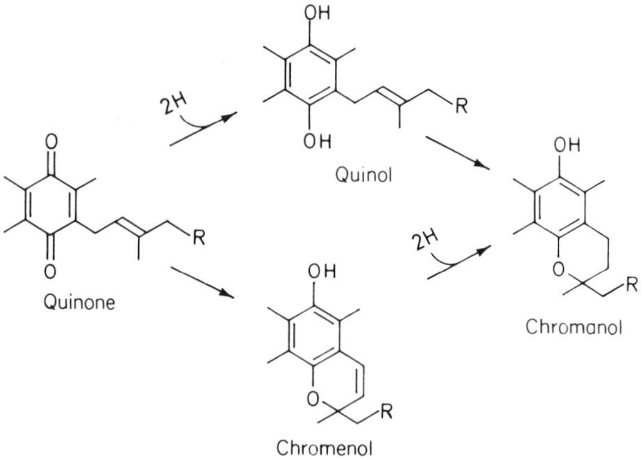

Fig. 13. Possible pathways for the formation of a chromanol ring.

decorative rubber plant, indicating the involvement of either an NADPH-dependent reductase capable of hydrogenating all the double bonds in the tetraprenyl group or several NADPH-dependent reductases each of which is specific for a given double bond. In this connection, it is worth pointing out that if the chromanol ring is formed from a tetraprenyl- or phytylbenzoquinol then the 2',3'-double bond will not need to be reduced by an NADPH-dependent reductase, since it will be saturated in the course of the cyclization reaction (Fig. 13). However, if it is formed via a chromenol from tetraprenyl- or phytylbenzoquinone, then a reductase will be required to hydrogenate the 3,4-double bond of the chromenol (Fig. 13).

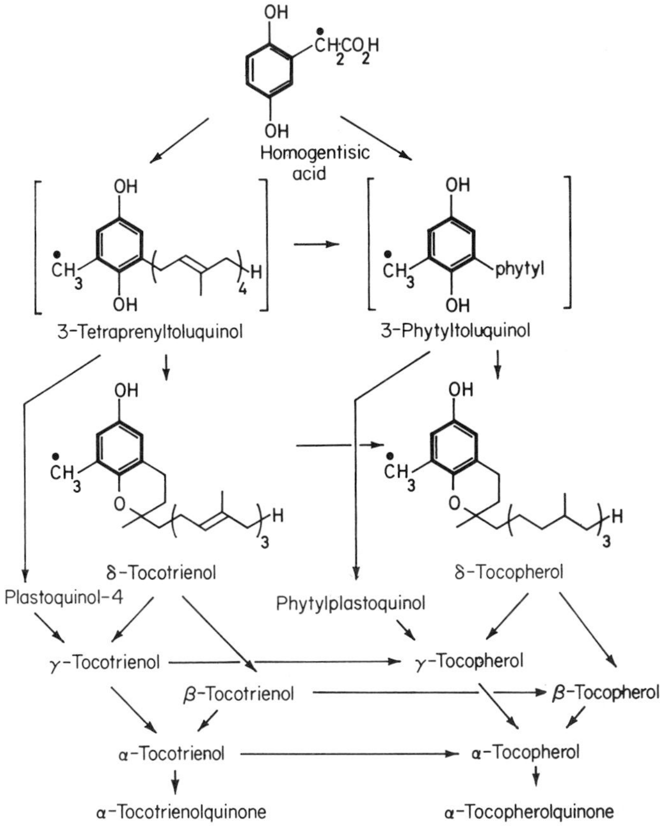

Fig. 14. Possible pathways for the biosynthesis of tocochromanols and toco-quinones from homogentisate.

E. Pathways from Homogentisic Acid

1. Tocochromanols and Tocoquinones

The details of the pathway leading from homogentisate to the toco-chromanols and tocoquinones have still to be worked out. It is almost certain, however, that C_6–C_1 compounds such as gentisic acid, gentisalde-hyde, gentisyl alcohol, and toluquinol or their glucosides are not involved (Section III,B,3). The simplest explanation that can be invoked to account for the noninvolvement of these compounds is that the first step on the pathway is the concomitant tetraprenylation and decarboxylation of homogentisate to form 3-tetraprenyltoluquinol (Fig. 14). Cyclization of 3-tetraprenyltoluquinol would give δ-tocotrienol, a compound that can be regarded as the parent member of both the tocotrienol and tocopherol series. Thus, the tocochromanols can be arranged to form a metabolic grid providing six alternative pathways of hydrogenation and methylation for the formation of α-tocopherol from δ-tocotrienol (Fig. 14). An alternative possibility is that methylation and, in the case of tocopherol biosynthesis, hydrogenation could precede cyclization, as it would if plastoquinone-4 and phytylplastoquinone were precursors of γ-tocotrienol and γ-tocopherol, respectively (Fig. 14). Again, in the case of tocopherol biosynthesis it may be that phytylation rather than tetraprenylation of homogentisate takes place to form 3-phytyltoluquinol (Fig. 14).

In all the proposals outlined above it is assumed that in the formation of dimethyl and trimethyl tocochromanols from homogentisate, prenylation will take place before methylation. It is possible, however, that methylation could take place before prenylation. If this is the case, then the sequence of reactions must be of such a nature that the assymetry of the aromatic nucleus with respect to the carbon atoms carrying oxygen functions is preserved (Section III,B,2), i.e., the sequential or concomitant methylation and decarboxylation of homogentisate to form 2,3-dimethylquinol is excluded.

At the experimental level the investigations carried out so far have been concerned solely with the possibility that dimethyl and trimethyl tocochromanols are formed by the methylation and, if necessary, hydrogenation of monomethyl and dimethyl tocochromanols, respectively. In 1964 Pennock et al. suggested the final stages in α-tocopherol biosynthesis involved the methylation of δ-tocotrienol to β-tocotrienol or γ-tocotrienol, further methylation to α-tocotrienol, followed by hydrogenation to α-tocopherol; other tocopherols are formed by the hydrogenation of the corresponding tocotrienols. Biogenetic studies with Hevea latex and latex-containing leaves of decorative rubber, two systems that contain tocotrienols, have provided results which are consistent with the pathway:

δ-Tocotrienol → γ-tocotrienol → α-tocotrienol → α-tocopherol

(Section III,B,3). However, similar studies with maize shoots, French bean shoots, red-veined dock leaves, ivy leaves and rubber leaves, tissues which do not contain tocotrienols, have provided some evidence that γ-tocopherol is a precursor of α-tocopherol, but that δ-tocopherol is not a precursor of γ-tocopherol or α-tocopherol (Section III,B,3).

Tocotrienolquinones and tocopherolquinones are probably formed by the oxidation of the corresponding tocochromanols. Specific radioactivity data from biogenetic studies with a variety of radioactive substrates has indicated that in maize shoots, French bean shoots, and ivy leaves α-tocopherol and α-tocopherolquinone are in equilibrium (Dada *et al.*, 1968; Threlfall *et al.*, 1968; Whistance and Threlfall, 1970a).

2. *Plastoquinones and Plastochromanols*

As in the case of the tocochromanols and tocoquinones, it appears that no C_6–C_1 compounds or their glucosides are involved in the formation of plastoquinones and plastochromanols from homogentisate (Section III,B,3). It is tempting to propose that the first step on this pathway also is the concomitant polyprenylation and decarboxylation of homogentisate to form 3-all-*trans*-polyprenyltoluquinol (Fig. 15). Methylation and oxidation of 3-nonaprenyl-, 3-octaprenyl-, 3-tetraprenyl-, and 3-triprenyltoluquinol could give plastoquinone-9, -8, -4, and -3, respectively (Fig. 15). Plastoquinone-9 could then be converted into plastoquinones-B, -C, and -Z by the pathways proposed by Wallwork and Pennock (Fig. 15). Some evidence to support the view that plastoquinone-9 is a precursor of plastoquinones-B, -C and -Z is the fact that in ^{14}C-tracer experiments with higher plants plastoquinones-B, -C, and -Z have always been found to have specific activities appreciably lower than those of plastoquinone-9 (Griffiths *et al.*, 1968; Whistance and Threlfall, 1968b, 1970d). Plastochromanol-8 can be seen as arising from 3-nonaprenyltoluquinol (Fig. 15); however, biogenetic studies with ^{14}C]homogentisic acid have provided some evidence that it is probably formed by cyclization of plastoquinol-9 (Whistance and Threlfall, 1970d). The other types of plastochromanols could be formed from either plastochromanol-8 by reactions similar to those involved in the formation of plastoquinones-B, -C, and Z or by cyclization of the appropriate·plastoquinols (Fig. 15).

F. INTRACELLULAR SITES OF SYNTHESIS

Investigations have been carried out to determine the intracellular sites of synthesis of the isoprenoid quinones and chromanols found in photosynthetic cells. In the early 1960's it was becoming increasingly apparent that chloroplasts have a high degree of biochemical autonomy, and that they very probably carried out the complete synthesis of many of their components. It was not surprising, therefore, that Goodwin and Mercer (1963) should propose that there are two sites for the biosynthesis of terpenoids in the photosynthetic plant cell, an intrachloroplastidic site responsible for the synthesis of carotenoids and the polyprenyl groups of chlorophylls, phylloquinone, plastoquinones, tocopherols, and tocopherolquinones, and an extrachloroplastidic site where 4-demethylsterols, pentacyclic triterpenes, and the polyprenyl groups of ubiquinones are synthesized. These proposals were later extended by

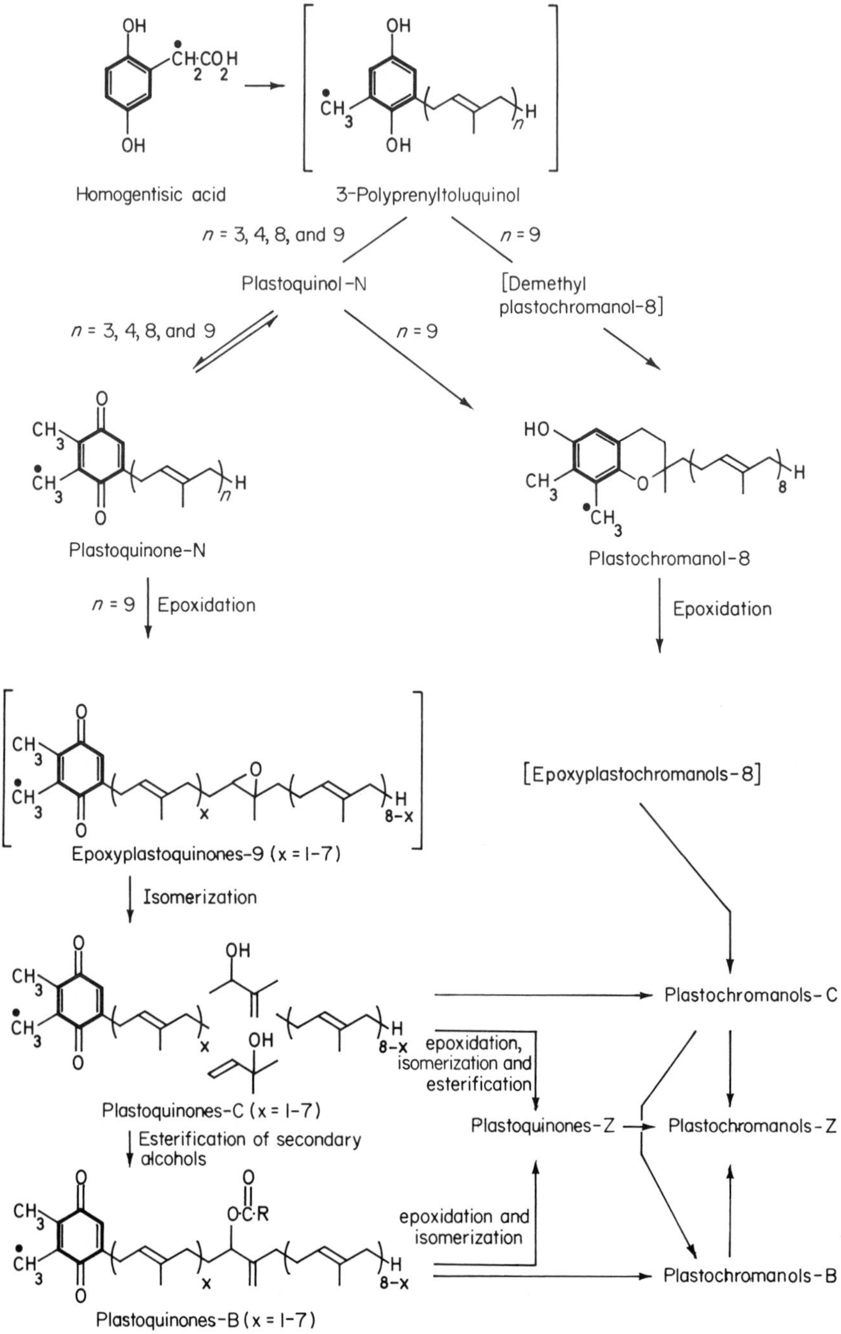

Homogentisic acid

3-Polyprenyltoluquinol

n = 3, 4, 8, and 9

n = 9

Plastoquinol -N

[Demethyl plastochromanol-8]

n = 3, 4, 8, and 9

n = 9

Plastoquinone-N

Plastochromanol-8

n = 9 | Epoxidation

Epoxidation

Epoxyplastoquinones-9 (x = 1-7)

[Epoxyplastochromanols-8]

Isomerization

Plastoquinones-C (x = 1-7)

Plastochromanols- C

epoxidation, isomerization and esterification

Esterification of secondary alcohols

Plastoquinones-Z

Plastochromanols-Z

epoxidation and isomerization

Plastoquinones-B (x = 1-7)

Plastochromanols-B

Threlfall and Griffiths (1967), who suggested that the overall biosynthesis of phylloquinone, plastoquinones, tocopherols, and tocopherolquinones takes place within the chloroplast and that that of ubiquinone occurs elsewhere within the cell.

The evidence in support of these proposals has come mainly from experiments on the incorporation of radioactivity from $^{14}CO_2$, DL-[2-^{14}C]-mevalonic acid, L-[Me-^{14}C]methionine, D-[G-^{14}C]shikimic acid, and L-[U-^{14}C]tyrosine into the intrachloroplastidic components phylloquinone, plastoquinone-9, plastoquinones-C, α-tocopherol, γ-tocopherol [the precise intracellular distribution of this compound is not known with certainty (see Section III,A,1)] and α-tocopherolquinone. The levels of radioactivity entering the above lipids have been compared with those incorporated into the extrachloroplastidic components ubiquinone-9 and -10 by greening etiolated maize and French bean shoots and young tobacco seedlings (Dada et al., 1968; Griffiths et al., 1968; Threlfall and Griffiths, 1967; Threlfall et al., 1967b, 1968; Whistance et al., 1967). The results of these experiments showed that radioactivity from $^{14}CO_2$ is incorporated well into the intrachloroplastidic components, but only poorly into the extrachloroplastidic component. Conversely, radioactivity from the other substrates is incorporated well into extrachloroplastidic component, but relatively poorly into the intrachloroplastidic components. These findings were interpreted as showing that after fixation of the $^{14}CO_2$ in the chloroplast radioactivity is incorporated more rapidly to the intermediates on the intrachloroplastidic pathways leading to the formation of phylloquinone, plastoquinones, tocopherols, and tocopherolquinones than to those on the extrachloroplastidic pathways leading to the formation of ubiquinone. In the case of the other ^{14}C-labeled substrates, the reverse situation holds. Further support for these proposals is the demonstration that on illumination of etiolated maize shoots or dark-grown cells of Euglena gracilis the synthesis of phylloquinone, plastoquinone-9, α-tocopherolquinone, and, in the case of the alga, α-tocopherol parallels the formation of chloroplasts from proplastids, whereas that of the extrachloroplastidic ubiquinone does not (Griffiths et al., 1967; Threlfall and Goodwin, 1967). Direct evidence for the intrachloroplastidic synthesis of plastoquinone-9 is the demonstration that

---

FIG. 15. Possible pathways for the biosynthesis of plastoquinones and plastochromanols from homogentisate. The interrelationships of the plastoquinones and plastochromanols is based on the proposals of Wallwork and Pennock (1968) and Peake et al. (1970b). The plastochromanols-B, -C, and -Z could be formed either from plastochromanol-8 in a manner identical to the formation of plastoquinones-B, -C, and -Z from plastoquinone-9 or from plastoquinones-B, -C, and -Z in a manner identical to the formation of plastochromanol-8 from plastoquinone-9.

horse chestnut chloroplasts are capable of incorporating radioactivity from DL-[2-¹⁴C]mevalonic acid into plastoquinone-9 (Wellburn and Hemming, 1967).

The above results taken together provide evidence that phylloquinone and the homogentisate derived compounds plastoquinone, α-tocopherol, γ-tocopherol, and α-tocopherolquinone are made inside the chloroplast and the p-hydroxybenzoate-derived compound ubiquinone is made outside. They do not, however, provide a clear indication as to the site of synthesis of those tocopherols which are found outside the chloroplast [δ-, half to all of the γ-, and possibly some α- (Section III,A,1)]. The question which must be answered in the case of these compounds is: Are there tocopherol synthesizing sites outside as well as inside the chloroplast, or are δ-, γ-, and α-tocopherol synthesized inside the chloroplast and then transported out?

REFERENCES

Allen, C. F., Franke, H., and Hirayama, O. (1967). *Biochem. Biophys. Res. Commun.* **26**, 562.
Allen, C. M., Alworth, W., MacRae, A., and Bloch, K. (1967). *J. Biol. Chem.* **242**, 1895.
Azerad, R., Bleiler-Hill, R., Catala, F., Samuel, O., and Lederer, E. (1967). *Biochem. Biophys. Res. Commun.* **27**, 253.
Barr, R., and Arntzen, C. J. (1969). *Plant Physiol.* **44**, 591.
Barr, R., and Crane, F. L. (1967). *Plant Physiol.* **42**, 1255.
Barr, R., Magree, L., and Crane, F. L. (1967). *Amer. J. Bot.* **54**, 365.
Bartlett, K. (1968). B.Sc. Thesis, University College of Wales, Aberystwyth.
Baszynski, T. (1961). *Acta Soc. Bot. Pol.* **30**, 307.
Baszynski, T., Dudziak, B., and Arnold, D. (1969). *Ann. Univ. Mariae Curie-Sklodowska, Sect. C* **24**, 1.
Bertel, R. (1903). *Chem. Zentralbl.* **1**, 178.
Bishop, D. H. L., and King, H. K. (1962). *Biochem. J.* **85**, 550.
Bishop, D. H. L., Pandya, K. P., and King, H. K. (1962). *Biochem. J.* **83**, 606.
Booth, V. H. (1963). *Phytochemistry* **2**, 421.
Brown, B. S., Whistance, G. R., and Threlfall, D. R. (1968). *FEBS Lett.* **1**, 323.
Bucke, C. (1968). *Phytochemistry* **7**, 693.
Campbell, I. M. (1969). *Tetrahedron Lett.* **54**, 4777.
Campbell, I. M., Coscia, C. J., Kelsey, M., and Bentley, R. (1967). *Biochem. Biophys. Res. Commun.* **28**, 25.
Catala, F., Azerad, R., and Lederer, E. (1970). *Int. Z. Vitaminforsch.* **40**, 363.
Christenson, J., Gross, S. K., and Robbins, P. W. (1969). *J. Biol. Chem.* **244**, 5436.
Clayton, R. B. (1965). *Quart. Rev., Chem. Soc.* **19**, 168 and 201.
Cox, G. B., and Gibson, F. (1964). *Biochim. Biophys. Acta* **93**, 204.
Cox, G. B., and Gibson, F. (1966). *Biochem. J.* **100**, 1.
Dada, O. A. (1968). M.Sc. Thesis, University College of Wales, Aberystwyth.
Dada, O. A., Threlfall, D. R., and Whistance, G. R. (1968). *Eur. J. Biochem.* **4**, 329.
Dansette, P., and Azerad, R. (1970). *Biochem. Biophys. Res. Commun.* **40**, 1090.
Dilley, R. A., and Crane, F. L. (1963). *Plant Physiol.* **38**, 452.

Dolin, M. I., and Baum, R. H. (1965). *Biochem. Biophys. Res. Commun.* **18**, 202.

Dunphy, P. J., Whittle, K. J., Pennock, J. F., and Morton, R. A. (1965). *Nature (London)*, **207**, 521.

Dunphy, P. J., Whittle, K. J., and Pennock, J. F. (1966). *In* "The Biochemistry of Chloroplasts" (T. W. Goodwin, ed.), Vol. 1, p. 165. Academic Press, New York.

Dunphy, P. J., Gutnick, D. L., Phillips, P. G., and Brodie, A. F. (1968). *J. Biol. Chem.* **243**, 398.

Dunphy, P. J., Peake, I. R., and Pennock, J. F. (1969). *Biochem. J.* **113**, 35P.

Eck, H., and Trebst, A. (1963). *Z. Naturforsch. B* **18**, 446.

Egger, K. (1965). *Planta* **64**, 41.

Ellis, J. R. S., and Glover, J. (1968). *Biochem. J.* **110**, 22P.

Fuller, R. C., Smillie, R. M., Rigopoulos, N., and Yount, V. (1961). *Arch. Biochem. Biophys.* **95**, 197.

Gale, P. H., Arison, B. H., Trenner, N. R., Page, A. C., Jr., and Folkers, K. (1963). *Biochemistry* **2**, 200.

Geissman, T. A. (1967). *In* "Biogenesis of Natural Compounds" (P. Bernfeld, ed.), p. 743. Pergamon, Oxford.

Gibson, F. (1964). *Biochem. J.* **90**, 256.

Gibson, F., and Pittard, J. (1968). *Bacteriol. Rev.* **32**, 465.

Gibson, M. I., and Gibson, F. (1964). *Biochim. Biophys. Acta* **65**, 160.

Goodwin, T. W., and Mercer, E. I. (1963). *Biochem. Soc. Symp.* **24**, 37.

Graebe, J. E. (1967). *Science* **157**, 73.

Green, J. (1958). *J. Sci. Food Agr.* **9**, 801.

Green, J. (1970). *In* "Fat Soluble Vitamins" (R. A. Morton, ed.), Vol. 9, p. 71. Pergamon, Oxford.

Griffiths, W. T., Threlfall, D. R., and Goodwin, T. W. (1964). *Biochem. J.* **90**, 40P.

Griffiths, W. T., Threlfall, D. R., and Goodwin, T. W. (1967). *Biochem. J.* **103**, 589.

Griffiths, W. T., Threlfall, D. R., and Goodwin, T. W. (1968). *Eur. J. Biochem.* **5**, 124.

Guérin, M., Azerad, R., and Lederer, E. (1965). *Bull. Soc. Chim. Biol.* **47**, 2105.

Guérin, M., Leduc, M. M., and Azerad, R. G. (1970). *Eur. J. Biochem.* **15**, 421.

Gullis, R. J. (1971). B.Sc. Thesis, University College of Wales, Aberystwyth.

Hall, G. S., and Laidman, D. L. (1968). *Biochem. J.* **108**, 475.

Hall, R. A. (1970). B.Sc. Thesis, University College of Wales, Aberystwyth.

Hammond, R. K., and White, D. C. (1969a). *J. Chromatogr.* **45**, 446.

Hammond, R. K., and White, D. C. (1969b). *J. Bacteriol.* **100**, 573.

Hemming, F. W. (1970). *In* "Natural Substances formed Biologically from Mevalonic Acid" (T. W. Goodwin, ed.), p. 105. Academic Press, New York.

Henninger, M. D., Dilley, R. A., and Crane, F. L. (1963). *Biochem. Biophys. Res. Commun.* **10**, 237.

Hurd, D. M. (1970). B.Sc. Thesis, University College of Wales, Aberystwyth.

Inoue, H., Arai, T., and Takano, Y. (1958). *Chem. Pharm. Bull.* **6**, 653.

IUPAC-IUB Commission of Biological Chemistry. (1967). *Biochem. J.* **102**, 15.

Jackman, L. M., O'Brien, I. G., Cox, G. B., and Gibson, F. (1967). *Biochim. Biophys. Acta* **141**, 1.

Jacobsen, B. K., and Dam, H. (1960). *Biochim. Biophys. Acta* **40**, 211.

Jauréguiberry, G., Lenfant, M., Das, B. C., and Lederer, E. (1966). *Tetrahedron, Suppl.* **8**, Part 1, 27.

Jeffries, L., Cawthorne, M. A., Harris, M., Diplock, A. T., Green, J., and Price, S. A. (1967). *Nature (London)* **215**, 257.

Jungalwala, F. B., and Porter, J. W. (1967). *Arch. Biochem. Biophys.* **119**, 209.

Kandutsch, A. A., Paulus, M., Levin, E., and Block, K. (1964). *J. Biol. Chem.* **239**, 2507.

Krishnamurthy, S., and Bieri, J. G. (1963). *J. Lipid Res.* **4**, 330.

Lederer, E. (1969). *Quart. Rev., Chem. Soc.* **23**, 453.

Leduc, M. M., Dansette, P. M., and Azerad, R. G. (1970). *Eur. J. Biochem.* **15**, 428.

Leistner, E., and Zenk, M. H. (1968a). *Z. Naturforsch. B* **23**, 259.

Leistner, E., and Zenk, M. H. (1968b). *Tetrahedron Lett.* **7**, 861.

Leistner, E., Schmitt, J. H., and Zenk, M. H. (1967). *Biochem. Biophys. Res. Commun.* **28**, 845.

Lester, R. L., White, D. C., and Smith, S. L. (1964). *Biochemistry* **3**, 949.

Lichtenthaler, H. K. (1968a). *Planta* **81**, 140.

Lichtenthaler, H. K. (1968b). *Z. Pflanzenphysiol.* **59**, 195.

Lichtenthaler, H. K. (1969). *Z. Naturforsch. B* **24**, 1462.

Lichtenthaler, H. K., and Tevini, M. (1970). *Z. Pflanzenphysiol.* **62**, 33.

McKenna, M., Henninger, M. D., and Crane, F. L. (1964). *Nature (London)* **203**, 524.

Maroc, J., DeKlerk, H., and Kamen, M. J. (1968). *Biochim. Biophys. Acta* **162**, 621.

Maroc, J., Azerad, R., Kamen, M. D., and Le Gall, J. (1970). *Biochim. Biophys. Acta* **197**, 87.

Martius, C. (1962). *Vita. Horm. (New York)* **20**, 457.

Martius, C., and Furer, E. (1962). *Biochem. Z.* **336**, 106.

Martius, C., and Leuzinger, W. (1964). *Biochem. Z.* **340**, 304.

Matschiner, J. T., and Amelotti, J. (1968). *J. Lipid Res.* **9**, 176.

Matsumura, U., and Shibata, Y. (1964). *Chem. Abstr.* **61**, 2104d.

Meister, A. (1965). "Biochemistry of the Amino Acids," Vol. 2, pp. 894–908. Academic Press, New York.

Mellors, A., and Barnes, M. McC. (1966). *Brit. J. Nutr.* **20**, 69.

Misiti, D., Moore, H. W., and Folkers, K. (1965). *J. Amer. Chem. Soc.* **87**, 1402.

Nandi, D. L., and Porter, J. W. (1964). *Arch. Biochem. Biophys.* **105**, 7.

Neish, A. C. (1964). *In* "Biochemistry of Phenolic Compounds" (J. B. Harborne, ed.), p. 295. Academic Press, New York.

Nickerson, W. J., Falcone, G., and Strauss, G. (1963). *Biochemistry* **2**, 537.

Noll, H., Ruegg, R., Gloor, U., Ryser, G., and Isler, O. (1960). *Helv. Chim. Acta* **43**, 433.

Osnitskaya, L. K., Threlfall, D. R., and Goodwin, T. W. (1964). *Nature (London)* **204**, 80.

Oster, M. O., and West, C. A. (1968). *Arch. Biochem. Biophys.* **127**, 112.

Peake, I. R., Audley, B. G., and Pennock, J. F. (1970a). *Biochem. J.* **119**, 58P.

Peake, I. R., Dunphy, P. J., and Pennock, J. F. (1970b). *Phytochemistry* **9**, 1345

Pennock, J. F. (1966). *Vitam. Horm. (New York)* **24**, 307.

Pennock, J. F., Hemming, F. W., and Kerr, J. D. (1964). *Biochem. Biophys. Res. Commun.* **17**, 542.

Phillips, P. G., Dunphy, P. J., Servis, K. L., and Brodie, A. F. (1969). *Biochemistry* **8**, 2856.

Plack, P. A., and Bieri, J. G. (1964). *Biochim. Biophys. Acta* **84**, 729.

Pollard, C. J., Bonner, J., Haagen-Smit, A. J., and Nimmo, C. C. (1966). *Plant Physiol.* **41**, 66.

Popják, G. (1970). *In* "Natural Substances formed Biologically from Mevalonic Acid" (T. W. Goodwin, ed.), p. 17. Academic Press, New York.

Porter, J. W. (1969). Carotenoids other than Vitamin A, *In* "I.U.P.A.C., Division of Organic Chemistry Symposium," Vol. 2, p. 449. Butterworth, London.

Powls, R. (1970). *FEBS Lett.* **6**, 40.

Powls, R., and Hemming, F. W. (1966). *Phytochemistry* **5**, 1249.

Powls, R., and Redfearn, E. R. (1967). *Biochem. J.* **104**, 24C.

Powls, R., and Redfearn, E. R. (1968). *Biochim. Biophys. Acta* **172**, 429.

Powls, R., Redfearn, E. R., and Trippet, S. (1968). *Biochem. Biophys. Res. Commun.* **33**, 408.

Raman, T. S., Sharma, B. V. S., Jayaraman, J., and Ramasarma, T. (1965). *Arch. Biochem. Biophys.* **110**, 75.

Raman, T. S., Rudney, H., and Buzzelli, N. K. (1969). *Arch. Biochem. Biophys.* **130**, 164.

Ramasarma, T., and Ramakrishnan, T. (1961). *Biochem. J.* **81**, 303.

Redfearn, E., and Powls, R. (1967). *Biochem. J.* **106**, 56P.

Rietz, P., Gloor, U., and Wiss, O. (1970). *Int. Z. Vitaminforsch.* **40**, 351.

Robins, D. J., Campbell, I. M., and Bentley, R. (1970). *Biochem. Biophys. Res. Commun.* **39**, 1081.

Samuel, O., and Azerad, R. (1969). *FEBS Lett.* **2**, 336.

Sanderman, H. W., and Simatupang, M. H. (1962). *Angew. Chem.* **74**, 782.

Sanderman, H. W., and Simatupang, M. H. (1967). *Naturwissenschaften* **54**, 118.

Sarikabuhti, B. (1968). M.Sc. Thesis, University of Liverpool.

Sasarman, A., Surdeanu, M., Portelance, V., Dobardzic, R., and Sonea, S. (1969). *Nature (London)* **224**, 272.

Schiefer, H. G., and Martius, C. (1960). *Biochem. Z.* **333**, 454.

Seward, C. R., and Corwin, L. M. (1963). *Arch. Biochem. Biophys.* **101**, 71.

Snyder, C. D., and Rapoport, H. (1970). *Biochemistry* **9**, 2033.

Stevenson, J., Hemming, F. W., and Morton, R. A. (1963). *Biochem. J.* **88**, 52.

Stoffel, W., and Martius, C. (1960). *Biochem. Z.* **333**, 440.

Sun, E., Barr, R., and Crane, F. L. (1968). *Plant Physiol.* **43**, 1935.

Threlfall, D. R., and Goodwin, T. W. (1967). *Biochem. J.* **103**, 573.

Threlfall, D. R., and Griffiths, W. T. (1967). *In* "The Biochemistry of Chloroplasts" (T. W. Goodwin, ed.), Vol. 2, p. 254. Academic Press, New York.

Threlfall, D. R., Whistance, G. R., and Goodwin, T. W. (1967a). *Biochem. J.* **102**, 49P.

Threlfall, D. R., Griffiths, W. T., and Goodwin, T. W. (1967b). *Biochem. J.* **103**, 831.

Threlfall, D. R., Whistance, G. R., and Goodwin, T. W. (1968). *Biochem. J.* **106**, 107.

Tornabene, T. G., Kates, M., Gelpi, E., and Oro, J. (1969). *J. Lipid Res.* **10**, 294.

Wallwork, J. C., and Pennock, J. F. (1968). *Chem. Ind. (London)* p. 1571.

Weber, M. M., Matschiner, J. T., and Peck, H. D. (1970). *Biochem. Biophys. Res. Commun.* **38**, 197.

Wellburn, A. R. (1968). *Phytochemistry* **7**, 1523.

Wellburn, A. R. (1970). *Phytochemistry* **9**, 743.

Wellburn, A. R., and Hemming, F. W. (1967). *Biochem. J.* **104**, 173.

Whistance, G. R., and Threlfall, D. R. (1967). *Biochem. Biophys. Res. Commun.* **28**, 295.

Whistance, G. R., and Threlfall, D. R. (1968a). *Biochem. J.* **109**, 482.

Whistance, G. R., and Threlfall, D. R. (1968b). *Biochem. J.* **109**, 577.

Whistance, G. R., and Threlfall, D. R. (1970a). *Biochem. J.* **117**, 593.

Whistance, G. R., and Threlfall, D. R. (1970b). *Phytochemistry* **9**, 213.

Whistance, G. R., and Threlfall, D. R. (1970c). *Phytochemistry* **9**, 737.

Whistance, G. R., and Threlfall, D. R. (1970d). Unpublished observations.

Whistance, G. R., and Threlfall, D. R. (1971). *Phytochemistry* (in press).

Whistance, G. R., Threlfall, D. R., and Goodwin, T. W. (1966a). *Biochem. J.* **85**, 14P.

Whistance, G. R., Threlfall, D. R., and Goodwin, T. W. (1966b). *Biochem. Biophys. Res. Commun.* **23**, 849.

Whistance, G. R., Threlfall, D. R., and Goodwin, T. W. (1967). *Biochem. J.* **105**, 145.

Whistance, G. R., Dillon, J. F., and Threlfall, D. R. (1969). *Biochem. J.* **111**, 461.

Whittle, K. J., Audley, B. G., and Pennock, J. F. (1967). *Biochem J.* **103**, 21C.

Winrow, M. J., and Rudney, H. (1969). *Biochem. Biophys. Res. Commun.* **37**, 833.

Yoshida, S. (1969). *Annu. Rev. Plant Physiol.* **20**, 41.

Zenk, M. H., and Leistner, E. (1967). *Z. Naturforsch. B* **22**, 460.

The Excretion of Steroid Hormone Metabolites in Bile and Feces

W. TAYLOR

Department of Physiology, The Medical School, The University,
Newcastle upon Tyne, England

I. Introduction

The presence of steroid hormone activity in bile was first demonstrated nearly fifty years ago. Progress in the analysis of bile was slow compared to that of urine because of the technical problems associated with the qualitative and quantitative analysis of the small amounts of steroids excreted in bile and feces. The availability of labeled steroid hormones greatly facilitated investigations. More recently, the use of gas–liquid chromatography, particularly when associated with mass spectrometry, has facilitated research in this field, and in the last few years a vast amount of data has been accumulated. This review deals mainly with this more recent work, but earlier work is also considered to maintain chronological continuity and to illustrate the progress that may be expected in future investigations. For a fuller account of earlier work, the following reviews should be consulted: Adlercreutz (1962, 1965), Peterson (1965), and Taylor (1965b).

II. The Biliary System and Bile Secretion

An understanding of the significance of biliary excretion of steroid hormone metabolites requires some knowledge about the structure of the biliary system and of current ideas on the formation and secretion of bile. Therefore, a brief outline of this subject is given in this section.

The primary units of the biliary system are the bile canaliculi. They are formed as very fine tubules between adjacent pairs of parenchymal cells, each cell contributing one half of the canaliculus. The canaliculi can be seen only by electron microscopy. The membrane of that part of the cell which forms the canaliculus has numerous microvilli which project into the lumen of the canaliculus. The microvilli are about 0.2 μ in diameter, and the membrane is about 100 Å thick. The Golgi apparatus of the cell is close to the canaliculus, and strong ATPase activity can be demonstrated around the canaliculus. This organization indicates that the canaliculi are regions in which active secretory processes occur.

Adjacent parenchymal cells are usually tightly bound together, and so the junction between the cells is impervious to water and to solutes. Therefore, under normal conditions, transfer of substances from blood to the bile canaliculi must occur by movement of water and solutes across the parenchymal cells. Consequently, this transfer may be controlled by the cell, and may be disturbed if cellular organization and function are abnormal.

The small bile ducts (15–20 μ in diameter) are formed by anastomoses of bile canaliculi. The ducts increase in size and the cuboidal epithelium thickens as the diameter of the ducts increases.

The blood supply of parenchymal cells differs from that of most other cells in the body. The smallest blood vessels, which are larger than capillaries, are called sinusoids. The sinusoids are formed from either of two types of cells. The first are typical endothelial cells. The second are the

Kupffer cells, which are part of the reticuloendothelial system, are highly phagocytic, and avidly take up and store particulate materials injected into the blood. These cells may also store blood-borne substances for considerable periods of time. The membranes of the parenchymal cells adjacent to the sinusoids show abundant microvilli which project into the space between the sinusoids and parenchymal cells (the perisinusoidal space of Disse). The presence of these microvilli suggests that this is a region of high absorptive and secretory activity. The sinusoids do not have the same structure throughout the whole liver. In large regions of the liver the gaps between the sinusoids and parenchymal cells are sufficiently large to permit direct contact between blood (except the formed elements) and the parenchymal cells. Figure 1 shows a diagram of the

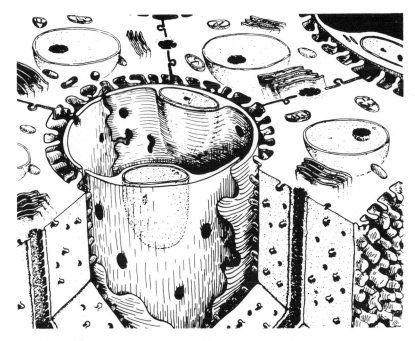

FIG. 1. Schematic representation of the ultrastructure of the liver. The large central tube is a sinusoid, lined by Kupffer cells, surrounded by hepatic cells which are held together by a "snap fastener" mechanism. Between the hepatic cells and the outer surface of the Kupffer cells is the perisinusoidal space of Disse. The canaliculi lie between the hepatic cells and contain many microvilli, as seen in the cut-away portion in the foreground, which shows canaliculi in longitudinal section. Microvilli also project from the hepatic cells into the space of Disse. Nuclei, nucleoli, mitochondria, and endoplasmic reticulum in the hepatic cells are also shown. Note the presence of "holes" in the Kupffer cells and the loose overlapping of these cells. From Elias (1965).

major features of the microanatomy of the biliary system, and Fig. 2 is an electron micrograph of normal cat liver showing mainly the structures associated with the canaliculus.

From this brief account of the microstructure of the liver, it will be apparent that the processes involved in the transport of steroid metabolites into bile are markedly different from the mechanism of transport of steroids into urine. The liver is a major site of steroid metabolism and conjugation, and the metabolites may be transferred back into the blood to be excreted by the kidney, or may cross the membrane of the canaliculus to be excreted in the bile.

A considerable area exists in the liver for the transport of solutes from the hepatocytes into bile. Wheeler (1968) has calculated that the total surface of the canaliculi in 1 gm of liver is about 70 cm^2, but this is probably an underestimate because no account was taken of the elaborate system of microvilli which project into the lumen of the canaliculi. However, variations among animal species in the relationship between the canaliculi and the sinusoids exist. In man, cat, and dog there are usually at least eight hepatocytes surrounding the sinusoid, whereas in rodents and the horse there are usually only four (Elias, 1965).

The larger bile ducts are associated with blood and lymph vessels in the portal triads. It is still a matter of dispute whether the major bile ducts are simply tubes for carrying bile, or whether water and organic solutes can enter and leave the bile as it passes down the ducts. However, it is accepted that transport of water and some ions does occur in the smaller bile ducts (Wheeler, 1968).

Bile eventually passes into the small intestine either as hepatic bile or, in those animals which have a gallbladder, as a mixture of gallbladder and hepatic bile. (It is worth noting that the rat does not have a gallbladder, whereas most other common laboratory animals do.) The rate of secretion of hepatic bile and the release of gallbladder bile are under the control of gastrointestinal hormones. It is also probable that secretion may be partially controlled, directly or indirectly, by the vagus and splanchnic nerves. The continuous production of hepatic bile is very much dependent on the reabsorption of bile salts from the intestinal tract and transport of these salts back to the liver in the portal circulation. Therefore, removal of bile for analysis will result in depletion of bile salts in the liver with consequent decrease in bile production.

Because of the minute size of the bile canaliculi, the composition of primary bile is not known, and so an exact explanation of the processes involved in bile secretion is not possible at this stage. Therefore the factors that influence the excretion of steroid hormones in bile are obscure. [The microanatomy of the biliary system and theories of the mechanisms

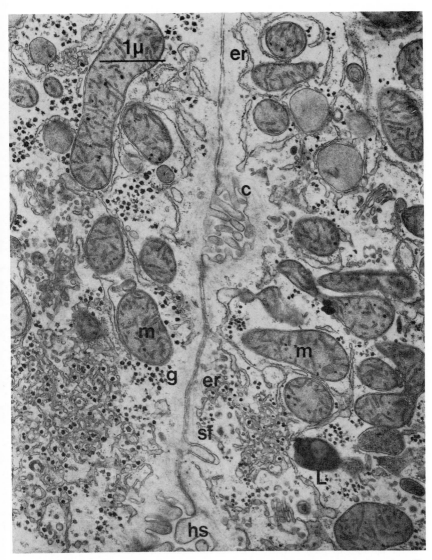

FIG. 2. Electron micrograph of cat liver showing the junction of two hepatic cells to form the canaliculus (c) with its numerous microvilli. er = endoplasmic reticulum, g = glycogen granules, L = lysosome, m = mitochondrion, sf = "snap fastener" holding hepatic cells together; hs = microvilli of hepatic cells projecting into space of Disse.

involved in bile secretion have been comprehensively reviewed (Rouiller, 1963; Taylor, 1965a; Ericsson, 1969; Schanker, 1968; Wheeler, 1968).]

III. Difficulties in Interpreting Results of Analyses of Steroids in Bile and Feces

From what has been described in Section II, it will be apparent that interpretation of the results obtained by analysis of steroids in bile is more complex than analysis of urine. The significance of the results is complicated by the fact that removal of bile for analysis will markedly influence the overall production of bile. Therefore, a sample of bile collected over 24 hours cannot be equated with a 24-hour urine sample. Also, the collection of bile, whether it be by cannulation of the bile duct, from the gallbladder, or by duodenal intubation does not provide an accurate assessment of the role of bile as an excretory route for steroid metabolites. In the intact animal the steroids excreted in bile undergo metabolic changes in the intestinal tract due to the enzymatic activity of the intestinal microflora. Also, enterohepatic recirculation of steroid metabolites, with possible further metabolic changes in the liver, is known to occur in many species. The reabsorbed metabolites may be excreted in the bile again or pass into urine. Removal of bile for analysis prevents these processes from occurring.

The analysis of feces for steroid metabolites is technically more difficult than analysis of urine. Fecal steroids do not necessarily reflect accurately the steroids initially excreted in bile, because the steroids are subject to metabolic changes caused by the intestinal microflora and some metabolites may be reabsorbed as described above. Also, even with the use of fecal markers, it is not reasonable to equate a 24-hour feces collection with the urine collected over the same period.

IV. Excretion of Metabolites Associated with Radioactivity after Administration of Labeled Free Steroids

Table I summarizes work done on the distribution in bile, urine, and feces of metabolites associated with radioactivity after administration of labeled free steroids to experimental animals and man. All investigators do not use the same experimental techniques, and so the column heading "Type of preparation" provides only a guide to the techniques used. In general, "chronic bile fistula" refers to an animal in which a fistula has been prepared, and the steroid was not administered until the animal had recovered from the operation. With such animals bile can be collected for several days, provided that the intestinal tract is not completely deprived of bile for that time, or bile salts are administered to maintain bile flow. The term "acute, cannulated bile duct" means that the animals were anesthetized during the whole period of the experiment and bile was collected for only a few hours. The human subjects from whom bile was collected usually had been fitted with a T-tube in the common bile duct, a common practice after surgery on the biliary system, usually cholecystectomy. The T-tube is constructed so as to allow bile to flow to an external collection vessel or to pass into the intestine as required. Therefore it must be borne in mind that the distribution of radioactivity might have been affected by the particular operative technique used.

Another limitation to the type of experiment described in Table I is that the amount of steroid administered to the animal, although small compared with studies with nonradioactive steroids, is still relatively large. This applies particularly to those experiments in which the steroid is administered as a single intravenous injection. It is assumed that the doses given are within the "physiological range," and that the administered steroid mixes freely with endogenous steroids in the body pool. Neither assumption can be proved to be correct. Indeed, it can be said with some certainty that, for example, 20 μg of a particular steroid administered to an animal weighing 1 or 2 kg is not a physiological dose.

However, in spite of the limitations of these experiments some consistent patterns do emerge from the results. Metabolites of the less polar steroids tend to be excreted in bile to a greater extent than metabolites of polar steroids; e.g., progesterone metabolites are present in bile (and feces) of rats and human subjects. In contrast, hydrocortisone is almost completely excreted as urinary metabolites by human subjects, and the proportion of the dose of this steroid appearing in bile of rats is much less than when progesterone is given.

In a number of the investigations shown in Table I, attempts were made to isolate metabolites from bile after the administration of labeled steroids. It will become apparent from later sections that such investigations could not have yielded a great deal of information because of the state of knowledge about steroid metabolism and of the limited technical facilities and reference steroids available at the time that these studies began. Therefore, no attempt will be made here to describe the few metabolites which were detected in bile. Instead, the evolution of new concepts which arose from the early studies will be illustrated.

A. METABOLITES OF PROGESTERONE IN BILE

Before labeled steroids became available, little was known about the metabolic fate of endogenous or exogenous progesterone in man. Small amounts of pregnanediol had been found in bile and feces after administration of massive doses of progesterone (e.g., Rogers and McLellan, 1951). In 1958 A. A. Sandberg and Slaunwhite administered [4-^{14}C]progesterone

TABLE I

EXCRETION OF METABOLITES ASSOCIATED WITH RADIOACTIVITY AFTER
ADMINISTRATION OF LABELED FREE STEROIDS

Species and steroid	Type of preparation	Percent of dose in			Reference
		Bile	Urine	Feces	
Progesterone					
Rat	Normal	—	27	56 ⎫	
	Chronic bile fistula	73	22	2 ⎬	Shen et al. (1954)
	Ligated bile duct	—	80	10 ⎭	
Rabbit	Normal	—	15–37	—	Cooke et al. (1963)
	Acute, cannulated bile duct	35–41	22–44	—	Taylor and Scratcherd (1963)
		31–44	13–31	—	Senciall and Thomas (1970)
Cat	Normal	—	0.6–3.0	53–59	Taylor and Scratcherd (1962)
	Acute, cannulated bile duct	26–27	0.5	—	Taylor and Scratcherd (1961)
Ewe	Normal	—	21	— ⎫	Stupnicki et al.
	Chronic bile fistula	70	26	— ⎭	(1969)
Baboon	Normal	—	34–41	14–17	Kulkarni et al. (1970)
Human	Normal	—	46–59	8–17 ⎫	A. A. Sandberg and
	T-tube drainage	20–35	38–70	3 ⎭	Slaunwhite (1958)
20α-Dihydroprogesterone					
Rabbit		30–51	15–23	— ⎫	Senciall and Thomas (1970)
20β-Dihydroprogesterone					
Rabbit		21–31	10–15	— ⎭	
Pregnenolone					
Rat	Normal, male	—	50	45 ⎫	
	female	—	45	50 ⎪	Eriksson and
	Germfree, male	—	40	55 ⎪	Gustafsson (1970a)
	female	—	40	55 ⎭	
17α-Hydroxyprogesterone					
Human	Normal	20	55	— ⎫	Slaunwhite and
	T-tube drainage	—	55	— ⎬	Sandberg (1961) Vermeulen et al. (1961)
17α-Acetoxyprogesterone					
Human	T-tube drainage	40	35	—	Slaunwhite and Sandberg (1961)
6α-Methyl-17α-acetoxyprogesterone					
Human	T-tube drainage	40	35	—	Peterson (1965)
Testosterone					
Mouse	Normal	—	34–49	33–65 ⎫	Barry et al. (1952)
Rat	Normal	—	7–12	32–59 ⎭	
Guinea pig	Normal	—	83	3	Burstein et al. (1955)

TABLE I (*Continued*)

Species and steroid	Type of preparation	Percent of dose in			Reference
		Bile	Urine	Feces	
Cat	Acute, cannulated bile duct	69–80	3	—	Archer *et al.* (1965)
Rabbit	Normal	—	80–95	3–5	Taylor (1971)
	Acute, cannulated bile duct	41	25	—	Taylor and Scratcherd (1967)
Baboon	Normal	—	78–92	5	Kulkarni *et al.* (1970)
Human	Normal	—	89	6 ⎫	A. A. Sandberg and
	T-tube drainage	11–14	50–90	2 ⎬	Slaunwhite (1956)
	Normal	10	70	—	Peterson (1965)
	Normal	—	57	5	Fukushima *et al.* (1954)
Androstenedione					
Human	T-tube drainage	5	75	—	Peterson (1965)
11β-Hydroxyandrostenedione					
Human	Normal	—	95	Trace ⎱	A. A. Sandberg and
	T-tube drainage	2	95	Trace ⎰	Slaunwhite (1957a)
	T-tube drainage	5	90	—	Peterson (1965)
Dehydroepiandrosterone					
Human	T-tube drainage	5	75	—	Peterson (1965)
17α-Methyl-5-androstene-3β,17β-diol					
Rat	Normal	—	32–43	50–63 ⎫	
	Chronic bile fistula: bile collected				⎬ Hyde *et al.* (1954)
	(1) in glass tubes	74–93	8–17	0–3	
	(2) via plastic tube	46–67	12–24	5–15 ⎭	
Corticosterone					
Rat	Normal	87	5	—	Lowy *et al.* (1969)
	Normal, male	—	25	70 ⎫	
	female	—	40	50 ⎬ Eriksson and	
	Germfree, male	—	40	55 ⎪ Gustafsson (1970a)	
	female	—	15	80 ⎭	
Dog	Normal	—	55	20	Willoughby *et al.*
	Chronic bile fistula	25–50	30–65	—	(1959)
Cat	Normal	—	2	53–65	Taylor and Scratcherd (1962)
	Acute, cannulated bile duct	84–92	1	—	Taylor and Scratcherd (1963)
Human	Normal	—	80	—	Migeon *et al.* (1956)
	T-tube drainage	11	80	—	
	Normal	—	70	—	Pasqualini (1969)
11-Deoxycorticosterone					
Human	T-tube drainage	26	70	—	Peterson (1965)

(*Continued*)

TABLE I (*Continued*)

Species and steroid	Type of preparation	Percent of dose in			Reference
		Bile	Urine	Feces	
Hydrocortisone					
Rat	Normal	—	31–36	61 ⎫	Hyde and Williams
	Chronic bile fistula	79–91	6–15	1 ⎬	(1957)
Baboon	Normal	—	80–96	—	Kulkarni et al. (1970)
Human	Normal	—	70–83	9	Hellman et al. (1954)
	Normal	—	79–94	—	Romanoff et al. (1961)
	T-tube drainage	5	90	—	Peterson (1965)
Cortisone					
Cat	Acute, cannulated bile duct	68–89	0.5–7.1	—	Taylor (1969)
Rabbit	Acute, cannulated bile duct	42	42	—	Taylor (1970)
Human	Normal	—	90	—	Peterson et al. (1957)
	T-tube drainage	4	90	—	
11-Deoxycortisol					
Human	T-tube drainage	10	80	—	Peterson (1965)
Estrone					
Rat	Normal	—	7.4	10.8 ⎫	
	Actue, cannulated bile duct	58	4.2	—	
Rabbit	Normal	—	69	16	A. A. Sandberg et al.
	Acute, cannulated bile duct	17	36	— ⎬	(1967)
Guinea pig	Normal	—	64	8	
	Acute, cannulated bile duct	59	20	— ⎭	
Golden hamster	Normal	—	84	—	Collins et al. (1967)
Dog	Acute, cannulated bile duct	1.3–8	6.4–16	—	Longwell and McKay (1942)
Human	Normal	—	85	7 ⎫	A. A. Sandberg and
	T-tube drainage	75	15	— ⎬	Slaunwhite (1957b)
Estradiol					
Golden hamster	Normal	—	94	—	Collins et al. (1967)
Bull	Catheter in gall bladder	53	4	—	Pearson and Martin (1966)
Cat	Acute, cannulated bile	54–56	1	—	Karim and Taylor (1970a)
	Ligated bile duct	—	1	—	Karim and Taylor (1970b)
Baboon	Normal	—	54–78	0–4	Kulkarni et al. (1970)

TABLE I (*Continued*)

Species and steroid	Type of preparation	Percent of dose in			Reference
		Bile	Urine	Feces	
Human	Normal	—	85	7 ⎫	A. A. Sandberg and
	T-tube drainage	50	15	— ⎬	Slaunwhite (1957b)
	Normal	—	63	—	Hobkirk *et al.* (1969)
Estriol					
Rat	Normal	—	11	17 ⎫	
	Acute, cannulated bile duct	36	5.4	— ⎪	
Rabbit	Normal	—	69	4 ⎪	
	Acute, cannulated bile duct	45	11.4	— ⎬	A. A. Sandberg *et al.* (1967)
Guinea pig	Normal	1	51	16.3 ⎪	
	Acute, cannulated bile duct	72	17	— ⎭	
Human	Normal	—	81–88	0–4.4	A. A. Sandberg and
	T-tube drainage	17–38	70–83	0–2	Slaunwhite (1965)
Ethynylestradiol					
Human	Normal	—	40.5	—	Abdel-Aziz and Williams (1970)
	T-tube drainage	26	28	—	Cargill *et al.* (1969)
Ethynylestradiol-cyclopentyl ether					
Human	T-tube drainage	2–10	8–14	—	Cargill *et al.* (1969)
3-Hydroxy-19-norpregna-1,3,5(10)-trien-20-one					
Rabbit	Normal	—	3.3–6.5	71–79 ⎫	Schulster and Kellie
	Normal (gut and contents, bile)	73	6	9 ⎬	(1967)

to human subjects from some of whom bile could be collected by T-tube drainage. Intact subjects excreted about 52% of the dose in the urine and about 13% in feces. The subjects with T-tube drainage excreted 30% of the dose in the bile, 53% in urine, and about 3% in feces. This was one of the first indications that such a large proportion of a dose of steroid could be excreted into the bile, and helped to explain the well-known fact that after administration of progesterone to human subjects only about 10–20% of the dose could be accounted for as known urinary metabolites, mainly pregnanediol (e.g., Klopper *et al.*, 1957).

Wiest *et al.* (1958) carried out a fuller investigation of the radioactive metabolites in bile and urine of a woman given labeled progesterone. This particular subject excreted 42% of the radioactivity in the bile and 20% in urine in 24 hours. By means of paper chromatography and reverse isotope dilution techniques applied to steroids rendered soluble in organic solvent by standard hydrolytic techniques, they found that

about 50% of the radioactivity in urine was hydrolyzed by β-glucuroni-
dase whereas 70% was hydrolyzed in bile. Both pregnanediol and pregnanolone were isolated from this hydrolyzed fraction of bile and urine.
These steroids were present in the same proportions in both bile and urine,
pregnanediol accounting for about 50% of the radioactive glucuronides
and pregnanolone about 12%. A considerable proportion of the radioactivity remained at the origin of the chromatograms and was described
as "highly polar." The nature of this radioactivity will be discussed later
in this section. Chang *et al.* (1960) extended these investigations and
identified pregnanediol as a major metabolite, and 5α-pregnanediol,
pregnanolone, and progesterone as minor metabolites in bile. The same
steroids, and 5β-pregnane-3,20-dione were also found in urine. The
[14]C-labeled progesterone used in these investigations had a low specific
activity compared to the ^{14}C-labeled progesterone currently available,
and the counting equipment was not very sensitive. Also current knowledge about metabolic products of progesterone was limited, and many
possible reference compounds were not available.

Thus, under the experimental conditions used, only slight differences
in the type of conjugate and steroid in both bile and urine were found.
Therefore it would seem that in man, and possibly other species, the
routes by which steroid metabolites are excreted are not determined by
the specific nature of these metabolites.

Taylor (1965a) investigated the metabolites of [4-^{14}C]progesterone
in cat bile after standard hydrolytic procedures. However, the bewilder-
ing array of substances revealed by autoradiography of paper chromatograms precluded any systematic investigation of the great number of
radioactive metabolites. Pregnanediol and pregnanolone were not detectable by reverse isotope dilution. In experiments with rabbits, Taylor
and Scratcherd (1963) found the same array of metabolites, but pregnanediol and pregnanolone were identified by reverse isotope dilution. It
was evident to the author that the progress then being made in gas
chromatography–mass spectrometry was about to make obsolescent identification of these metabolites by other means.

The normal procedure for extracting metabolites of neutral steroids is
to wash the organic solvent with sodium hydroxide and water to provide
a neutral extract. However, Allen and Thomas (1967) found that as
much as 70% of the radioactivity in hydrolyzed urine from rabbits dosed
with labeled progesterone could be extracted from organic solvent into
sodium bicarbonate solution. They found that these "acidic metabolites"
of progesterone are also present in urine of pregnant rabbits (Allen and
Thomas, 1968). Such metabolites would, of course, be removed by washing solvent extracts with sodium hydroxide. Senciall and Thomas (1970)

studied the metabolites of progesterone in bile and urine of rabbits given [4-^{14}C]progesterone. After hydrolysis of bile with Ketodase, the neutral metabolites accounted for about 83% of the dose, and "acidic metabolites" about 15%. In urine the corresponding values were 19–33% (neutral) and 7–10% ("acidic"). The patterns of neutral Ketodase-hydrolyzed metabolites after thin-layer chromatography were different for bile and urine. The values for bile and urine in the fractions corresponding to (a) highly polar compounds were 34% and 68%, (b) pregnanediols, 55% and 11%, (c) pregnanolones, 7% and 16%, and (d) pregnanediones, 4% and 5%, respectively. This pattern for both biliary and urinary pregnanediols and pregnanolones differs markedly from that observed in human subjects by Wiest et al. (1958). However, these experiments with rabbits throw some light on the possible nature of the "highly polar" metabolites of progesterone in human bile. Senciall and Thomas (1970) oxidized the polar metabolites from rabbit bile and urine with chromic acid, and chromatography of the products showed the presence of a complex mixture of 5α/β-pregnane-3,6,20-triones.

Therefore it seems highly probable that the polar metabolites of progesterone found in the bile of man and other animals are pregnane derivatives with an hydroxyl group at C-6 and possibly at other positions in the steroid nucleus. Such hydroxylated products have been found in human bile and feces by mass spectrometry, but there is no current evidence that these are derived exclusively from progesterone. The "acidic metabolites" of rabbit bile have not as yet been detected in human excreta.

Therefore, the most promising approach to obtaining a fuller understanding of the source(s) of steroid metabolites in bile and feces seems to lie in a combined operation involving administration of labeled steroids and analyses by gas chromatography–mass spectrometry, and radio–gas chromatography. It would be highly advantageous if ^{14}C-labeled metabolites could be differentiated from ^{12}C-labeled metabolites by high-resolution mass spectrography (Section VI).

The validity of a wide variety of chemical and physical methods for the identification and assay of steroids has been discussed by Brooks et al. (1970). The proposals put forward by those authors should be carefully studied before claims of identity of steroids in biological media are made.

B. CONJUGATED METABOLITES OF STEROIDS IN BILE

Other aspects of steroid metabolism of great interest and importance were also revealed by these early studies with labeled steroids. A. A. Sandberg and Slaunwhite (1958) used standard hydrolytic techniques to liberate metabolites of progesterone excreted in human bile. These were the hydrolytic procedures in routine use for isolation of steroids from urine, i.e., enzyme hydrolysis of "glucuronides," cold-acid solvolysis of "sulfates," and finally hot-acid hydrolysis. The "neutral steroid fraction" was obtained in the usual way. However, it was found that a considerable proportion of the radioactivity present in bile (and urine) samples remained water soluble after these hydrolysis procedures. The nature of this "unaccounted for" radioactivity remains a mystery to this day, although some may be present as the "acidic metabolites" of Allen and Thomas (1967, 1968). This "unaccounted for" radioactivity was subsequently found to be excreted in bile (and urine) after the administration of other labeled steroids to man and other animals. Also, the amount of this radioactivity excreted in bile varies from species to species for a steroid, and from steroid to steroid for a particular species.

When bile and urine samples were collected over short time intervals, it was found that the patterns of conjugates in the successive samples differed in the proportions of particular conjugates and "unaccounted for" radioactivity. Specific examples of these variations are shown below. The histograms show the percentages of radioactivity present in the particular bile or urine samples as conjugated and "unaccounted for" radioactivity. In cats dosed with progesterone (Fig. 3), there is (1) a marked decrease in the proportion of radioactivity excreted as glucuronides in bile, (2) an increase in cold-acid solvolyzed conjugates, (3) little or no change in hot-acid hydrolyzed conjugates, and (4) an increase in "unaccounted

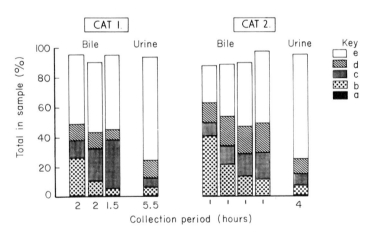

Fig. 3. Proportions of "conjugates" in bile and urine of male cats after a single intravenous dose of [4-^{14}C]progesterone. The values are shown as a percentage of the total amount of radioactivity present in the particular sample. a, "free steroids"; b, "glucuronides"; c, "sulfates"; d, hot-acid hydrolyzed metabolites; e, "unaccounted for" radioactivity. From Taylor (1965b).

for" radioactivity. In urine the radioactivity is excreted mainly as "unaccounted for" radioactivity (Fig. 3). The pattern after administration of
corticosterone differs in some respects: a smaller proportion of the dose is
excreted as glucuronides, a smaller and constant proportion as cold-acid
solvolyzed conjugates, and a larger and decreasing proportion of hot-acid
hydrolyzed metabolites. The proportion of "unaccounted for" radioactivity increases with time and forms a larger proportion of the excreted
radioactivity (Fig. 4).

The pattern in rabbits dosed with progesterone is quite different. Most
of the dose is excreted in the glucuronide fraction, which shows a tend-
ency to decrease with time. The cold- and hot-acid hydrolyzed metabolites show no marked changes with time, and the amount of "unaccounted

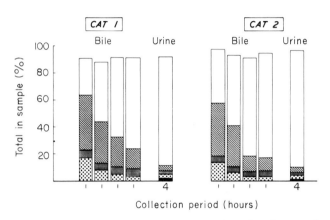

Collection period (hours)

Fig. 4. Proportions of "conjugates" in bile and urine of male cats after a single
intravenous dose of [4-¹⁴C]corticosterone. Details as in Fig. 3. From Taylor (1965b).

for" radioactivity is small in bile but larger in urine. There is no significant sex difference in the amounts of conjugates excreted by male and
female animals (Fig. 5).

The distribution of radioactivity in fractions from bile of male cats
given [4-¹⁴C]estradiol is shown in Fig. 6, and this differs from the pattern seen in bile of female cats (Fig. 7). In male cats there is a marked
decrease in the glucuronide fraction with time, whereas in female cats
this decrease is not seen. Male cats excrete significantly more cold-acid
solvolyzed metabolites than do female cats. There is no significant sex
difference in cats in the excretion of hot-acid hydrolyzed or "unaccounted
for" radioactivity (Karim and Taylor, 1970a).

These few examples (see also Fig. 8, Section V,B,1) show the marked
species–steroid differences which exist in biliary excretion of exogenous

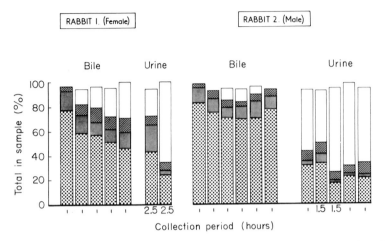

FIG. 5. Proportions of "conjugates" in bile and urine of male and female rabbits after a single intravenous dose of [4-^{14}C]progesterone. Details as in Fig. 3. From Taylor (1965b).

steroids. The value of such studies in elucidating the mechanism of biliary excretion of steroids is discussed in Section XI.

C. ENTEROHEPATIC CIRCULATION OF STEROID METABOLITES

In Table I there are many studies in which the excretion of radio-activity by normal and bile fistula (or bile duct cannulated) animals is compared. Allowing for the reservations about the care which needs to

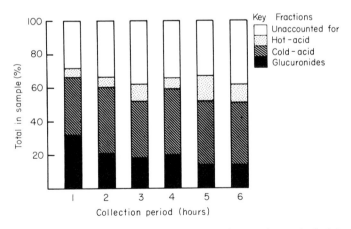

FIG. 6. Proportions of "conjugates" in bile of a male cat after a single intravenous dose of [4-^{14}C]estradiol. From Karim and Taylor (1970a).

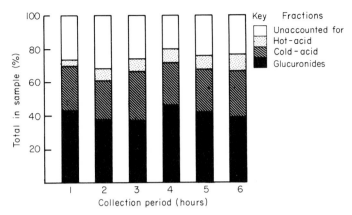

Fɪɢ. 7. Proportions of "conjugates" in bile of a female cat after a single intravenous dose of [4-¹⁴C]estradiol. From Karim and Taylor (1970a).

be taken in drawing firm conclusions from such studies, information about the enterohepatic circulation of steroid metabolites can be obtained. A few examples are chosen to illustrate this.

A. A. Sandberg and Slaunwhite (1958) suggested that enterohepatic circulation of progesterone metabolites either does not occur in human subjects or that any metabolites which may be reabsorbed from the gut are excreted again in the bile and are not excreted by the kidney. The liver is a major excretory organ for progesterone metabolites in man. In contrast, metabolites of 11β-hydroxy-4-androstenedione (Peterson, 1965; A. A. Sandberg and Slaunwhite, 1957a), hydrocortisone (Hellman et al., 1954; Romanoff et al., 1961; Peterson, 1965), and cortisone (Peterson et al., 1957) are excreted almost entirely by the kidney. There is evidence that biliary excretion of metabolites of these steroids occurs to a small extent, but the reabsorbed metabolites are excreted in urine.

A. A. Sandberg et al. (1967) made a systematic study of the biliary excretion and enterohepatic circulation of metabolites of estrone and estriol in rats, rabbits, and guinea pigs. They discussed the results of this work in relation to the situation pertaining in man, and calculated the extent of enterohepatic reabsorption of the estrogen metabolites initially excreted in bile. They found that reabsorption of estriol metabolites in rabbits and man was about 90%, in guinea pigs about 72%, and in rats only 36%. The values for estrone metabolites were different: man, 92%; guinea pig, 87%; rat, 81%, and rabbit only 4.7%. This great difference between rabbits and the other species was attributed to the ability of rabbits to form single and double conjugates containing N-acetylglucosamine (Layne et al., 1964). However, this cannot be the only explanation since estrogens conjugated with N-acetylglucosamine have now been found in bile and urine of human subjects (Section V).

Other points of interest arise from Table I. The cat seems to be unique among the animals so far studied in its ability to excrete steroid metabolites almost entirely in the bile or feces. Even when the bile duct is ligated, metabolites of estradiol are not excreted in the urine, whereas ligation of the bile duct of rats diverts metabolites of progesterone from the biliary to the renal excretory route. Another point of importance, and one to which too little attention has been paid, is that the method of collecting bile may greatly affect the proportion of metabolites excreted by the liver. Hyde *et al.* (1954) administered 17α-methyl-5-androstene-3β,17β-diol to rats with chronic bile fistulas. When bile was collected in glass tubes, 74–93% of the administered radioactivity was excreted in bile; but when collections were made through plastic tubes, excretion of radioactivity by this route fell to 46–67%.

Other factors that may influence the excretion of steroids in bile of anesthetized animals are the nature of the anesthetic and the time allowed to elapse between the surgical procedure and administration of the steroid (Doisy, 1965).

D. GENERAL CONCLUSIONS

The major conclusions to be drawn from Table I are: (a) different steroids are excreted to different extents in the urine and bile (or feces) of the same species; (b) the same steroid is excreted to different extents in the urine and bile (or feces) of different species; (c) species differences are found in the extent of enterohepatic circulation of metabolites of a particular steroid; (d) in the same species there are differences in the extent of enterohepatic circulation of metabolites of different steroids; (e) the proportions of conjugated metabolites in bile (and urine) samples vary with the period of collection of the sample.

V. STEROID EXCRETION PATTERNS AFTER ADMINISTRATION
OF LABELED CONJUGATES

It is now generally recognized that conjugation of steroid hormones and their metabolites does not necessarily represent an "inactivation" process. Indeed, conjugated steroids are now known to participate in biosynthetic pathways, at least partly, in the conjugated form, usually as sulfate esters. Adlercreutz (1962) administered 5 mg of estradiol-3-sulfate intramuscularly to one male subject and orally to another male subject. He measured the amounts of estradiol, estrone, and estriol in the "sulfate" and "glucuronide" fractions in samples of bile collected at intervals of about 2 hours. It was found that the estrogen sulfates were more rapidly excreted than were glucuronides, and that estradiol and estrone conjugates were more rapidly excreted than those of estriol. These results have been fully discussed by Adlercreutz (1962, 1965).

In recent years the availability of labeled steriods combined with ^{14}C-labeled glucuronic acid or ^{35}S-labeled sulfate has greatly stimulated interest in the fate of exogenous steroid conjugates in man and animals. Much of the work has been concerned mainly with the urinary excretion of metabolites. Not all this work is recorded here, but a selection has been made of investigations that directly or indirectly provide information about biliary excretion of steroid conjugates. The results are summarized in Table II. However, it must be pointed out that this summary does not deal comprehensively with the many interesting aspects of steroid metabolism revealed by this work. It is strongly recommended that the original papers be consulted.

A. Neutral Steroids

Few investigations with neutral steroid conjugates have been carried out. It is apparent from Table II that in human subjects radioactive metabolites of dehydroepiandrosterone sulfate are excreted in bile and feces, possibly to a greater extent than are metabolites of the free steroid. Patients with T-tube drainage were given a mixture of the sulfate labeled with tritium and the free steroid labeled with ^{14}C. An average of 3% of ^{14}C was excreted in bile, but much more ^{3}H (9–16%) was excreted by this route. There was less difference in the urinary excretion of ^{3}H and ^{14}C. It was also concluded that enterohepatic circulation, with subsequent excretion of the reabsorbed substances, occurs in man when this steroid is metabolized and excreted. Androgens in general are excreted in bile to only a small extent by human subjects (Slaunwhite et al., 1967).

The results obtained by Pasqualini (1969) indicate that in man the major part of a dose of corticosterone or its sulfate is excreted in urine. However, some excretion of metabolites of this steroid into bile and feces probably occurs (Table I). Some workers have claimed that up to 25% of corticosterone metabolites may be excreted in the bile of human subjects (Migeon et al., 1956; Peterson, 1959). If this be so, then considerable enterohepatic circulation of these metabolites must occur in man.

It is probable that the exogenous sulfates of neutral steroid hormones are not completely hydrolyzed before being metabolized and excreted. Such sulfates are generally considered to be resistant to hydrolysis in the body (Calvin et al., 1963; K. D. Roberts et al., 1964; E. Sandberg et al., 1964). Sulfates of phenolic steroids, however, are readily hydrolyzed in vivo (Twombly and Levitz, 1960; see also Section V,B,1).

TABLE II

STEROID EXCRETION PATTERNS AFTER ADMINISTRATION OF LABELED CONJUGATES

Steroid conjugate and species	Type of preparation	Percent of dose as metabolites in			Reference
		Bile	Urine	Feces	
Dehydroepiandrosterone-3-sulfate (4-^{14}C] or (7α-^{3}H])					
Human males	Normal	—	—	28–45	Hellström et al. (1969)
Human males and females	Normal	—	55	—	Slaunwhite et al
	T-tube drainage	11	—	—	(1967)
[4-^{14}C]Corticosterone-21-sulfate					
Human males	Normal	—	77–85	—	Pasqualini (1969)
[6,7-^{3}H]Estrone-3-[^{35}S]sulfate		(Excretion of ^{3}H)			
Human female	T-tube drainage	32	65	—	Jirku and Levitz (1969)
		(Excretion of ^{35}S)			
		3	62	—	
		(Excretion of ^{3}H)			
Female rabbit		—	84	—	Collins and Layne (1969)
		(Excretion of ^{35}S)			
		—	45	—	
[15-^{3}H]Estriol-3-[^{35}S]sulfate		(Excretion of ^{3}H)			
Human females	T-tube drainage	13	71	—	Emerman et al. (1967)
		(Excretion of ^{35}S)			
		1.5	72	—	
[16-^{14}C]Estriol-16α-glucuronide		(Excretion of ^{14}C)			A. A. Sandberg and Slaun- white (1965)
Human females	Normal	—	86–92	—	
(single i.v. dose)					
	T-tube drainage	0	79–91	—	
[6,7-^{3}H]Estriol-16α-[^{14}C]glucuronide		(Excretion of ^{3}H)			
Human females (various	Normal (i.v.)	—	70	—	
conditions, different	Normal (oral)	—	45	—	
routes of	Pregnant (i.v.)	—	60	—	
administration)	Normal (infusion)	—	85	—	Inoue et al. (1969a)
	Normal (portal vein)	—	50	—	
	Normal (instillation into ileum)	—	60	—	
[6,7-^{3}H]Estradiol-17-glucuronide		(Excretion of ^{3}H)			
Human females (one given	Normal	—	89	—	Hobkirk and Nilsen (1969a)
labeled glucuronide with		(Excretion of ^{3}H ^{14}C)			
[4-^{14}C]estradiol)		—	72	63	—	

TABLE II (*Continued*)

Steroid conjugate and species	Type of preparation		Percent of dose as metabolites in			Reference
			Bile	Urine	Feces	
Human female	Normal		(Excretion of ³H)			Hobkirk and Nilsen (1969b)
			—	85	—	
[6,7-³H] or [3-¹⁴C]Estriol-3-glucuronide						
Human females	Normal	[³H]	—	107	—	
(normal)(23 yr)(mixture		[¹⁴C]	—	104	—	
of both given i.v.)						
(After cholecystectomy)	T-tube	[³H]	0	106	—	Kirdani *et al.* (1969)
(83 yr)(mixture of both	drainage	[¹⁴C]	0	99	—	
given i.v.)						
Carcinoma of cervix)	Normal	[³H]	—	46	—	
(age 48 yr)([³H] conju-		[¹⁴C]	—	45	—	
gate into cubital vein,						
[¹⁴C]estriol into portal vein)						
[15-³H]Estriol-3-sulfate-16α-glucuronide			(Excretion of ³H)			
Human subjects (sex not	1. Normal		—	95	—	
specified)(mixture of			(Excretion of ³H)			
double conjugate and [¹⁴C]	2. Normal		—	68	—	Levitz and Katz (1968)
estriol-16α-glucuronide)			(Excretion of ¹⁴C)			
			—	87	—	
	3. 2-T-tube		21, 25	60, 45	—	
	drainage					
[6,7-³H]Estradiol-17α-3-[¹⁴C]glucuronide			(Excretion of ³H)			
Female rabbit	Normal		—	89	—	
			(Excretion of ¹⁴C)			D. G. Williamson and Layne (1970)
			—	70	—	
[6,7-³H]Estradiol-17α-3-[14ᶜ]glucoside			(Excretion of ³H)			
Female rabbit	Normal		—	79	—	
			(Excretion of ¹⁴C)			
			—	0	—	

B. PHENOLIC STEROIDS

1. *Estrogen Sulfates*

Jirku and Levitz (1969) administered doubly labeled estrone-3-sulfate to a woman with a T-tube drainage and determined the distribution of the tritium label in the conjugated metabolites in bile and urine. More metabolites of estrone are excreted in bile (32% of dose) than when estriol sulfate is administered (13% of dose).

Comparison of the ³⁵S:³H ratios showed that some of the administered conjugate had been excreted unchanged in the bile, but the greatest amount of estrone sulfate in bile had been produced by hydrolysis and subsequent sulfoconjugation (Fig. 8). However, the ^{35}S:^{3}H ratios of urinary metabolites indicated that more of the original conjugate was excreted by the kidney than by the liver. Figure 8 shows that the major conjugates in bile were sulfates and sulfoglucuronides, whereas in urine glucuronides and sulfates were the major conjugates. Of particular interest is the presence in bile of considerable quantities of the double conjugate, sulfo-N-acetylglucosaminide. Another finding of great importance was that about 26% of the metabolites in bile were the 15α-hydroxy derivatives of estrone and estradiol, and that these compounds were con-

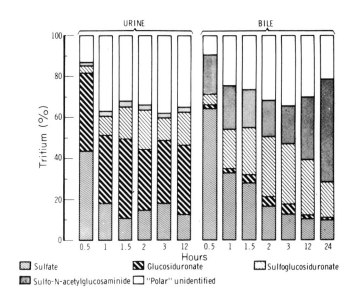

FIG. 8. Patterns of ^{3}H-labeled conjugates in urine and bile after the administration of [6,7-^{3}H]estrone-3-[S^{35}]sulfate to a woman with a bile fistula. From Jirku and Levitz (1969).

jugated mainly with N-acetylglucosamine and sulfate. This suggests that double conjugates are more avidly taken up by the liver and secreted into the bile canaliculi than are single conjugates.

The steriods isolated after hydrolysis of bile and urine are shown in Table III. The relative amounts are indicated: the original paper should be consulted for the actual amounts.

The fate of estrone-3-sulfate in the rabbit is discussed in Subsection 4.

Emerman *et al.* (1967) administered doubly labeled estriol sulfate to women, but the bile and urine samples were not thoroughly investigated.

TABLE III
METABOLITES IDENTIFIED IN BILE AND URINE IN 24 HOURS AFTER
ADMINISTRATION OF ESTRONE SULFATE TO A
HUMAN FEMALE SUBJECT[a]

Steroid	Present in bile[b]			Present in urine[b]		
	S	G	SG	S	G	SG
2-Methoxyestrone	+	++	0	+	+	+
Estrone	+++	+	0	++	+	0
15α-Hydroxyestrone	+	+	0	?	?	0
16-Epiestriol	?	+	+	++	+	++
Estriol	+	++	++	+++	+++	+++
15α-Hydroxyestradiol	+	0	0	+	0	0
"α-Ketols"	++	+	0	+	+	0
Estradiol	0	+	0	0	+	0
2-Hydroxyestrone	0	0	0	0	++	0
16α-Hydroxyestrone	0	0	+	0	0	++
16β-Hydroxyestrone	0	0	+	0	0	+

[a] From Jirku and Levitz (1969).
[b] S = sulfate: G = glucuronide: SG = sulfoglucuronide.

A striking feature of the results is that the proportion of the dose excreted in bile was less than half that excreted after administration of estrone sulfate. It can be seen from Table III that estriol was the major metabolite found in urine.

Examination of bile showed the presence of estriol-3-sulfate and estriol-16-glucuronide. These each accounted for only about 3% of the ^{3}H in bile: the major metabolite (75% of biliary ^{3}H) was estriol-3-sulfate-16-glucuronide. Urine contained the same metabolites of estriol but in different proportions, the values being sulfate, 22%; glucuronide, 47%; and double conjugate, 19%. Comparison of [35]S:[3]H ratios indicated that part of the originally administered estriol sulfate was excreted unchanged in bile and urine, particularly in the early samples.

It is of interest that the sulfoglucuronide double conjugate was excreted to a much greater extent in bile than in urine, thus providing further evidence for the suggestion that double conjugates are more selectively and/or more rapidly secreted into the bile canaliculi.

The failure to detect estriol-3-glucuronide in bile or urine is surprising, but this illustrates a drawback of studies of this kind since removal of bile for analysis prevented possible hydrolysis, conjugation with glucuronic acid, and reabsorption of estriol in the intestine. This cannot be the only explanation, since Adlercreutz (1962) found appreciable amounts of estriol glucuronide in human bile after administration of estriol. Therefore, the conjugation of the estriol with sulfate at C-3 may prevent the addition of glucuronic acid at this and other positions.

2. Estrogen Glucuronides

A. A. Sandberg and Slaunwhite (1965) studied the fate of ^{14}C-labeled estriol conjugated with unlabeled glucuronic acid in normal subjects and in patients with T-tube drainage of bile. In both groups radioactive metabolites were excreted almost completely in urine: no radioactivity was found in bile. This is in marked contrast to the distribution of radioactivity when free estriol is administered to human subjects (Table I). Radioactivity was excreted more rapidly in urine after administration of the conjugate than after administration of the free steroid. The patients with T-tube drainage also excreted 80% of the conjugate as urinary glucuronides, whereas the normal subjects excreted only 60–70% in this form. The major urinary metabolite was estriol-16α-glucuronide in both groups, suggesting that the administered glucuronide had undergone little metabolism or hydrolysis before excretion.

Inoue et al. (1969a) carried out a more extensive study using doubly labeled estriol glucuronide administered by different routes. No analyses of bile or feces were carried out. A full discussion of the results is outside the scope of this review, but some data relevant to the present discussion were obtained. When the conjugate was given orally the ^{3}H:^{14}C ratios of the urinary metabolites differed from those found after intravenous administration. In both instances the same two metabolites (estriol-16α-glucuronide and estriol-3-sulfate-16α-glucuronide) were major constituents of urine. However, the ^{3}H:^{14}C ratios in these metabolites indicated that more than 90% of the ingested estradiol glucuronide had been hydrolyzed, reconjugated, reabsorbed, and then excreted by the kidney. When the conjugate was injected into the portal venous system the ^{3}H:^{14}C ratios in the urinary estriol glucuronide and sulfoglucuronide were much the same as in the administered conjugate. Only 45% of the dose was recovered in this experiment. Støa and Levitz (1968) administered ^{14}C-labeled estriol into the duodenum and ^{3}H-labeled estriol almost simultaneously into the antecubital vein of a male patient; bile and urine were collected at intervals for 30 hours. They found that the excretion of ^{3}H (i.e., intravenously administered) radioactivity was more rapid in bile and urine than was ^{14}C, and that 20% of ^{3}H and 17% of ^{14}C were excreted in bile while 55% of ^{3}H and 76% of ^{14}C were excreted in urine. These findings support the results of Inoue et al. (1969a) in that metabolites were excreted mainly in urine despite the different routes of administration. In bile, about 80% of the radioactive metabolites were present as estriol-3-sulfate-16α-glucuronide, but in urine only a small amount of this double conjugate was excreted. This supports the view expressed above that double conjugates of estrogens may be more readily excreted into bile than single conjugates.

When Inoue et al. (1969a) instilled the doubly labeled estradiol conjugate into the intestine, radioactive metabolites slowly appeared in urine and the $^3H:^{14}C$ ratio remained unchanged for about 24 hours. In the next 24 hours the ratio suddenly increased, the excretion of estriol-3-sulfate-16α-glucuronide ceased, and estriol-3-glucuronide containing ^{14}C in the glucuronic acid moiety appeared. Such hydrolysis of estriol-16α-glucuronide and reconjugation at C-3 has also been reported by Goebelsmann et al. (1965). This transconjugation occurs in the intestine.

Inoue et al. (1969a) have suggested that the slow rate of formation of estriol-3-glucuronide is due to a slow secretion of estrogen metabolites into the intestine via the bile or succus entericus, and they have also suggested that the passage of estrogens into intestinal secretions (other than bile) may play an important role in the overall metabolism and excretion of estrogens.

The results further indicate that the liver is the main site for sulfoconjugation at C-3, and this is not affected by the presence of a hydroxy group at the 16α-position. However, the experiments also show that the liver is not the site of formation of estriol-3-glucuronide. When the original conjugate was administered via the portal vein, estriol-3-glucuronide could not be detected in urine.

Hobkirk and Nilsen (1969a,b) investigated the urinary estrogen conjugates after administration of the singly labeled [6,7-^3H]estradiol-17β-glucuronide to young women. The major compounds isolated were estrone-3-glucuronide, estradiol-17β-glucuronide and estradiol-3-glucuronide. Very small amounts of estrone-3-sulfate and estradiol-3-sulfate-17β-glucuronide were also detected. Since the glucuronic acid in the administered conjugates was unlabeled no conclusions can be drawn about the transfer of glucuronic acid from C-17 to C-3 of estrone or estradiol. Nor can it be concluded that sulfoconjugation at C-3 of the original conjugate occurred without prior hydrolysis of the glucuronic acid at C-17. Experiments with a doubly labeled conjugate are required to clarify these problems. It does seem, however, that conjugation of estradiol with glucuronic acid prevents the further metabolism of this steroid to estriol.

Kirdani et al. (1969) administered mixtures of ^3H- and ^{14}C-labeled estriol-3-glucuronide to 3 women. From one of these subjects bile was collected by T-tube drainage, but no radioactivity was found in her bile. In this subject and another, the mixture of estriol conjugate was given intravenously. The $^3H:^{14}C$ ratio in the metabolites in urine was much the same as that in the administered mixture. However, a third subject was given ³H-labeled conjugate in a peripheral vein and at about the same time free [16-¹⁴C]estriol was injected into the portal venous system during major abdominal surgery. The low total recovery of both ³H and ¹⁴C from the urine of this patient was attributed to the stress of surgery. A wide range of ³H:¹⁴C ratios (1.2–13.2) was found in the urinary metabolites. This indicated that metabolites of the free estriol and its conjugate were excreted by the kidney at different rates. Analysis of the estrogen conjugates in urine of the first two subjects showed that the ³H:¹⁴C ratios in successive urine samples remained virtually constant and were about the same as in the administered mixture. Therefore it was concluded that no appreciable hydrolysis and reconjugation of the estriol-3-glucuronide had occurred.

Thus, both the 16α- and 3-glucuronides of estriol do not undergo hydrolysis and reconjugation and are not excreted in bile to any appreciable extent when administered intravenously to human subjects (Kirdani et al., 1969; Inoue et al., 1969a). This is in marked contrast to the fate of estrone and estriol sulfates which are hydrolyzed and reconjugated and are excreted in bile (Jirku and Levitz, 1969; Emerman et al., 1967). The results of Hobkirk and Nilsen (1969a,b) do not provide sufficient evidence for firm conclusions to be drawn about the fate of estradiol-17-glucuronide. However, the information available at this time suggests that estrogen glucuronides tend to be protected from further metabolism by the presence of the glucuronic acid moiety, and such monoglucuronides are preferentially excreted by the kidney. The reasons for these observations require further investigation.

3. Estrogen Sulfoglucuronide

Levitz and Katz (1968) administered [15-³H]estriol-3-sulfate-16α-glucuronide to two groups of human subjects. In an intact subject 95% of the radioactivity was excreted in the urine in 24 hours. A second normal subject was given a mixture of the tritium-labeled double conjugate and [¹⁴C]estriol-16α-glucuronide. Two other subjects were given the double conjugate which was passed into the intestine via the T-tube carried by these subjects. The T-tube was clamped for 30 minutes to permit the conjugate to pass down the intestine so as not to contaminate subsequently collected bile samples. The radioactivity in bile and urine of these subjects is shown in Table II. Bile and urine were analyzed for estrogen conjugates, and the conjugates were hydrolyzed and the steroid moiety identified.

The patterns of excretion of conjugates in bile and urine were different in some ways and similar in others. Estriol-16α-glucuronide was present in both bile and urine in significant amounts. However, estriol-3-glucuronide was present only in urine, and estriol-3-sulfate-16α-glucuronide only in bile. The presence of this double conjugate in bile in significant amounts adds more support to the view expressed above that bile is the preferred route of excretion of double conjugates of estrogens.

The results show that enterohepatic circulation of the double conjugate administered to the patients had occurred, since about 80% of the intra-intestinal dose had been reabsorbed and excreted in bile and urine within 24 hours. Considerable metabolism of the conjugate had occurred during this time. Labeled estriol-3-glucuronide appeared in the urine only about 6–8 hours after the administration of the double conjugate. Administered estriol-3-glucuronide is rapidly and completely excreted in urine (Kirdani et al., 1969). The delay in the urinary excretion after intraintestinal administration is presumably due to the slow rate of the enterohepatic circulation and the hydrolysis and reconjugation of the estriol. The estriol-3-glucuronide must have been formed by hydrolytic removal of the 3-sulfate and 16α-glucuronide, but these experiments do not provide information about which position is hydrolyzed first nor whether trans-conjugation from the 16α- to the 3-position had occurred.

A puzzling feature of these results is that estriol-3-sulfo-16α-glu-curonide was not found in urine of the patients fitted with T-tubes, although it was found in the urine of the intact subjects. It was also found in urine after administration of free estriol and estriol-3-sulfate (Jirku and Levitz, 1969) and estriol-16α-glucuronide (A. A. Sandberg and Slaunwhite, 1965) to intact subjects. Levitz and Katz (1968) were also surprised when they were unable to detect estriol-3-glucuronide in bile or urine of subjects given estriol-3-sulfate. These two puzzling aspects of estrogen metabolism may be connected, and further work is required to resolve this problem.

4. Estrogen Glucoside

In rabbits estradiol-17α is a major urinary metabolite of estradiol-17β and estrone (see Velle, 1963, for references), and the major conjugate of this estrogen found in rabbit urine is estradiol-3-glucuronide-17α-N-acetylglucosaminide (Collins and Layne, 1969). Since the 3-glucosides of estrogens are formed by rabbit tissues in vitro, Williamson and Layne (1970) administered the 3-glucoside and 3-glucuronide of estradiol-17α to rabbits. As shown in Table II most of the administered tritium radioactivity was excreted in the urine in 24 hours. The animal given the glucuronide excreted most of the ^{14}C in urine, but no ^{14}C was detected in the urine of rabbits given the glucoside. After administration of the glucuronide the estradiol-3-glucuronide-17α-N-acetyl glucosaminide excreted in urine had a much higher $^{3}H:^{14}C$ ratio than the injected conjugate. Therefore, about half of the dose of conjugate was not hydrolyzed at C-3 prior to conjugation at C-17. After administration of the glucoside no ^{14}C was found in the urinary double conjugate, indicating that removal of the glucose at C-3 and reconjugation with glucuronic acid took place. The authors suggested that little, it any, unhydrolyzed glucoside was excreted in bile.

When doubly labeled estrone-3-sulfate was administered to a female rabbit the major conjugate in urine was estradiol-3-glucuronide-17α-N-glucosaminide which accounted for 60% of the urinary conjugates. Thus, the estrone sulfate had been hydrolyzed at C-3, a view supported by the excretion of ^{35}S in urine, and reduced and conjugated at C-17. Estradiol-3-sulfate-17α-N-acetylglucosaminide accounted for 25% of urinary conjugates, and had the same ^{3}H:^{35}S ratio as the original estrone-3-sulfate. Therefore, reduction and conjugation occurred without disturbance of the C-3 sulfate. Other conjugates, which accounted for 10% of the total in urine, were isolated; these were the 3-sulfates of estrone, estradiol-17α and estradiol-17β which had the same ^{3}H:^{35}S ratio as the injected conjugate.

C. General Conclusions

The work described in this section has revealed that considerable enterohepatic circulation, further metabolism and reconjugation of steroid conjugates occurs in man and probably other species. As yet only a few experiments with conjugates of neutral steroids have been carried out, and the results of future work with these conjugates will add much to an overall understanding of the biliary and fecal excretion of steroids.

The results obtained with the estrogen conjugates are of great interest. It is apparent from these results that the ultimate fate of estrogens secreted by the ovary, placenta, and adrenal cortex will depend on the nature of the steroid produced by hepatic and extrahepatic metabolism and on the type of conjugates formed. For instance, part of any estrone-3-sulfate formed in the liver (from estradiol) could return to the peripheral circulation and be excreted in urine, or it could be excreted directly into the bile. However, the greatest part would undergo further metabolism and conjugation; some of these metabolites would be excreted into the bile and some into the urine. That part excreted into bile could undergo deconjugation and/or transconjugation in the intestine during enterohepatic circulation. The reabsorbed metabolites might then undergo further metabolism in the liver, and the products could reenter the peripheral circulation to be excreted by the kidney or be reexcreted into bile (see for example Table III and Fig. 8). The possible ramifications of these metabolic and excretory pathways are extensive, and much thought will be required to sort out this complex and fascinating problem. As yet, little is known about the mechanism(s) which determines which steroid conjugates and what proportion of a particular conjugate will be excreted by the liver or the kidney.

At the present time knowledge about the excretion of estrogens in feces is so scanty as to be nonexistent. When feces are analyzed for phenolic steroids further complications will be introduced as a result of the metabolism of these steroids by the intestinal microflora.

VI. Steroids in Bile

The results of experiments with labeled steroids shown in Table I and discussed in Section IV proved that steroid metabolites are excreted, mainly in the conjugated form, in bile. The extent of this biliary excretion varies from species to species and is dependent also on the particular steroid administered. Experiments with labeled conjugates of steroids have confirmed and extended the results of work with free steroids (Table II, Section V). However, until recently only a few neutral steroids had been isolated from bile, and no quantitation of those steroids which are present in bile had been attempted (Section IV,A; see Taylor, 1965a, for references to early work).

The development of gas–liquid chromatography associated with mass spectrometry completely revolutionized the approach to the identification and quantitation of the small amounts of the large number of steroid metabolites present in biological media. These techniques have been brilliantly applied by Scandinavian workers to the study of steroids in bile and other biological media in subjects not dosed with steroids.

A. Neutral Steroids in Human Bile

Laatikainen and his colleagues have made an intensive study of the C_{19}- and C_{21}-steroids in the bile of human adult male and nonpregnant female subjects. The results obtained are summarized in Table IV. However, this table provides only an indication of the steroids which have been detected and fully characterized. The data on the quantitative aspects of this work are too extensive to be summarized here. The original papers should be consulted for the full details. As an example of the extent of the work, the investigations of Laatikainen (1970c) will be discussed in some detail. He measured the amounts of many of the steroids shown in Table IV in bile obtained by T-tube drainage from 5 males and 5 nonpregnant females, and also in bile from the gallbladder of 5 nonpregnant females.

A variety of neutral steroids was found in these bile samples, but there was a wide individual variation in the amounts of particular steroids. For

TABLE IV
NEUTRAL STEROIDS IN FISTULA AND GALLBLADDER BILE OF ADULT HUMAN MALE AND NONPREGNANT FEMALE SUBJECTS: NO EXOGENOUS STEROID ADMINISTERED[a]

Steroid	Present as[b]		
	MoS	DiS	Gluc
$C_{19}O_2$			
Dehydroepiandrosterone	+	−	+
3α-Hydroxy-5-androsten-17-one	+	−	+
Androsterone	+	−	+
Etiocholanolone	+	−	+
5α-Androstanediols: 3α,17α	+	+	−
3α,17β	+	+	+
5β-Androstanediol: 3α,17β	−	−	+
5-Androstenediols: 3β,17α	+	+	−
3β,17β	+	+	−
$C_{19}O_3$			
16α-Hydroxydehydroepiandrosterone	+	+	−
16β-Hydroxydehydroepiandrosterone	+	+	−
18-Hydroxyandrosterone	+	+	−
5α-Androstane-3α,16α,17β-triol	+	+	−
5-Androstenes: 3β,16α-diol-17-one	+	+	−
3β,16β-diol-17-one	+	+	−
3α,16α,17β-triol	+	+	−
3β,16α,17β-triol	+	+	−
3β,16β,17α-triol	−	+	−
$C_{21}O_2$			
Pregnenolone	+	−	+
5-Pregnene-3β,20α-diol	+	+	+
Pregnanolone			+
5α-Pregnane-3α,20α-diol	+	+	+
5β-Pregnane-3α,20α-diol	+	+	+
$C_{21}O_3$			
5α-Pregnanetriol: 3α,17α,20α	+	−	−
3α,16α,20α	?	?	?
5β-Pregnanetriol: 3α,17α,20α	+	−	+
3α,21-Dihydroxy-5β-pregnan-20-one	+	+	+
5-Pregnenetriols: 3α,17α,20α	+	−	−
3β,17α,20α	+	+	+
$C_{21}O_4$			
3α,11β,21-Trihydroxy-5α-pregnan-20-one	+	−	−
3α,11β,21-Trihydroxy-5β-pregnan-20-one	+	−	−
3α,11β-Dihydroxy-5β-pregnan-11,20-dione	+	−	−

[a] Data from Laatikainen (1970a,b,c); Laatikainen and Víhko (1969a,b); Laatikainen *et al.* (1968).
[b] MoS = monosulfate; DiS = disulfate; Gluc = glucuronide.

example, the amounts of etiocholanolone per 100 ml of bile excreted as glucuronide ranged from 4.0 to 24.4 μg in males, from 1.4 to 32.2 μg in fistula bile from females, and from 60 to 220 μg in gallbladder bile. (The higher amounts of steroids found in gallbladder bile are to be expected because of the concentration of bile which occurs in the gallbladder.) Less etiocholanolone was excreted as monosulfate in the 3 types of bile; the values were $<$1–5.7 for males, $<$1–6.5 for female fistula-bile and 3.8–46.0 for gallbladder bile. It is of interest that there did not appear to be any statistical difference between the amounts of etiocholanolone excreted by the male and female subjects. However, there appeared to be a sex difference in the amounts of androsterone excreted in fistula bile: the values were 2.9–10.7 μg (males) and 1.4–10.5 μg (females) as glucuronide and 5.7–37.0 μg (males) and $<$1–15.7 μg (females). The precursor of these two 17-oxosteroids in bile would presumably have been testosterone, at least in the male subjects. However, the major 17-oxosteroid in fistula bile was dehydroepiandrosterone, which was excreted mainly as the monosulfate. The values for males and females were 11.3–149 μg and 5.6–68.0 μg, respectively.

Another puzzling and interesting sex difference was observed in the amounts of the major $C_{21}O_2$ steroids (pregnanolone and "pregnanediols") in fistula bile. The mean concentrations per 100 ml were 210 μg (males) and 80 μg (females). Thus male bile contains nearly 3 times as much of these steroids, usually considered to be metabolites of progesterone, than does female bile. A possible explanation of this apparently anomalous finding is that in women those metabolites of progesterone are excreted to a greater extent by the kidney, whereas in men bile is the preferred route of excretion. Carefully controlled balance studies would be required to resolve this problem.

Assuming a normal bile production of about 1 liter per day, men excrete about 13 mg and women about 6.5 mg total neutral steroids in bile in 24 hours. Considerable amounts of $C_{21}O_4$ steroids are excreted in bile: these amount to about 1.5 mg/100 ml in fistula bile. However, these steroids are probably metabolites of adrenocortical hormones, the production of which may have been higher than normal because of the stress of the surgery undergone by the subjects with T-tube drainage. Nevertheless, the presence of these steroids in human bile is contrary to what might be expected from the results of administering labeled corticosteroids to human subjects (Table I). It is possible that the administered steroids did not equilibrate with the total body pool of endogenous corticosteroids and so were metabolized and excreted in slightly different but significant ways. Such discrepancies need to be borne in mind in interpreting the results of both types of experiments.

Laatikainen and Víhko (1969b) discussed the excretion of steroid sulfates in bile and urine. They concluded that sulfates of 17-oxosteroids are preferentially excreted in urine, those of androstanediols are excreted more or less equally in bile and urine, and those of 5-pregnene-3β,20α-diol are preferentially excreted in bile. Laatikainen (1970c) has suggested that 18-hydroxyandrosterone may be preferentially excreted into bile, since this steroid has not been detected in normal human urine. It is found in urine after administration of androsterone and during pregnancy. Several steroids which are excreted mainly as disulfates into bile are found in urine as glucuronides, and Laatikainen (1970c) has put forward the hypothesis that the formation of a sulfate diconjugate will favor biliary excretion whereas glucuronides will tend to be excreted by the kidney. He has also suggested that the structure of the steroid moiety to some extent determines the type of conjugate excreted in bile. Thus, $C_{19}O_2$ and $C_{21}O_2$ steroids with a 3α-hydroxy-5β structure are excreted mainly as glucuronides, while 3α-hydroxy-5α and 3β-hydroxy-Δ^5 steroids are excreted mainly as sulfates. These proposals are supported to some extent by experiments with labeled steroids, e.g., the isolation of pregnanediol and pregnanolone from the glucuronide fraction of human bile and urine after administration of progesterone (Section IV,A; Wiest et al., 1958).

B. PHENOLIC STEROIDS IN BILE OF ANIMALS AND MAN

Table V shows the estrogens isolated from bile of animals and man. Pearlman et al. (1947) isolated approximately 60 μg of estrone from 100 ml of gallbladder bile of pregnant cows, and estimated that 7 μg/ 100 ml of estradiol were also present. Adlercreutz et al. (1960) assayed the estrogen content of human pregnancy bile by the colorimetric method of Brown (1955). They found great individual variations among the different women, the estriol values ranging from 1.6 to 604 μg/100 ml. They estimated that the mean value was of the order of 72 μg/100 ml in pregnancy bile at term, and that there was at least 30 times as much estriol as estrone or 16-epiestriol. However, using gas–liquid chromatography, Adlercreutz and Luukkainen (1965a) identified estradiol-17α but not the 17β-epimer in human pregnancy bile. They suggested that the estrogenic activity observed by Pearlman et al. (1947) was due to estradiol-17α. The estrone present in the bile would also contribute to the estrogenic activity measured by bioassay.

Adlercreutz and Luukkainen (1965b) used gas–liquid chromatography–mass spectrometry to study the estrogen content of bile from a woman in the late stages of pregnancy and identified the 8 estrogens shown in Table V in the glucuronide fraction. No estrone was found in this fraction. Other investigations have shown that 16α-hydroxyestrone, 16-oxoestradiol, and 16-epiestriol are present in relatively large amounts in human bile

TABLE V

ESTROGENS IDENTIFIED IN BILE: NO EXOGENOUS STEROID ADMINISTERED

Source of bile	Type of conjugate	Steroid	Reference
Pregnant cow gallbladder	?	Estrone	Pearlman et al. (1947)
	Unconjugated	Estradiol-17α	Adlercreutz and Luukkainen (1965a)
	Unconjugated	Estrone	
Newborn calf gallbladder	?	Estradiol-17α	Rommel and Zschintzsch (1965)
Pregnant women, duodenal intubation	"Conjugates" hydrolyzed by hot acid	Estrone Estriol (Estradiol-17β) (16-Epiestriol)	Adlercreutz et al. (1960)
	Glucuronide and/or sulful- glucuronide	Estradiol-17α Extradiol-17β Estriol 16-Oxoestradiol 16α-Hydroxyestrone 16,17-Epiestriol 16-Epiestriol 17-Epiestriol	Adlercreutz and Luukkainen (1965b)
Human subjects T-tube drainage Men and postmeno- pausal women Nonpregnant women	Sulfate Glucuronide Glucuronide Sulfate Glucuronide Sulfate Glucuronide	Estrone Estriol Estradiol-17β Estrone Estriol (Estradiol-17β) (16-Epiestriol)	Adlercreutz (1962)

after administration of various estrogens (Adlercreutz and Luukkainen, 1967).

Estrone occurs in human bile mainly as the sulfate, estradiol mainly as glucuronide, and estriol mainly as the 3-sulfate-16α-glucuronide. Estriol-16α-glucuronide is the major urinary metabolite of estriol, but small amounts of this conjugate have also been detected in bile (Adlercreutz, 1970).

Adlercreutz and Luukkainen (1967) determined the amounts of estrone, estradiol, and estriol in fistula bile of men and nonpregnant women. In men only small amounts of estrogen were found. Estriol glucuronide was the major component (approximately 0.6 μg/100 ml) ; the amount in bile from a nonpregnant woman was about 1.6 μg/100 ml. The relative amounts of the 3 estrogens were the same for men and nonpregnant women, the ratios being estrone (1), estradiol (0.55), and estriol (7.1). The corresponding ratios for late pregnancy bile were 1, 0.32, and 54. The mean values for the 3 estrogens in late pregnancy bile were estrone 7, estradiol 1, estriol 375 μg/100 ml. The other estrogens were not determined in these women. However, for comparison of the excretion of estrogens in bile and urine, the following 8 steroids were determined after administration of estradiol to a male subject: estrone, 2-methoxyestrone, estradiol, 16α-hydroxyestrone, 16-oxoestradiol, estriol, 16-epiestriol, and 17-epiestriol. The excretion patterns in bile and urine were different. During the first 12 hours after administration of estradiol 30% of the total dose excreted was present in the bile, but in later samples the proportion of metabolites in bile became increasingly smaller. The most striking difference between the metabolites in bile and urine was with respect to the excretion of 16α-hydroxyestrone. Over the first 12 hours it was the major metabolite in bile, but was a relatively minor metabolite in urine. However, the proportion of this steroid in bile decreased and could not be detected after 36 hours. In urine, on the other hand, the steroid became a major metabolite between 36 and 48 hours. Other less dramatic changes were noted in the other steroids in bile and urine. A deficiency of this experiment was that only 19.3% of the administered estradiol could be accounted for as urinary and biliary metabolites in 48 hours. The inability to account for about 70–80% of the dose illustrates the value of the use of labeled steroids in this type of work. However, the results are in accord with those obtained using labeled steroids and conjugates (Sections IV and V,B).

C. GENERAL CONCLUSIONS

Biliary and enterohepatic circulation play a major role in the metabolism and ultimate excretion of estrogen metabolites. Therefore, it is very important to bear in mind the limitations imposed upon the interpretation of results obtained from analyses of steroids excreted in bile. The steroids listed in Tables IV and V are not necessarily eliminated from the body in the forms or in the amounts described. Enterohepatic circulation and the actions of enzymes in intestinal muscosa and microflora play a major role in determining the nature and amount of steroids excreted in the feces. The neutral steroids shown in Table IV should be compared with those in Table VI.

VII. STEROIDS IN FECES

The application of gas–liquid chromatography–mass spectrometry has provided a vast amount of data about the steroids excreted in feces of human adults and babies and of rats. Information about the role of enzymes of the intestine and of the gut microflora in steroid metabolism has also been obtained from these studies.

A. Neutral Steroids in Feces of Human Adults

The neutral steroids identified in feces are listed in Table VI and, formidable as the task may be, this table should be compared with Table IV.

1. Normal Males

Laatikainen and Víhko (1970a,b,c) have studied the steroids in pooled feces from 4 normal men. Eriksson and Gustafsson (1971) studied the steroids in separate samples of feces from 2 men. Some differences in the results of these investigations may be seen in Table VI. For example, Laatikainen and Víhko identified several steroids which were not found by Eriksson and Gustafsson; these include epiandrosterone, etiocholanolone, 5α-pregnane-3α,20α-diol and many others. Conversely, Eriksson and Gustafsson identified steroids which had not been found by Laatikainen and Víhko; e.g., 3 isomeric 5α-androstanetriols and a number of others. These differences probably represent variations between the groups of subjects. Eriksson and Gustafsson (1971) found that one of their male subjects excreted a number of steroids not excreted by the other. These steroids were 5α- and 5β-androstane-3α,16α,17β-triols, 5α-androstane-3β,16α,17β-triol, and 3α,20β-dihydroxy-5β-pregnan-11-one. The variation is probably at least partly the result of differences in the intestinal microflora of the subjects.

The most striking difference between steroids found in bile and feces is that no glucuronides are found in feces. Some of the steroids are excreted only in the free form, some as monosulfates and only one (5β-pregnane-3α,20α-diol) as disulfate, and some are excreted in both the free and conjugated state. This suggests that differential hydrolysis of steroid conjugates occurs as they travel down the gastrointestinal tract.

Another major difference between biliary and fecal steroids is that large amounts of 3β-hydroxy-Δ⁵ and 3α-hydroxy-5α and 3α-hydroxy-5β steroids are excreted in bile. In feces the steroids are mostly saturated and have the 3β-hydroxy-5α or 3α-hydroxy-5β conformation. These differences are due to the action of microbial enzymes. Schubert et al. (1962) found that, under anaerobic conditions, microorganisms of human feces were able to metabolize 17-oxosteroids. The 3β-hydroxy-Δ⁵ group was reduced to compounds with the 5β-conformation, and epimerizing enzymes tended to produce steroids with an equatorial hydroxyl group. Eriksson and Gustafsson (1971) incubated a number of steroids with the intestinal contents of the ileostoma of a colectomized patient. They found that enzymes were present which could produce the following changes: 16α-

TABLE VI

Neutral Steroids Identified in Feces of Adult Human Male and Nonpregnant and Pregnant Female Subjects: No Exogenous Steroid Administered[a]

Steroid	Present as[b]								
	(a)			(b)			Pregnant		
	Free	MoS	DiS	Free	MoS	DiS	Free	MoS	DiCon
$C_{19}O_2$									
Dehydroepiandrosterone	−	+	−	−	+(F)	−	−	−	−
Epiandrosterone	+	−	−	−	−	−	−	−	−
Etiocholanolone	+	−	−	−	−	−	−	−	−
5α-Androstanediols: 3α,17α	−	+	−	−	−	−	+	−	−
3α,17β	−	+	−	−	−	−	+	−	−
3β,17α	−	+	−	−	−	−	−	−	−
3β,17β	+	+	−	+(M)	+(M)	−	+	−	−
5β-Androstanediols: 3α,17α	−	+	−	+(M)	+(M)	−	+	−	−
3α,17β	−	−	−	+(M)	+(M)	−	−	−	−
3β,17β	−	−	+	−	−	−	+	−	−
5-Androstenediols: 3α,17β	−	+	+	+(M)	+(F)	−	−	−	−
3β,17α	−	+	−	+(M)	+(F)	−	−	−	−
3β,17β	−	+	−	+(M)	−	−	−	−	−
$C_{19}O_3$									
5α-Androstanetriols: 3α,16α,17β	−	−	−	+(M)	−	−	−	−	−
3β,16α,17β	−	−	−	+(M)	−	−	−	−	−
5β-Androstanetriol: 3α,16α,17β	−	−	−	+(M)	+(F)	−	−	−	−
5-Androstenetriol: 3β,16β,17α	−	−	−	−	−	−	−	−	−
$C_{21}O_2$									
Pregnenolone	−	+	−	+(F)	−	−	+	−	−
Pregnanol-20-ones: 5α(17α),3β-ol	−	−	−	−	−	−	+	−	−
5α(17β),3β-ol	−	−	−	−	−	−	+	−	−
5β(17α),3α-ol	−	−	−	+(F)	−	−	+	−	−
5β(17β),3α-ol	−	−	−	−	−	−	+	−	−
5α(17β),3α-ol	−	−	−	−	−	−	+	−	−

3α,20β		−						− +
3β,20α		+			+(M) −		+(M) −	+ +
3β,20β	+	−			−		−	+ −
5β-Pregnanediols: 3α,20α	+	+			+(M) (F)		+(M) (F) +(M)	+ + +
3β,20α	+ +	+ +			−		+(F)	+
5-Pregnanediols: 3α,20α	+ +	+			−		−	−
3β,20α	−				−		−	−
C₂₁O₃								
3α,20β-Dihydroxy-5β-pregnan-11-one					+(M)		−	−
5α-Pregnanediol-20-ones: 3α,16α					−		−	+
3β,16α					−		+(F)	+
5β-Pregnanediol-20-ones: 3α,16α					−		−	+
3β,16α					−		−	+
5α-Pregnanetriols: 3α,16α,20α	+				+(M) (F)		−	−
3β,16α,20β					−		−	+
3α,16α,20β					−		−	+
3β,16α,20β					−		−	+
3α,16α,20α	+				+(M)		−	−
3α,17α,20α					−		−	+ +
3α,20α,21					−		−	+
3β,20α,21					−		−	−
5β-Pregnanetriols: 3α,16α,20α	+				+(M) (F)		+(M) (F)	+
3β,16α,20α					−		+(F)	+
3α,16α,20β					−		+(F)	+
3β,16α,20β					−		−	+
3α,17α,20α					−		−	+
5-Pregnenetriols: 3β,16α,20β					−		−	−
3β,17α,20α					−		−	−

a (a) Laatikainen and Vihko (1970a,b,c), male subjects only; (b) Eriksson and Gustafsson (1971), male subjects (M) and nonpregnant female subjects (F); pregnant, Eriksson *et al.* (1970).

b Free = unconjugated; MoS = monosulfate; DiS = disulfate; DiCon = diconjugates, probably sulfates.

and 21-dehydroxylation; conversion of Δ^{16}-C_{21} steroids into 17α-pregnane derivatives; removal of the side chain of 17α,21-dihydroxy-$C_{21}O_5$ steroids to yield androstane-3,11,17-triols. The role of the intestinal microflora in metabolizing steroids is discussed more fully in Section VII,D, which is concerned with fecal steroids of germfree and conventional rats. However, it should be stressed that the microflora of rats are likely to be different from those of man. Indeed, the intestinal microflora of human subjects are probably different in different individuals and even vary from day to day in the same subject (Section VII,E).

Another possible reason for the differences between biliary and fecal steroids is that some of the metabolites, including glucuronides, are reabsorbed from the intestine. This has been discussed in Section IV,C. These considerations also apply to the fecal steroids of nonpregnant and pregnant women to be discussed below.

No data on the amounts of excreted steroids were reported.

2. Normal Female

Eriksson and Gustafsson (1971) studied the steroids in the feces of one nonpregnant woman. Some of the steroids identified were not found in feces of males, and some steroids present in male feces were not detected in female feces. The male subjects excreted most of the steroids in the free form, but the steroids in the feces of this female subject were present mainly as monosulfates. These differences are probably not the result of a sex difference, but are more likely to be due to the particular intestinal microflora of this subject.

No data on the amounts of excreted steroids were given.

3. Pregnant Women

Eriksson et al. (1970) studied the fecal steroids of 2 women, one of whom was in the 32nd week of pregnancy, the other in the 37th week. The steroids listed in the last column of Table VI were identified. It can be seen that the excretion pattern is markedly different from that of the males and nonpregnant female, particularly with respect to the $C_{21}O_2$ and $C_{21}O_3$ steroids. Partial quantitation of the steroids excreted by one subject was carried out; the results are shown in Table VII. The 5β:5α ratios were about 1.5 for pregnanediols, 2.4 for 17β-pregnanolones, and 3.9 for 17α-pregnanolones. Steroids with the 5α-conformation had mainly a 3β-hydroxyl group, and the 5β mainly a 3α-hydroxyl.

These results show that the fecal excretion plays an important role in the elimination from the body of steroids secreted by pregnant women. The 24-hour urinary excretion of pregnanediol isomers in the last tri-

TABLE VII
APPROXIMATE AMOUNTS OF DIFFERENT CLASSES OF STEROID IN FECES OF A
PREGNANT WOMAN (WEEK 37) (MG/24 HR)[a]

Steroids	Free[b]	MoS	Dicon
Androstanediols	1.4	—	—
Pregnanolones	4.3	—	—
Pregnanediols	18.7	0.5	0.3
Pregnanetriols	6.4	0.8	0.7
	30.8	1.3	1.0

[a] From Eriksson et al. (1970).
[b] Free = unconjugated; MoS = monosulfate; Dicon = diconjugates; probably sulfates.

mester of pregnancy is 30–40 mg (Wotiz, 1963). Table VII shows that about 20 mg of these isomers are excreted in feces over 24 hours. In the study of pregnancy feces glucuronides were not investigated, but in the light of current knowledge about fecal excretion of steroids it is unlikely that these conjugates will be found in large amounts in feces.

Calvin and Lieberman (1962) isolated 3α-hydroxy-5β,17α-pregnan-20-one from human urine and have shown that this steroid is a metabolite of 16α-hydroxyprogesterone. The 17α-pregnanolone is a major constituent of feces, and it is possible that the steroid undergoes partial enterohepatic circulation and subsequent renal excretion.

In pregnancy feces the two predominant isomers of the pregnanediols and pregnanolones have the 3α,5β- and 3β,5α-conformations. However, in bile (Table IV) the major isomers have the 3α,5α- and 3α,5β-conformations. Thus, the steroids excreted into the intestine in bile appear to undergo epimerization. A number of 5α- and 5β-pregnanetriols are found in pregnancy feces. In meconium (see also Section VII,C) 5α- and 5β-pregnane-3α,20α,21-triols have been found. However, only the 5α-epimers of these triols are found in pregnancy feces. Therefore it seems likely that the 5α-epimer is derived in the mother and the 5β-epimer in the fetoplacental unit.

The hepatic and biliary function, and possibly the intestinal microflora, will be affected to some extent by the large amounts of steroids produced during pregnancy. The extent of these effects may vary in different women and at different times in the same woman. This important finding that neutral steroids are excreted in human bile and feces and in feces of pregnant women in amounts approaching those found in urine must be taken into account in clinical assessment of pregnancy by analysis of urinary steroids.

B. Neutral Steroids of Human Infants

Table VIII shows the steroids which have been identified in feces of male and female human babies up to one year of age. A number of other steroids was also detected, but because of the small amounts present the

TABLE VIII

NEUTRAL STEROIDS IDENTIFIED IN FECES OF HUMAN MALE AND FEMALE INFANTS: NO EXOGENOUS STEROID ADMINISTERED[a]

Present as [b]			Steroid		Age of infants (weeks)[c]		
MoS	DiS	Dicon			2–8	9–24	25–52
			$C_{19}O_2$				
+			Dehydroepiandrosterone		ND	ND	ND
+			5-Androstene-3β,17β-diol	U	+	+	
+			5ξ-Androstane-3ξ,17ξ-diol		ND	ND	ND
			$C_{19}O_3$				
+	+	+	5-Androstenes: 3β,16α-diol-17-one	U	+	+	
	+	+	3β,16β-diol-17-one	U	+	+	
+			3β,17β,diol-16-one	U		ND	
+			3β,16β,17α-triol		+	+	
+	+	+	3β,16α,17β-triol	U		ND	
			3β,16β,17β-triol	U	+	+	
+			3ξ,16ξ-Dihydroxy-5ξandrostan-17-one			ND	
			$C_{21}O_2$				
+			Pregnenolone		+	+	
+			3β-Hydroxypregn-5,16-dien-20-one		+	+	
+	+	+	5-Pregnene-3β,20α-diol		+	+	+
+			3ξ-Hydroxy-5ξ-pregnan-20-one			ND	
+			3ξ-Hydroxy-5ξ,17α-pregnan-20-one			ND	
			$C_{21}O_3$				
+			3α,16α,Dihydroxy-5β-pregnan-20-one			ND	
+	+	+	5-Pregnenes: 3β,16α-diol-20-one	U	+	+	
+			3β,16β-diol-20-one			ND	
+			3β,16α,20α-triol		+	+	
	+		3β,17α,20α-triol		+	+	+
+			3β,20α,21-triol		+		
+			3ξ,20ξ-diol-16-one			ND	
+			5ξ-Pregnane-3ξ,16ξ,20ξ-triol			ND	
+			5ξ-Pregnane-3ξ,16ξ,20ξ-triol			ND	
			$C_{21}O_4$				
+			5-Pregnene-3β,16α,20α,21-tetrol		+		
+			5-Pregnene-3β,16ξ,17α,20ξ-tetrol			ND	

[a] J. A. Gustafsson et al. (1969, 1970). U: present in urine of infants (Mitchell, 1967).
[b] MoS = monosulfate: DiS = disulfate: Dicon = diconjugated, probably disulfate.
[c] ND, not determined.

confirmation of the substituents could not be ascertained. These steroids included: 5-androstane-3,17-diol(s);   3,16-dihydroxy-5-androstan-17-one(s);   3-hydroxy-5-pregnan-20-one(s);   3-hydroxy-5,17α-pregnan-20-one(s);   5-pregnane-3,16,20-triols (J. A. Gustafsson et al., 1969).

The predominant steroids found in infant feces are 5-androstenes and 5-pregnenes with a 3β-hydroxy and an α- or β-hydroxyl at C-16. This type of steroid is also predominant in the urine of human infants. The adrenal cortex of the human infant has a poor ability to convert Δ^5-3β-hydroxy steroids into Δ^4-3-oxo compounds. Also, the infant adrenal cortex and liver have high 16-hydroxylase activity, particularly for the 16α-conformation (Mitchell, 1967). Some steroids were found in infant feces which have been identified in urine: the principal steroids of this type were 5-pregnene-3β,20α,21-triol and 5-pregnene-3β,16α,20α,21-tetrol. The former compound could have been produced by further metabolism of the corresponding 20-oxo compound which is found in the urine of infants.

Insofar as fecal samples can be equated with 24-hr urine collections, quantitative studies on feces indicate that infants excrete almost as much steroid in the feces as in the urine. A comparison of Table IX and Table VIII shows a marked difference in excretion of steroids in meconium and in infant feces. Furthermore, qualitative and quantitative changes occur in the pattern of steroid as the age of the infant increases. J. A. Gustafsson et al. (1970) have studied the amounts of steroids shown in Table VIII in batches of infant feces: the batches were obtained from infants from 2–4, 4–6, to 20–24 weeks old.

Difficulties in obtaining comparable batches of feces and differences between babies do not permit any statistical analysis of the data, but some very marked differences were observed. In infants up to about 8 weeks old, the feces contain relatively large amounts (hundreds of micrograms) of most of the steroids listed in Table VIII. For example, 3β,16α-dihydroxy-5-pregnen-20-one is found in amounts ranging from 380 to 1620 μg per 100 gm feces (wet weight) up to the eighth week of life. After this, the amount of this steroid falls abruptly and is present at a level of 25 μg per 100 gm of feces from infants 20–24 weeks old. The urinary excretion of this steroid by infants follows a similar pattern (Mitchell, 1967), and the degree of change is of the same order as that found in fecal excretion. This change reflects the decreasing 16α-hydroxylase activity in tissues of older infants. As this activity decreases there is an increase in 17α-hydroxylation and in the reduction of the C-20 oxo to a 20α-hydroxyl group. Therefore, although the total amount of steroids found in feces in infants decreases with age, the ratio of 20α-hydroxy to 20-oxo compounds increases. A striking feature of these results is that in the first few weeks of life the baby excretes massive amounts of a wide variety of steroids, but in the second 6 months of life only two steroids are excreted in feces in detectable amounts.

Some of these changes may be due to metabolism in the intestinal tract of fecal steroids, but the extent of such metabolism cannot be assessed. Some hydrolysis of steroid metabolites by intestinal or microbial hydrolases does occur in infants, but it seems that such deconjugation is restricted to ring A saturated steroids, and these are present in only very small amounts in the free form.

Table VIII also shows the type of conjugate found in feces. In general, steroids conjugated in a particular manner are found in the same form in feces and urine. The steroids found in the feces (and urine) of infants are conjugated only with sulfuric acid. The absence of glucuronides may reflect the low capacity of the neonatal liver to form steroid (and other) glucuronides, and also may be due to the presence of steroids which are more readily converted into sulfates (Mitchell, 1967).

These qualitative and quantitative studies strongly indicate that fecal excretion of steroid metabolites is of major importance in very young babies, and so must be taken into account in assessment of urinary studies in diseases involving adrenal function in the baby.

The occurrence of such large quantities of steroids in feces raises the interesting question why so much steroid is excreted by this route by the young baby. There are a number of possible explanations. The structure of the infant liver and biliary system may favor biliary excretion of steroid metabolites; the immature infant intestine may not permit a sufficiently high degree of enterohepatic circulation of steroid metabolites to occur; the immature infant kidney may not be able to clear the large amounts of steroid metabolites presented to it and so the metabolites are diverted to the biliary system for excretion. Other factors may be involved, but further investigations will be required to answer these questions.

Another problem is to explain the function of the precursors of these metabolites which are secreted mainly by the adrenal cortex and presumably play an important role in the development of the infant. This problem has been well discussed by Mitchell (1967).

C. Steroids in Meconium of Human Babies

Table IX shows the steroids which have been identified in meconium, a medium which has not been so extensively studied as other excreta. The estrogens and pregnanediols are almost certainly derived from the mother and placenta since pregnanediol has not been found in feces of 2-week-old babies. Pregnant women excrete pregnanediol conjugated both as sulfate and glucuronide, but the steroid is found in meconium mainly as sulfate

TABLE IX
STEROIDS IDENTIFIED IN MECONIUM OF HUMAN BABIES: NO EXOGENOUS
STEROID ADMINISTERED TO BABY OR MOTHER

Steroid	Present as			Reference
	Free	MoS	Gluc	
Estrogens				
Estriol	+	+	+	Menini and Diczfalusy (1960, 1961) Eneroth and Gustafsson (1969)
Estrone				
Estradiol-17β				
Estradiol-17α				
11-Dehydroestradiol-17α	Free and "conjugated"			Luukkainen et al. (1970)
16α-hydroxyestrone				
16-Oxoestradiol				
15α-Hydroxyestrone				
Estriol				
16β-Hydroxyestrone	"Conjugated"			
Epiestriol				
$C_{19}O_2$				
Dehydroepiandrosterone	?			Francis et al. (1960)
$C_{19}O_3$				
Androstenes: 3β,16α-diol-17-one	—	+	—	Eneroth and Gustafsson (1969)
3β,16β,17α-triol	?			Shackleton et al. (1970)
$C_{21}O_2$				
5α-Pregnane-3α,20α-diol	+	—	+	Francis and Kinsella (1966)
5β-Pregnane-3α,20α-diol	+	—	+	
3α-Hydroxy-5β-pregn-16-en-20-one	—	—	+	Francis et al. (1962)
5-Pregnene-3β,20α-diol	—	+	—	Eneroth and Gustafsson (1969)
$C_{21}O_3$				
3β,16α-Dihydroxy-5-pregnen-20-one	—	+	—	Eneroth and Gustafsson (1969)
5α-Pregnane-3α,20α,21-triol	?			Gustafsson (in Eriksson et al., 1970)
5β-Pregnane-3α,20α,21-triol	?			

^{a} Free = unconjugated; MoS = monosulfate; Gluc = glucuronide.

(5.3 mg/kg wet wt of meconium) and only 0.17 mg/kg and 0.07 mg/kg can be detected as glucuronide in meconium from male and female babies, respectively. A steroid which also has been isolated in large amounts from meconium is 3α-hydroxy-5β-pregn-16-en-20-one: hydrolysis of meconium by β-glucuronidase yielded 1.3 mg of this steroid per kilogram. This steroid may originate from the baby, initially as 3α,16α-dihydroxy-5β-

pregnan-20-one, a major component of the feces of young babies (Table VIII). However, the latter steroid is present in infant feces as the sulfate, whereas the former is present mainly as the glucuronide in meconium. The major 5-androstenetriol, accounting for 90% of epimeric androstenetriols in meconium, is the 3β,16β,17α-triol. The other epimers are present only in trace amounts. However, the pattern changes when the baby begins to produce feces, presumably due to microbial enzymes. The major androstenetriol then becomes the 3β,16α,17β epimer, which accounts for 66% of these triols in infant feces. The cis-isomers (16α,17α and 16β,17β) found in feces are undoubtedly formed by microbial epimerizing enzymes, since these isomers are not found in the blood, urine, or meconium of babies.

In addition to the steroids listed in Table IX, Eneroth and Gustafsson (1969) found that various isomers of pregnane-3,20-diols, 3,16α-dihydroxypregnan-20-ones and pregnane-3,20,21-triols were present in meconium.

Most of the estrogens identified by Luukkainen et al. (1970) have also been found in pregnancy urine, cord plasma, amniotic fluid, and maternal plasma by Adlercreutz and Luukkainen (1970).

Further investigations are required to establish the site of production and metabolic changes undergone by steroids found in meconium.

D. Steroids in Feces of Germfree and Conventional Rats

1. Steroids in Bulked Feces of Male and Female Germfree and
Conventional Rats

B. E. and J. A. Gustafsson and co-workers have investigated the role of the intestinal microflora in the excretion of neutral steroid hormone metabolites in feces by comparing the pattern of steroids excreted by germfree and conventional rats (Table X). Gas–liquid chromatography and mass spectrometry of steroid silyl ethers were used for qualitative and quantitative analyses. The use of the rat for such investigations has both advantages and disadvantages, apart from the technical problem of maintaining the animals in a germfree condition.

In this species the bile is the major route of excretion for steroid hormone metabolites (Table I). The rat adrenal cortex secretes corticosterone as the major glucocorticoid, and so the absence of metabolites of hydrocortisone reduces the number of metabolites which might be expected to be present. In vitro studies with rat liver have shown that many Δ⁴-3-oxo steroids are converted to metabolites with only the 5α-conformation (e.g., Taylor, 1954; Shirley and Cooke, 1968), and steroid C-20 reductases are absent from the tissues of this animal (Schneider, 1952; Taylor, 1954,

TABLE X

NEUTRAL STEROID[a] IDENTIFIED IN POOLED FECES OF MALE AND FEMALE
GERMFREE AND CONVENTIONAL RATS: NO EXOGENOUS
STEROID ADMINISTERED[b]

Steroid	Germfree	Conventional
$C_{19}O_2$ Dehydroepiandrosterone	0	+
5α-Androstanediols: 3α,17β	(+)U	+U
3β,17β	0	+
$C_{19}O_3$		
5α-Androstanediol-17-ones: 3α,7α	+++U	+U
3α,11β	+++U	+U
3α,15α	(+)	0
3α,19	+	+U
3β,19	0	+
5α-Androstanetriols: 3α,7α,17β	++U	+U
3α,15α,17β	+	+
$C_{21}O_2$		
3α-Hydroxy-5α-pregnan-20-one	0	+U
3α-Hydroxy-5α,17α-pregnan-20-one	0	+U
3α-Hydroxy-5α-pregn-16-en-20-one	0	(+)
$C_{21}O_3$		
5α-Pregnanediol-20-ones: 3α,15α	+U	+U
3β,15α	(+)	+U
3α,16α	+++U	+U
3β,15α	(+)	+
3α,19	0	+
3β,19	0	+
$C_{21}O_4$		
5α-Pregnanes: 11β,21-diol-3,20-dione	+U	0U
3α,21-diol-11,20-dione	(+)	0
3α,11β,21-triol-20-one	+U	0U
$C_{21}O_5$		
5α-Pregnanes: 3α,15α,21-triol-11,20-dione	++U	0U
3α,11β,15α,21-tetrol-20-one	++U	0U
5-Pregnenes: 3α-hydroxy-20-one	0	+
3β,16α-diol-20-one	+	(+)

[a] All steroids present mainly as sulfates. (+): present in very small amounts or presence not fully established. U: also present in urine of female rats (J. A. Gustafsson, 1970).

[b] From J. A. Gustafsson (1968): J. A. Gustafsson and Sjövall, 1968a,b; Eriksson et al., 1968; B. E. Gustafsson et al., 1968a,b).

1956). The steroids shown in Table X all have the 5α-conformation, but no C-20 hydroxy compounds are found. Therefore the results in Table X support the *in vitro* studies.

Some steroids are present in feces of germfree rats but absent from feces of conventional rats and vice versa. For instance, no steroids with a

C-21 hydroxyl group are found in the feces of conventional rats, although such compounds are present in the urine of both the germfree and conventional animals. Therefore, it would appear that C-21 hydroxylated steroids are produced by rat tissues, but the microflora in the conventional rats convert such steroids to as yet unidentified products. It has been suggested that steroids with a C-20 oxo group may undergo dehydroxylation by intestinal microflora at C-16 or C-21, and that steroids with the $16\alpha,20$- or $20,21$-dihydroxy structure are resistant to this dehydroxylation (Eriksson, 1971). Also, steroids with the $5\alpha,3\beta$-hydroxy conformation (e.g., $3\beta,15\alpha$-dihydroxy-5α-androstan-17-one) are found in only very small amounts in feces of germfree rats, and such steroids are not found in the urine or feces of either type of rat. This suggests that the intestinal microflora contain enzymes which convert 3α- to 3β-hydroxyl groups. However, these enzymes appear to act only on steroids saturated in ring A, since $3\beta,16\alpha$-dihydroxy-5-pregnen-20-one is present in the feces of germfree rats, but not to any appreciable extent in feces of conventional rats.

The results shown in Table X are not entirely reconcilable with those shown in Table I. From the results of experiments with labeled steroids it has been inferred (Section IV) that metabolites of the less polar steroids do not undergo enterohepatic circulation and subsequent urinary excretion to any appreciable extent. However, the $C_{19}O_3$ and $C_{21}O_3$ compounds shown in Table X form the largest part of the less polar metabolites in rat feces. The major compound in this group is $3\alpha,6\alpha$-dihydroxy-5α-pregnan-20-one, and this steroid is present in feces and urine of both types of animal. Its most likely precursor is 3α-hydroxy-5α-pregnan-20-one, derived from progesterone, but the former steroid is absent from both feces and urine of germfree rats, although present in feces and urine of conventional animals. The reason for the presence of this hydroxylated pregnanolone in germfree rat feces remains obscure.

The microflora of conventional rats are able to convert the side chain of 3α-hydroxy-5α-pregnan-20-one ($C_{21}O_2$) into the 17α-conformation, since this steroid is not found in the feces of germfree rats. It is of interest that the 17α-epimeric steroid is also found in the urine of conventional rats, since, presumably, this steroid is reabsorbed from the intestine to some extent and subsequently excreted in the urine.

The results shown in Table X indicate that there is some selectivity in the route of excretion and the extent of enterohepatic circulation of steroid metabolites in rats, and that germfree animals exhibit a different specificity from conventional animals in this respect. Three steroids are found in the urine, but not feces, of germfree rats: these steroids are 3α- and $3\beta,17\alpha$-dihydroxy-5α-pregnan-20-one and 5α-pregnane-$3\alpha,6\alpha,20\alpha$-

triol. The first two steroids are the only C_{21} steroids with a C-17 hydroxyl group found in germfree rats, and the parent steroid of these metabolites is not known. Other examples of selectivity in excretion and possible enterohepatic circulation can be seen in Table X. Thus, of the $C_{19}O_3$ steroids, $3\alpha,19$-dihydroxy-5α-androstan-17-one is present in feces and urine of conventional animals, but not in the urine of germfree animals. However, the 3β-epimer is absent from feces and urine of germfree rats but present in the feces of conventional animals. The $C_{21}O_4$ steroids are absent from the feces of conventional animals, but two of these steroids occur in urine. Therefore, it seems probable that these C_{21} steroids are completely converted to other metabolites by intestinal microflora. However, it is possible that those two steroids which appear in urine are completely reabsorbed via the enterohepatic circulation and then excreted by the kidney.

A number of other speculations could be made from the results in Table X. The general impression is that no firm conclusions can be drawn from these results with respect to the important question as to what factors determine whether a particular steroid will be excreted mainly in the feces or the urine. J. A. Gustafsson (1970) found that the urine of conventional rats contains three major steroids which are not found in urine of germfree rats, viz. 3α-hydroxy-$5\alpha,17\alpha$-pregnan-20-one, 3α-hydroxy-5α-pregnan-20-one, and 3α-hydroxy-5α-pregn-16-en-20-one. He suggests that these steroids pass into urine after enterohepatic circulation. The C-16 unsaturated compound has been detected only tentatively in feces, and it must be supposed that almost complete reabsorption of this steroid from the intestine occurs, whereas the reabsorption of the other two steroids is not so extensive. The available evidence supports his view, and is further supported by the work of Eriksson and Gustafsson (1970a) in which labeled pregnenolone and corticosterone were administered to rats (see below).

A most surprising aspect of the work of the Gustafssons described above is their finding that no steroid glucuronides were excreted in feces or urine of germfree or conventional rats. Steroids from pooled feces of male and female rats were present almost entirely as sulfoconjugates. In urine, metabolites of labeled pregnenolone and corticosterone were excreted in the free form by male rats, but mainly as monosulfates by female rats. These findings are difficult to reconcile with *in vitro* experiments with rat liver. Rao and Taylor (1965) found that at high tissue: steroid ratios rat liver converts progesterone into metabolites hydrolyzed by β-glucuronidase (male 70%; female 52% of substrate) and by solvolysis (male 7%; female 12%). Similar experiments have been carried out with rabbits which convert Δ^4-3-oxo steroids to metabolites conjugated with glucuronic acid *in vitro* (Rao and Taylor, 1965), and which excrete steroid glucuronides in both bile and urine (Taylor, 1965c, 1970, 1971).

The absence of steroid glucuronides from rat feces and urine could be due to hydrolysis of these conjugates in the cecum. Eriksson and Gustafsson (1970b) found sulfatase activity of microbial origin in the cecal contents of conventional rats. In germfree rats glucuronidase activity was present: since this could not be of microbial origin, it was assumed that this enzymatic activity originated in mucosal cells of the intestine. The absence of steroid glucuronides from rat feces therefore could be due to hydrolysis of these conjugates by glucuronidases in the cecum, but the absence of steroid glucuronides in rat urine requires further investigation. It is unlikely, on the basis of the evidence cited above, that the rat does not produce steroid glucuronides *in vivo*. It is also unlikely that all the steroids present in rat urine have undergone enterohepatic circulation after prior hydrolysis to free steroids. Therefore the role of steroid glucuronides in steroid metabolism and excretion in the rat remains obscure. One possible explanation of the discrepancy in the results of these investigations is that different strains of rats were used by different workers. Long-Evans rats were used by Gustafsson and his associates. It has been observed that the liver of some batches of "Wistar albino" rats failed to produce conjugated metabolites of progesterone *in vitro*, whereas the livers from another batch of animals were very active in their ability to conjugate steroid metabolites (Rao and Taylor, 1964). Lowy *et al.* (1969) also used rats of the Wistar strain and found that corticosterone was metabolized partly to steroids with the 5β-conformation. Migeon *et al.* (1956) administered labeled corticosterone to human subjects and found that approximately 24% of the dose was excreted in bile as metabolites conjugated with glucuronic acid. Human subjects also convert corticosterone to metabolites predominantly with the 5β-conformation (Engel *et al.*, 1955).

Therefore, the overall metabolism and excretion of metabolites of corticosterone (and other steroids) are different in man and the rat.

2. Sex Differences in the Excretion of Steroid Metabolites by Germfree and Conventional Rats after Administration of Labeled Pregnenolone and Corticosterone

Female rats excrete urinary steroids mainly as monosulfates, whereas male rats excrete steroids almost entirely in the unconjugated form (J. A. Gustafsson, 1970). Because of this difference the distribution of metabolites of [4-^{14}C]pregnenolone and [1,2-^{3}H]corticosterone was investigated in male and female germfree and conventional rats (Eriksson

and Gustafsson, 1970a) and in germfree and conventional male rats
(Eriksson, 1971).

Eriksson and Gustafsson (1970a) studied the amount of radioactivity
in various organs, feces, and urine at various times after intraperitoneal
injection of the steroids. In germfree rats given labeled pregnenolone
approximately 50% of the radioactivity was excreted in the feces and
35% in the urine over 15 days. No sex difference in excretion was noted.
When conventional rats were treated in the same way fecal excretion of
metabolites was much more rapid than excretion in germfree rats, but the
total amount of radioactivity in feces was less and in urine more in conventional animals than in germfree rats. Also, conventional rats showed a
sex difference in the amounts of radioactivity excreted in feces (male,
38%; female 42%) and in urine (male, 45%; female 38%). Essentially

TABLE XI

STEROIDS IDENTIFIED IN FECES OF GERMFREE AND CONVENTIONAL MALE RATS
AFTER ADMINISTRATION OF [4-^{14}C]PREGNENOLONE
AND [4-^{14}C]CORTICOSTERONE[a]

| | Germfree | | Conventional |
Steroid	MoS[b]	DiS	F
$C_{19}O_3$			
5α-Androstanes: 3α,7α-diol-17-one	+		
3α,11β-diol-17-one	+		
3α,16α-17β-triol	+		
$C_{21}O_3$			
5α-Pregnanes: 3α,16α-diol-20-one	+		
3α,20β-diol-11-one			+*
3β,20β-diol-11-one			+*
$C_{21}O_4$			
5α-Pregnanes: 3α,11β,21-triol-20-one		+*	
3β,11β,21-triol-20-one		+*	
3α,11β,20β,21-tetrol	+*	+*	+*
3β,11β,20β,21-tetrol	+*	+*	+*
$C_{21}O_5$			
5α-Pregnanepentols: 3α,11β,16α,20β,21			+* U
3α,11β,16β,20β,21			+* U
3β,11β,16α,20α,21			+* U
3β,11β,16α,20β,21			+* U
3β,11β,16β,20α,21			+* U
3β,11β,16β,20β,21			+* U
(Epimers of			+*) U
3,11,16,21-tetrol-20-one			

[a] From Eriksson (1971).
[b] MoS = monosulfate; DiS = disulfate; F = free; * = radioactive.

the same results were obtained when labeled corticosterone was administered.

Differences in the mode of conjugation were also noted. The results are summarized in Table XI. The most striking features are (a) there were no marked sex differences in metabolites in the fecal excretion patterns, but there were differences between germfree and conventional rats; (b) slight differences were found between the excretion of metabolites of pregnenolone and corticosterone; (c) there was a difference in the amounts of metabolites in the free and monosulfate fractions between germfree and conventional animals for both steroids; and (d) marked differences existed between fecal and urinary patterns, especially the excretion of metabolites of both steroids in the free form by both germfree and conventional male rats. The presence of the intestinal microflora resulted in a change in the ratio of conjugated:free steroids because of the presence of sulfohydrolases. Also, conventional rats excreted greater amounts of metabolites in urine.

Eriksson (1971) extended these studies to attempt to identify the metabolites of the labeled steroids in male rats by gas–liquid chromatography, mass spectrometry, and radio–gas chromatography. The steroids isolated are shown in Table XII. In germfree animals all steroids identified were present as mono- and/or disulfates, whereas in the conventional rats all steroids were unconjugated. The steroids marked with an asterisk were radioactive metabolites of corticosterone. In the experiments with labeled pregnenolone and germfree rats several peaks of radioactivity were

TABLE XII

DISTRIBUTION OF RADIOACTIVITY IN FECES AND URINE OF RATS AFTER
ADMINISTRATION OF [4-^{14}C]PREGNENOLONE AND [4-^{14}C]CORTICOSTERONE[a]

Type of rat and steroid	Feces			Urine		
	F[b]	MoS	DiS	F	MoS	DiS
Pregnenolone						
Germfree: male	++	++	+	+++	0	0
female	++	++	+	+	+++	0
Conventional: male	+++	+	Trace	+++	0	0
female	+++	+	Trace	++	++	0
Corticosterone						
Germfree: male	+	+++	+	+++	0	0
female	+	+++	+	+	+++	0
Conventional: male	+++	++	+	+++	0	0
female	++	++	+	++	++	0

[a] From Eriksson and Gustafsson (1970[a]).
[b] F = free, MoS = monosulfate, DiS = disulfate.

obtained from the free steroid fraction, but corresponding mass peaks were absent. The polarity of these radioactive compounds corresponded to trihydroxymonooxo and tetrahydroxy steroids, and also to steroids with more than 4 oxygen substituents. This is an unexpected finding. It is reasonable to assume that at least part of the pregnenolone might be converted to progesterone and metabolized to $C_{21}O_2$ derivatives. Such compounds have been found in the feces of conventional, but not of germ-free, rats. The 16α-hydroxy derivative of pregnenolone has been tentatively identified in feces of both types of rat (Table X). If this steroid is present in rat feces, the precursor is presumably not pregnenolone.

The corticosterone was converted into a number of highly polar epimeric $C_{21}O_5$ pentols and a tetrolone and two $C_{21}O_3$ diolones. None of these steroids has been isolated from feces or urine of rats not previously dosed with corticosterone. Therefore, the source of the $C_{21}O_4$ and $C_{21}O_5$ 11-oxygenated steroids in Table X remains obscure.

These studies emphasize the great technical problems associated with attempts to use tracer doses of steroids to determine the precursors of metabolites found in bile, feces, and urine.

However, these extensive studies with germfree and conventional rats have provided valuable information on the role of the intestinal microflora on the metabolism and excretion of neutral steroid hormones. Differences in the metabolism of estrogens by germfree and conventional rats remain to be studied. The intestinal flora of other animals (and particularly man) almost certainly differ markedly from those of laboratory rats. The results of experiments with other germfree animals, particularly rabbits, will be awaited with great interest.

E. GENERAL CONCLUSIONS

The steroids excreted in feces differ in many respects from those present in bile, and most of these differences can be attributed to the action of the intestinal microflora (however, see Section VIII), and microorganisms present in feces. The role of these microorganisms can be investigated by comparing the fecal excretion of steroids by conventional and by germfree animals. It would also be of interest to observe the fecal excretion of steroids by human subjects treated with antibiotics, and in germfree animals other than rats. Care must be taken in the interpretation of the results of fecal steroid analyses. It is not valid to extrapolate conclusions about changes caused by fecal microorganisms found in one species to changes in another species. Nor is it valid to draw specific conclusions about human subjects from analyses of feces from a few subjects investigated for a few days. Variations in the patterns of fecal microorganisms between different subjects and between different samples in the same subject are well documented (e.g., Emslie-Smith, 1965). Also, as Luckey (1965) has pointed out, germfree animals differ from conventional ones with respect to certain aspects of general morphology, the size of the cecum, ability to reproduce, nutrition, and food utilization. The presence or absence of intestinal microflora may also have an indirect effect on biliary secretion, since intestinal bacteria produced marked changes in the lipids, sterols, and acids in the intestinal tract. For example, cholic acid is transformed into deoxycholic acid, and chenodeoxycholic acid is dehydroxylated to lithocholic acid (B. E. Gustafsson et al., 1957). Since reabsorbed bile acids exert a controlling effect on bile secretion by the liver, alterations in the composition of reabsorbed bile acids may affect bile production and hence steroid secretion into bile.

However, even when these factors are taken into account, the results recorded in this section show that considerable amounts of steroid hormone metabolites are excreted in feces. So far in man attention has been largely focused on neutral steroid excretion; the fecal excretion of phenolic steroids remains to be investigated.

VIII. Steroid Metabolism and Absorption in the Intestine

In earlier sections of this review metabolism of steroids and conjugates in the intestine has been mentioned. This section deals with further examples of metabolism and absorption of steroids in the intestine, excluding any effects resulting from the enzymatic action of the intestinal microflora.

The extent to which steroids and conjugates are altered by intestinal metabolism undoubtedly plays a part in determining the ultimate fate of particular steroid metabolites. Some steroids excreted into bile and then into the intestine may be metabolized to products that can be absorbed by the intestine to a greater or lesser extent than the original steroid. The reabsorbed metabolite may undergo further metabolism at hepatic and/or extrahepatic sites, and the product(s) may be excreted again in the bile or eliminated from the body by the kidney. On the other hand, some other steroids may be metabolized in the intestine to products which are not readily reabsorbed and so would be eliminated in the feces.

Some examples of the changes which are brought about in the intestine are described below. The subject has been reviewed by Sandberg et al. (1970).

Estrogens are readily conjugated in the intestine of the rat (Lehtinen et al., 1958a,b), and estriol glucuronides were identified in the intestinal wall and the venous blood of isolated loops of human intestine after free estriol was introduced into the lumen (Diczfalusy et al., 1961). When estradiol was introduced into the lumen the steroid was partially converted to estrone glucuronide in the intestinal wall, but estriol was not formed from either estrone or estradiol (Diczfalusy *et al.*, 1962). Lisboa *et al.* (1965) used everted portions of rat small intestine to study the transport of estrogens across the intestinal wall. They did not find any evidence for the formation of sulfoconjugates, but the 3-glucuronides of both estradiol and estrone were formed from free estradiol. No active transport of free or sulfated estrogens was observed, whereas estrogen glucuronides do appear to be actively transported across the intestinal wall. There is also evidence from all the investigations described here that free estrogens may be transported from the intestine to the liver partly in the free form. However, Twombly and Levitz (1960) have shown that estrone sulfate is much more readily absorbed from the intestine than is free estrone.

A number of experiments have shown that steroid conjugates passing into the intestine in bile may be hydrolyzed, reconjugated in the intestinal wall, and transported into the intestinal venous blood. However, this appears to be a selective process depending on the nature of the steroid and the conjugate. For instance, A. A. Sandberg and Slaunwhite (1965) have provided evidence to show that estriol-16α-glucuronide administered intravenously to human subjects is excreted in urine almost entirely unchanged. However, this conjugate may not have been excreted in bile to any appreciable extent and so would have escaped the action of intestinal processes. Inoue *et al.* (1969a) instilled the doubly labeled 16α-glucuronide of estriol directly into the intestine of human subjects. Radioactive metabolites appeared slowly in the urine over the first 24 hours, but in the next 24 hours estriol-3-glucuronide, containing ^{14}C in the glucuronic acid, was excreted in urine. Thus hydrolysis of the 16α-glucuronide had occurred, and the glucuronic acid was transferred to C-3 by transconjugation. It was suggested that this transconjugation occurs in the intestine during reabsorption. Other examples of changes undergone by steroid conjugates, particularly those of estrogen, have been described in Section V.

Inoue *et al.* (1969b) have studied the fate of free estriol administered to human subjects by various routes: cubital vein, portal vein, oral ingestion, and instillation into the terminal ileum. The purpose of this investigation was to obtain supporting evidence for the view of Inoue *et al.* (1969a) that there exists a pool for estrogen metabolites which does not readily equilibrate with the vascular circulation. They suggested that the succus entericus comprises this pool (Section V,B,2). The results obtained from the intravenous injections (cubital or portal vein) are mainly in accord with those obtained by Inoue *et al.* (1969a) and Emerman *et al.* (1967) and need not be considered further. When the estriol was given orally the urinary excretion of estriol-16α-glucuronide and estriol-3-sulfate-16α-glucuronide was much the same as when the estriol was given by the portal vein. Therefore it is probable that these conjugates are formed in the liver. However, there was a marked difference in the distribution of metabolites of estriol and of estriol-16α-glucuronide when these substances were given as a single injection or as an infusion over 5 hours. No difference in the distribution of metabolites of the free estriol was observed, whereas Inoue et al. (1969a) observed a great difference when the glucuronide was given in these two ways. Inoue et al. (1969b) suggest that estriol is so rapidly cleared by the liver that it does not enter the intestinal pool, or that free estriol is transported across the intestinal wall more readily than the conjugate.

On the basis of their results with the conjugated and free estriol they have come to a number of conclusions about the fate of estrogens in the intestine. In the upper part of the small intestine estriol conjugates are not hydrolyzed. Intestinal reabsorption of estriol and its conjugates is passive, although free estriol could be absorbed into the lipoidal face of the intestinal mucosa in a manner similar to that in which progesterone (Schedl, 1965) and hydrocortisone (Schedl and Clifton, 1963) are absorbed. Estriol-3-sulfate-16α-glucuronide is not readily absorbed from the intestine since its size (6 Å diameter, 13 Å long) is greater than the pore size of the mucosal membrane (3–6.5 Å). Therefore this conjugate probably reaches the terminal ileum to be hydrolyzed by the intestinal flora and then reconjugated to the 3- or 16α-glucuronides which are reabsorbed and then excreted in the urine. [However, this may not be a normal physiological route for excretion of estriol since the patterns of excretion of metabolites when estriol was instilled into the terminal ileum differed markedly from the patterns observed when the steroid was given by other routes (Inoue et al., 1969b).] The upper part of the small intestine forms mainly the 16α-glucuronide of estriol in vitro, but the lower part forms the 16α- and 3-glucuronides of estriol in the ratio 2.5:1. Therefore it is probable that the lower small intestine is mainly responsible for the formation of estriol-3-glucuronide. Some estriol-3-sulfate-16α-glucuronide is secreted directly into the succus entericus and slowly released, and eventually is excreted in urine by the processes of hydrolysis and reconjugation in the terminal ileum described above.

Conjugation of steroids, other hormones and many drugs has for many years been considered to be a process of "inactivation" of these substances prior to their elimination from the body. The work discussed in this section poses the puzzling question why elaborate metabolic changes in the steroid molecule accompanied by conjugation and subsequent biliary excretion occur, only for many of these changes to be reversed in the intestine. Free bilirubin is readily reabsorbed from the intestine but the glucuronide is not. It has been suggested by Lester (1965) that the reason why bilirubin is conjugated (mainly with glucuronic acid) before excretion into bile is to prevent the reabsorption of this toxic substance from the intestine. So, in teleological terms, the metabolism of steroids in the intestine appears to provide no biological advantage, and the physiological role of the enterohepatic circulation of steroid metabolites remains obscure.

IX. Effects of Steroids on Bile Secretion

Previous sections of this review have provided conclusive evidence that a wide range of exogenous and endogenous steroids is excreted into the bile of many species, including man. The possible mechanisms of secretion of steroids into bile will be discussed in Section XI.

It is also well established that many steroids which are excreted to an appreciable extent in bile may have a marked influence on bile formation and the secretion of nonsteroidal substances for which bile is the normal route of excretion.

Lathe and Walker (1958a,b) studied the conjugation of bilirubin by liver slices of rats, rabbits, and monkeys. Higher rates of conjugation were obtained when human male serum was added to the incubation medium. However, serum obtained from pregnant women and newborn babies reduced the level of conjugation. Since the inhibitory factor was found to be diffusible, it seemed possible that this factor was a free steroid or was competing with bilirubin for glucuronide conjugation. However, sera containing the inhibitory factor(s) did not affect conjugation of bilirubin in broken cell preparations. Therefore, it is unlikely that the effects of the sera were due to competition for the bilirubin conjugating mechanism. Several steroids acted as inhibitors of bilirubin conjugation in liver slices; these inhibitory steroids appeared to have the following basic structures: 5β-pregnane, 5β-androstane, 4-pregnene, 3α-hydroxy, 3β-hydroxy, 3-oxo, 17α-hydroxy, 17β-hydroxy, 17-oxo, 20α-hydroxy, 20β-hydroxy, 20-oxo and 21-hydroxy. The inhibitory effect was reversed by steroids with the following structures: 5α-androstane, 4-androstene, 5-androstene, 5α-pregnane, 5-pregnene, 11α-hydroxy, 11β-hydroxy, and a phenolic A-ring. The effect of these steroids seems to be on the permeability of the hepatic cell for bilirubin. If such an effect is present in the intact animal, then hepatic disposal of bilirubin and transport of the pigment into bile might be impaired. However, the high capacity of the liver for excreting bilirubin almost certainly precludes such interference with biliary excretion of bile pigments in normal subjects.

More direct evidence that steroids influence biliary function has been obtained. In man, administration of Norethandrolone (17-ethyl-19-nortestosterone) causes a delay in hepatic clearance of bromosulfalein (BSP) (Scherb et al., 1963; Schoenfield and Foulk, 1964), although conflicting claims about the effects of this steroid on hepatic function in animals have been made. In rats the excretion of bilirubin is decreased after administration of Norethandrolone (Arias, 1963; Hargreaves, 1965). Various effects of Norethandrolone on hepatic function of rabbits, rats, and dogs have been reported (see R. J. Roberts et al., 1968, for references).

R. J. Roberts et al. (1968) studied the effects of a wide range of doses of Norethrandolone and methyltestosterone on the excretion of exogenous bilirubin in 2 strains of rats and in mice (note that these animals excrete steroid metabolites almost exclusively in bile). They found that the steroid did not impair the removal of bilirubin from the plasma of mice; indeed, there was some evidence of an increase in the ability of the liver to dispose of the bilirubin. Increasing the dose of the steroid did not decrease the ability of mice and rats to dispose of the exogenous bilirubin. These findings, which conflict with those of others mentioned above, could have been due to species and strain variation, but two strains of rat (Simonsen Sprague-Dawley and Wistar) gave essentially the same results. Body temperature was found to have a marked effect on the results. Decreasing the rectal temperature of the animals by 4° caused a decrease in bile flow and a decrease in the output of bilirubin. At normal body temperature methyltestosterone produced a markedly decreased bile flow and a decrease in bilirubin concentration in bile. The reasons for the different actions of these two anabolic steroids cannot as yet be explained, but the effect of hypothemia on biliary secretion is discussed in Section XI.

A number of clinical observations (Section X) indicate that estrogens, particularly at high concentrations, have a pronounced effect on bile formation. Large doses of estrogen result in impaired BSP elimination in rats (Gallagher et al., 1966) and in man (Mueller and Kappas, 1964). In those experiments conjugation of BSP was normal, and so it is probable that the estrogen was interfering with the secretion of BSP into the bile canaliculus. Forker (1969) attempted to study the effects of estrogens on the passive permeability of the canalicular membrane. When female rats were given large doses of estrone there was an increased permeability of the biliary system as judged by an increased excretion of sucrose and mannitol. However, the estrogen treatment caused an increase in liver weight and a decrease in bile production. Forker (1969) quotes the work of others to show that sucrose and mannitol enter bile by passive transport, and therefore he ascribes the effect of estrone to its effect(s) on the parenchymal cells rather than on transport processes lower down the biliary tree. Lanman and Schanker (1970) studied the biliary excretion of mannitol in rats and found that the mannitol reached maximal concentrations in bile and liver in the very short time of about 1 minute. They concluded that the liver cell membrane contains aqueous pores much larger than those thought to exist in membranes of most other cells, or that the liver takes up mannitol by some form of specialized transport mechanism. They pointed out that the speed at which mannitol enters the liver and bile was not appreciated by Forker (1969) whose experiments were of long duration. They also found that mannitol can readily equilibrate with water in hepatic parenchymal cells, but certain nonparenchymal cells are relatively impermeable to this compound. However, the work of Forker (1969) showed that the estrone undoubtedly affected at least some of the biliary secretory mechanisms.

The impairment of liver function by large doses of estrogens in rats has been reported by other workers (e.g., Mueller and Kappas, 1964; Gallagher et al., 1966). Endogenous hormones, presumably estrogens, produced during pregnancy may produce cholestasis or affect liver function in other ways (Svandborg and Ohlsson, 1959; Kreek et al., 1967a,b) (but see Section XI). The effects of treating rats with ethynylestradiol for several days on several aspects of biliary function have been studied by Kreek et al. (1969). The excretion of labeled estradiol, estradiol glucuronide, BSP in bile, and total bile production were compared in treated and control animals. Bile production was almost halved and BSP excretion in bile was delayed in the treated animals. The metabolites of labeled estradiol were more completely excreted in the control animals than in the treated animals. All of these differences were statistically significant. The biliary excretion of administered estradiol glucuronide was also impaired in the treated animals, but radioactivity appeared in bile more rapidly in both groups of animals than when free estradiol was given.

These authors have suggested that because of the decreased bile flow in the treated animals the ethynylestradiol acts on the mechanism of bile salt secretion, which is considered to be a primary mechanism in bile secretion. It would have been interesting to attempt to restore the bile secretion of the treated animals to normal by administering bile salts, but such experiments were not carried out.

The decreases in excretion of metabolites of labeled estrogens in bile of treated animals in unit time was greater than the decrease in bile flow, and thus the mechanism for excretion of estrogen metabolites in bile appears to have been affected more than the primary mechanism(s) of bile production. Such a deduction implies that specific secretory mechanisms for steroid metabolites into bile exist, but at the present time there is no firm evidence that such a specific mechanism exists.

Kreek *et al.* (1969) have also suggested that the effect of ethynylestradiol on steroid excretion in bile acts mainly on the mechanism for transferring conjugated estrogen from the hepatocyte into the canaliculus. This suggestion is based on the finding that metabolites of exogenous estradiol glucuronide are more rapidly excreted into bile in both groups of animals than are metabolites of administered estriol. However, another possible explanation is that ethynylestradiol affects steroid metabolizing and conjugating systems in the liver and the metabolism of estradiol is more affected than the metabolism of the glucuronide.

Another possible explanation of all these results is that damage to the hepatocytes or the canalicular system was caused by the very large doses of ethynylestradiol administered: such changes would not have been observed by the light microscopic examination of liver sections carried out by Kreek *et al.* (1969). Electron microscope studies of livers of the treated rats would have provided useful information about the mechanism of action of ethynylestradiol on the liver and biliary system.

Another possible explanation for the effects of ethynylestradiol described above arises from the work of Heikel and Lathe (1970a,b). They found that 17α-ethynyl-substituted estrogens greatly decreased bile production in rats, and that many of these and other steroids inhibited ATPase, and especially the $Na^+ + K^+$-stimulated ATPase of the plasma membrane of rat liver *in vitro*. The inhibition of the *in vitro* system and inhibition of bile production by particular steroids were not absolutely parallel, but it is probable that the differences are due to metabolic changes undergone by the steroids in the *in vivo* system.

This work raises the interesting suggestion that cation transport may be one of the mechanisms involved in bile production. Such a view is supported by the finding that ouabain, a potent inhibitor of $Na^+ + K^+$-stimulated ATPase, causes decreased bile production *in vivo* (Erlinger *et al.*, 1969).

When corticosteroids are given to patients with hyperbilirubinemia there is a dramatic decrease in jaundice and a fall in plasma bilirubin, particularly in patients with viral hepatitis (e.g., Katz *et al.*, 1957; R. Williams and Billing, 1961). The mechanism of this process is uncertain, but it is almost certainly not due to an increase in bile flow since corticoids do not exert a choleretic effect (e.g., Clifton *et al.*, 1958). However, the ameliorative action of the corticoids on jaundice need not be directly on the biliary system, since there are many other possible ways in which the corticoids could cause a decrease in plasma bilirubin. It is currently thought that the corticoids may be acting on the enzyme systems responsible for the production of bilirubin (Aach, 1969). However, a possible action of corticoids on the liver and biliary system cannot be entirely ruled out.

Progesterone affects liver weight, the liver:body weight ratio, and hepatic function when administered in large doses to rats (Fahim and Hall, 1970), but the effect of this steroid on bile production does not seem to have been studied.

Some women develop jaundice when taking oral contraceptives, and many of these women have a previous history of intrahepatic cholestasis of pregnancy (Haemmerli and Wyss, 1967). This suggests that the contraceptive steroids, particularly the estrogen component, can severely affect hepatic and biliary function. Application of the standard BSP test to women taking oral contraceptives has revealed that BSP retention occurs only occasionally, but the effect appears to be related to the amounts of the contraceptives taken (Allan and Tyler, 1967). However, Kleiner et al. (1965) used an infusion technique to study the storage and maximal excretory capacity of the liver for BSP in women taking preparations containing Norethynodrel and Mestranol. After several months of treatment the storage capacity of the liver for BSP was unchanged but the maximal excretory capacity was markedly reduced. When treatment with the steroids was stopped the hepatic function returned to normal within about a week. It is of interest that there is circumstantial evidence that synthetic estrogens and progestins may be excreted in bile and/or retained in the body for long periods. For instance, K. I. H. Williams (1969) studied the urinary excretion of tritium-labeled Mestranol metabolites in normal women after oral administration. After 3 days, and even after 9 days in one subject, only 29–43% of the dose was excreted in urine. This low recovery of radioactivity was probably not due to incomplete absorption since Fotherby et al. (1968) recovered about 50% of an intravenous dose of labeled synthetic progestins as urinary metabolites in 4 days.

The effects of estrogen, progestins, and pregnancy on physiological and biochemical processes in liver have been reviewed by Song and Kappas (1968).

Although much of the evidence is equivocal, it appears reasonable to accept that steroid hormones can markedly affect certain aspects of hepatic and biliary function. However, most of the effects have been observed only when massive doses of steroids have been administered. Therefore the possibility that steroid hormones influence biliary secretion under physiological conditions must remain an open question until further work is carried out.

X. Disturbances of Steroid Metabolism and Excretion in Liver Disease and Pregnancy

When it became apparent that the liver is the major site of steroid catabolism in animals and man, the effects of liver disease on steroid metabolism were soon investigated with the hope that the results would be useful in diagnosis and prognosis. The association of liver dysfunction and pregnancy was also well known, and investigations to establish a possible cause of this association have also been carried out.

A. Excretion of Steroid Hormone Metabolites in Liver Disease

There are many processes concerned with the biliary (and urinary) excretion of steroid hormones that may be affected by liver disease. These processes include the uptake, storage, and metabolism of steroids by hepatocytes (and possibly also the Kupffer cells); conjugation of free steroids or further conjugation of partially conjugated steroids with glucuronic and sulfuric acids, N-acetylglucosamine and glutathione, and possibly with other substances such as amino acids in the liver cells; the transport of final metabolic products into the blood (or lymph) or into the bile canaliculi; the extent of enterohepatic circulation.

Other processes not directly involving steroids may also be affected; secretion of bile salts into the bile canaliculi; the availability of bile salts from the enterohepatic circulation and *de novo* biosynthesis from cholesterol; the formation of bilirubin conjugates and the transport of these into bile; the general biochemical processes within the liver cell resulting in deficiency of energy production for conjugation and active transport of substrates and metabolites into and out of the cell; the biosynthesis of plasma proteins, some of which are involved in binding of steroids (and other substances). The net effect of disturbance of some or all of these processes accounts for many of the symptoms associated with "liver disease," viz. jaundice, cholestasis, formation of ascites. These disturbances may have severe consequences in systems of the body other than the liver and biliary tract. Therefore, in the study of disturbances of steroid metabolism and excretion in liver disease, the effects of disturbances on extrahepatic function must be taken into account. Furthermore, disturbance of pathways for the excretion of steroid metabolites could lead to a build-up of steroids in the body, and these could influence hepatic and biliary function by producing extra disturbances in the liver or aggravating those already present.

Another problem is the number of diseases of the liver and biliary system which have been described (e.g., Sherlock, 1963, 1965; Butt *et al.*,

1965). Some of these diseases may be the result of a specific metabolic deficiency. For example, the Crigler-Najjar syndrome, characterized by an elevated blood level of free bilirubin, has been attributed to a deficiency in the liver of the glucuronyl transferase system responsible for the formation of bilirubin glucuronides (Schmid and Hammaker, 1959). However, Butt *et al.* (1965) have suggested that this syndrome might also be caused by an impaired transport of bilirubin into the liver cells.

1. *Estrogens*

Gynecomastia and testicular atrophy are frequently observed in male patients with different types of liver disease, and menstrual irregularities are also sometimes observed in women. Therefore, it is natural to conclude that these conditions arise from a disturbance of estrogen metabolism in the damaged liver and/or an impaired biliary excretion of estrogen metabolites. Adlercreutz (1970) has recently reviewed the role of estrogen metabolism in liver disease. Because he has discussed this subject with great authority and clarity, only the major conclusions need be considered here.

In acute liver diseases the metabolism of estrogens, particularly hydroxylations, is disturbed, but it is not yet known whether this is due to enzyme deficiencies or to a defect in the uptake of estrogens by the liver cells. In chronic liver disease, especially in portal cirrhosis, without hypoproteinemia, edema, and ascites, urinary excretion of endogenous estrogens, mainly estriol, tends to be elevated. This is probably due to an interruption of enterohepatic circulation related to a general impairment of liver function. Administration of labeled estrogens shows that there is a decrease in 2-hydroxylation and possibly in 16α-hydroxylation. The impaired conversion of 16α-hydroxyestrone to estriol may be due to an interruption of enterohepatic circulation of estrogen metabolites. In chronic liver disease in which hypoproteinemia, edema, and ascites are present, free estrogens are excreted in the urine, and when estrogens are administered there is a decreased formation of estriol. A decrease in the ability of liver cells to take up estrogens seems to be a more likely explanation than that enzymatic deficiencies exist within the cells.

In liver disease associated with jaundice, the biliary excretion of estrogens is greatly reduced, particularly the polar conjugates. As might be expected from the experiments described in Section IX, the pattern of urinary estrogens is very different from normal.

The disturbances of estrogen metabolism in liver diseases are mainly attributable to decreased biliary excretion of estrogens, and so the metabolic changes in the intestine (Section VIII) and enterohepatic circulation of metabolites which normally appear in urine are much reduced. Changes in hepatic blood flow, decreased uptake of estrogens by the liver cells and decreased synthesis of plasma proteins, leading to edema and ascites, are major factors also. Many of the clinical signs of liver disease may be caused by disturbed estrogen metabolism, but other causative factors could be involved.

Estrogen determinations are of little or no value in the diagnosis of liver disease.

Further work carried out since the review of Adlercreutz (1970) has substantiated many of his conclusions. Hellman *et al.* (1970) studied the fate of intravenously administered [6,7-³H]estradiol in 2 male and 2 female patients with total biliary obstruction caused by occlusion of the common bile duct at its distal end by carcinomas. The total urinary excretion of metabolites was 70% (normal 57%); glucuronides were slightly below normal, but "nonglucuronide conjugates" were 39% (normal 12%). The steroids in the glucuronide fraction were abnormal; estriol was less than half the normal value whereas 16α-hydroxyestrone was increased by 2–3 times the normal level. This increase in 16α-hydroxylation is contrary to the conclusion of Adlercreutz (1970). Urinary estrone was slightly elevated, and 2 of the patients excreted less than normal amounts of 2-oxygenated estrones. The livers of the subjects were only very slightly or not at all affected by metastases. These alterations were similar in some respects to those observed in patients with liver cirrhosis, and so it seems that cholestasis is a major factor in abnormal estradiol metabolism in cirrhotic patients.

Feminization is often observed in cirrhosis, but not so frequently in patients with biliary obstruction. The latter condition tends to be more rapidly fatal than the former, and so the patients may not be exposed to estrogen for a sufficiently long time to become feminized. However, the metabolism of estradiol in cirrhosis is disturbed in two ways, 2-oxygenation and 16α-hydrolation, but in only one way in biliary obstruction, i.e., 16α-hydroxylation. Therefore, in cirrhosis of the liver estradiol would tend to be metabolized to a lesser extent than in biliary obstruction, and the retention of unmetabolized estradiol would tend to cause feminization more rapidly. Shaver *et al.* (1963) and Korenman *et al.* (1969) have shown that plasma estradiol levels are elevated in patients with cirrhotic livers. Hellman *et al.* (1970) reinforce the suggestion of Adlercreutz (1970) that specific and sensitive techniques should be applied to the study of plasma estrogen levels in liver disease.

2. Neutral Steroids

The metabolism and excretion of neutral steroids in liver disease have not been as extensively studied as have the estrogens.

Rogers (1956) found that some patients with liver disease excrete less urinary pregnanediol after progesterone administration than do normal subjects, presumably due to impaired metabolism in the liver. However, Marti *et al.* (1961) claimed that progesterone is metabolized more rapidly by women with liver disease than by normal women.

The urinary excretion of total 17-oxosteroids and of androsterone, etiocholanolone, dehydroepiandrosterone, and 11-oxoetiocholanolone are markedly decreased in some patients with liver disease (Birke, 1954).

Cronholm *et al.* (1970) have investigated the plasma levels of bile acids and steroid sulfates in patients with infective hepatitis. In the jaundiced phase the total bile acid levels were very much higher than normal. The increase for bile acids was about 50-fold and for bilirubin about 20-fold. The steroid sulfates did not increase to the same extent, but 5α-androstane-3α,17β-diol was present in the jaundiced phase and disappeared during convalescence. (This steroid is a major constituent of human bile, in which it occurs as sulfate and glucuronide, Table IV.) The other steroids determined, and an indication of the changes which occurred in passing from the jaundiced to the convalescent phases, are given below. The major changes in concentrations which were found in the jaundiced and convalescent phases are indicated thus: O = no change; R = rise; F = fall; conjugates present both as mono- and disulfates are indicated by MoS and DiS, respectively.

Dehydroepiandrosterone (O, R, and F)
5-Androstene-3β,17β-diol, MoS (O), DiS (F)
5-Androstene-3β,17α-diol, MoS (O), DiS (O)
Androsterone (F)
5α-Androstane-3α,17β-diol, MoS (O), DiS (F)
3β-Hydroxy-5α-androstan-17-one (F)
5α-Androstane-3β,17β-diol, DiS (O)
3β,16α-Dihydroxy-5-androsten-17-one, MoS (O)
Pregnenolone (O)
5-Pregnene-3β,20α-diol, MoS (R and F), DiS (F)
5-Pregnene-3β,17α,20α-triol, MoS (R)

The changes in plasma steroid sulfates could be due to different factors from those which affect the bile acids and bilirubin. Cholestasis might be responsible for the elevated levels of some steroids, many of which are present in human bile, but quantitative data on the biliary steroids are not available and so the bile:plasma ratios are not known. However, cholestasis cannot be the only factor since the concentration of dehydroepiandrosterone sulfate tended to decrease during the period of jaundice, but the presence in plasma of 16α-hydroxydehydroepiandrosterone indicates that alterations in steroid metabolism might also occur. [It is of interest that Hellman *et al.* (1970) found a 2- to 3-fold increase in the excretion of 16α-hydroxyestrone in patients with cirrhosis; see subsection 1 above.] The 16α-hydroxylation mechanism could have been stimulated by cell damage, and it is also possible that this mechanism was induced or stimulated by the drugs given to the patients.

Zumoff *et al.* (1967) found abnormal patterns of cortisol metabolites in urine of patients with liver cirrhosis; a decreased amount of these metabolites conjugated with glucuronic acid was also found. They attributed some of these abnormalities to the effect of cholestasis on the function of the smooth endoplasmic reticulum. Temporary induction of intrahepatic cholestasis by administration of Norethandrolone leads to the production of the same abnormal urinary metabolites of cortisol without alteration in the ability of the liver to form glucuronides (Zumoff *et al.*, 1968).

Since metabolites of neutral steroids are not extensively excreted in human bile, impairment of biliary function may not have the same dramatic effects as when estrogen excretion is disturbed. However, altered metabolism of neutral steroids by damaged liver could lead to marked pathological effects if these steroids are not rapidly excreted in the urine.

Bercovici and Mauvais-Jarvis (1970) have studied the metabolism of labeled testosterone in male patients with liver cirrhosis. The steroid was administered orally and intravenously. They calculated the contribution of the labeled testosterone metabolites to the urinary androsterone and etiocholanolone, and to the 5α- and 5β-androstane-3α,17β-diols in patients and normal male and female subjects. The amount of the 5α-androstanediol derived from an intravenous dose of testosterone was twice that obtained from an oral dose in male subjects. In cirrhotic patients, however, the route of administration did not affect the amount of the 5α-diol formed from the labeled testosterone. It was concluded from this evidence that testosterone does not undergo reduction to 5α-derivatives in the extrahepatic tissue of patients with cirrhosis. If this is so, the authors suggested that the hypogonadism observed in this liver disease might be partly the result of lack of conversion of testosterone to "5α-testosterone" in target tissues. Such a disturbance would not account for the gynecomastia observed in cirrhosis, but this novel concept is worthy of fuller investigation.

B. Disturbances of Steroid Hormone Metabolism and Excretion in Pregnant Women

In normal pregnancy there is no serious impairment of hepatic or biliary function. In the last trimester some liver function tests show minor abnormalities, but these are considered to be "normal" for pregnancy. In some complications of pregnancy the liver may be involved as a result of more generalized lesions, e.g., the marked changes in liver structure in eclampsia. Intrahepatic jaundice of pregnancy is rare, and minor attacks are probably responsible for the generalized pruritus of pregnancy (Sherlock, 1963). An obvious etiological factor in this latter condition is the large amounts of steroids produced during pregnancy.

1. Ultrastructure of the Liver

Adlercreutz et al. (1967a) have carried out studies on the ultrastructure of the liver and estrogen metabolism in late pregnancy. They quote earlier literature which has established that recurrent jaundice of pregnancy is due to an interference with bile flow. In one of the ten patients studied at laporotomy they found signs of intrahepatic cholestatic jaundice, but the amount, secretion pressure, and viscosity of the bile were within normal limits. Liver biopsies taken during a bout of jaundice were examined by electron microscopy and showed many abnormalities. Most of the bile canaliculi were dilated and in some areas there were no canalicular microvilli. Changes in mitochondrial structure and size were also observed. However, such changes have also been observed in extrahepatic cholestasis and in other pathological specimens of liver from nonpregnant patients. The changes seen in pregnancy are reversed after delivery, but tend to recur in subsequent pregnancies.

2. Estrogens

Adlercreutz et al. (1967b) quote many references to show that recurrent jaundice of pregnancy may be related to the cholestatic jaundice produced by administration of steroids such as methyltestosterone, anabolic steroids, contraceptive steroid preparations, and natural and synthetic estrogens (see also Section IX). The authors compared the urinary, and in one case the biliary, excretion of estrogens with that of normal pregnant women. The estrogens assayed were: estrone, estradiol, and estriol released by hydrolysis and their 3-sulfates. They found that the urinary excretion of the hydrolyzed estrogens was within the normal range, but the amounts of estradiol-3-sulfate were lower, and of estriol-3-sulfate higher, than normal. Also, there was a change in the pattern of conjugates of estrogens from 3-glucuronides and diconjugates to 16- or 17-glucuronides of estrogens more polar than estriol. In the bile of one patient there was a striking decrease in estrogen content toward the end of the pregnancy, and large amounts of the steroids were in the free form, but in blood and urine the levels of free estrogen were low. The conclusions drawn by Adlercreutz et al. (1967b) are as follows. In this condition there is a preferential formation of 16- or 17-glucuronides at the expense of 3-glucuronides or diconjugates. This could be due to impaired enterohepatic circulation and/or reduced biliary secretion leading to more rapid excretion of the conjugates into the urine. This view is supported by the finding of increased levels of estriol-3-sulfates in the urine of the patients. Since the urinary excretion of estrogens was within the normal range, the cholestasis is unlikely to have been caused by increased production of estrogens. There was some quantitative change in the pattern of estrogen sulfates which may have been due to impaired biliary excretion. The qualitative and quantitative changes in estrogen metabolites may be partly the result rather than the cause of the jaundice, and it is improbable that changes in estrogen metabolism are a major etiological factor in recurrent jaundice of pregnancy. Women who develop this condition may be abnormally sensitive to normal amounts of estrogen. This is supported by the fact that such women tend to develop jaundice when taking oral contraceptives. Evidence is quoted to suggest that progesterone and its metabolites might enhance the effect of estrogens on transport of bilirubin and its conjugates. Progesterone itself has no toxic effects on the normal adult human liver.

Therefore, although there is no definite evidence that estrogen metabolites are a primary factor in causing recurrent jaundice of pregnancy, the possibility remains that estrogens may have some etiological significance in this disease. Further studies of plasma estrogens by sensitive techniques, and the role of conjugates of estrogens other than glucuronides and sulfates in pregnancy are required.

3. Neutral Steroids

Many investigations of the excretion of neutral steroids during pregnancy have been carried out and need not be considered here. Recently, J. Sjövall and his co-workers developed a highly sensitive technique for the measurement in plasma of neutral steroid sulfates by gas chromatography–mass spectrometry (J. Sjövall and Víhko, 1968). Using this technique, K. Sjövall (1970) studied the concentrations of mono- and disulfates of $C_{19}O_2$, $C_{19}O_3$, $C_{21}O_2$, and $C_{21}O_3$ steroids in plasma during normal pregnancy and labor. The mean concentrations of total plasma steroids (per 100 ml) 1 week before delivery in the monosulfate fraction were 530 μg and in the disulfate fraction 350 μg. The predominant compounds were 5α-pregnane derivatives. The concentrations of many of the steroids investigated increased as the pregnancy progressed, but the rate of increase varied for different isomers and conjugates. Dehydroepiandrosterone sulfate, the predominant $C_{19}O_2$ steroid, decreased during pregnancy. The suggestion that this well-documented decrease in the concentration of this steroid is due to the utilization of the steroid by the fetoplacental unit cannot be entirely true, since the concentrations of the following monosulfates also decreased: androsterone, 3β-hydroxy-5α-androstan-17-one (epiandrosterone), 5-androstene-5β,17β- and -3β,17α-diols and 5-pregnene-3β,17α,20α-triol. Differences in the levels of other steroids between pregnant and nonpregnant women were also observed. It is of interest that 16α-hydroxydehydroepiandrosterone was present in pregnancy plasma but not in plasma of nonpregnant women. This steroid was also found in patients with infectious hepatitis by Cronholm et $al.$ (1970). Its presence in pregnancy plasma could be due to the high 16α-hydroxylating activity of the fetus, but the presence of the fetus is not essential since the steroid was found in the plasma of a patient with a nonviable fetus.

All of the $C_{21}O_2$ isomers were probably formed from progesterone, and many of these isomers were found in the plasma, bile, and urine after administration of large doses of progesterone to a pregnant woman with T-tube drainage (quoted from work of Adlercreutz and co-workers). The main urinary metabolites of progesterone have the 5β-conformation conjugated with glucuronic acid, but the 5α-epimers were predominant in plasma. The $C_{19}O_2$ and $C_{21}O_2$ steroids with 3α,5α, 3β,5α, and 3β-Δ^5 structures are conjugated with sulfuric acid. Steroid sulfates are less rapidly cleared than are glucuronides by the kidney, and this may explain the preponderance of 5α-steroid sulfates in plasma and bile (see K. Sjövall, 1970, for references).

J. Sjövall and Sjövall (1970) compared the levels of steroid sulfates in the plasma of healthy pregnant women and in 17 women with pruritus of pregnancy. Plasma bile acids and bilirubin were also determined. In some cases plasma bilirubin levels were normal when bile acid and steroid sulfate levels were elevated. This suggests that bilirubin may not be excreted by the same mechanisms as bile acids or steroid sulfates (see Section XI).

The main changes in steroid sulfates due to the intrahepatic cholestasis leading to the pruritus were: increased concentrations of C_{21}-3α,5α- and 3α,5β-steroids; a relative increase in 20α-hydroxy steroids, particularly of those present as disulfates, and a relative and sometimes absolute decrease of C_{21}-3β,5α-steroids. It seems likely that these changes are the result of impaired biliary excretion since many of these steroids are excreted in bile. However, there were some findings which cannot be entirely explained by impairment of bile flow. For example, the 3α,5α- and 3α,5β-epimers of pregnanediol are found as mono- and disulfates in bile (Table IV), but in patients with pruritus the monosulfate of the

$3\alpha,5\alpha$-epimer disappeared more rapidly after delivery than did the disulfate of this steroid.

In the patients with pruritus there were relatively low concentrations of $C_{21}O_2$-$3\beta,5\alpha$ steroids. Intestinal bacteria epimerize $3\alpha,5\alpha$-steroids to $3\beta,5\alpha$-compounds (Section VII), and decreased secretion of the $3\alpha,5\alpha$-steroids into bile might be the reason for this, since the steroids would not undergo epimerization and enterohepatic circulation.

The data presented indicate that pruritus of pregnancy results in a change in the metabolism of progesterone or in the conjugation of metabolites of this hormone. However, it cannot be concluded that these changes in metabolism are the cause or effect of the intrahepatic cholestasis. Song and Kappas (1968) have suggested that estrogens are mainly responsible for cholestatic jaundice of pregnancy (cf. Adlercreutz et al., 1967b, quoted in Section X,B,1 and IX). However, recent studies quoted by J. Sjövall and Sjövall (1970) indicate that progestins may also cause disturbed liver function.

Another possible explanation of cholestasis of pregnancy has been proposed by J. Sjövall and Sjövall (1970) because of a finding relevant to this review. The steroid 3α-hydroxy-$5\alpha(17\alpha)$-pregnan-20-one is structurally related to steroids which are hepatotoxic (Sherlock, 1963) and is found in plasma during pruritus of pregnancy and also in human feces (Table VI). Thus in pruritus an increased amount of this 17α-steroid may be formed by the intestinal microflora and be reabsorbed, enter the circulation, and exert toxic effects on the liver which lead to cholestasis. Thus the intestinal microflora may play a role in the development of intrahepatic cholestasis of pregnancy.

C. GENERAL CONCLUSIONS

Changes in urinary, biliary, and plasma levels of steroid hormones occur in various types of liver disease and in pregnancy. In liver disease the changes in metabolism and excretion of estrogens vary with the type and severity of the disease, but many of the findings can be explained on the basis that at least some of these changes result from impaired biliary excretion and enterohepatic circulation of estrogen metabolites. Gynecomastia and testicular atrophy, which are commonly found in many types of liver disease, are almost certainly due to the disturbance of estrogen metabolism and excretion. However, it is still an open question as to whether or not estrogens are an etiological factor in the disease of the liver itself. The role of neutral steroids in the development and symptomatology of liver disease is uncertain. Determinations of urinary steroids are of little or no value in the diagnosis of liver disease, but the analysis of plasma for estrogens, neutral steroids, and tropic hormones may provide useful information.

The same general conclusions apply to alterations in steroid metabolism and excretion in pregnancy complicated by liver disease. Determinations of neutral steroids in plasma of pregnant women have shown that both qualitative and quantitative changes are present when the pregnancy is complicated by intrahepatic cholestasis. It is not known whether estrogens or progestins or both groups of steroids are responsible for cholestasis in pregnancy.

Although studies of the type described have provided little information about the etiology of liver disease, the studies have yielded useful data about steroid metabolism, excretion, and enterohepatic circulation.

XI. The Mechanisms Involved in the Secretion of Steroids into Bile

Schanker (1968) began his review on "Secretion of organic compounds in bile" with this sentence: "Considering the number of studies dealing with biliary excretion of organic compounds, one might wonder why so few details of the processes have been learned." In spite of the great mass of extra information about the biliary excretion of steroids and other organic compounds which has been accumulated in recent years, the question asked by Schanker is no nearer to being solved. The reasons for this gap in our understanding have a number of bases, but one of the major reasons is that a great deal of effort and energy has been expended in determining what substances are excreted in bile. However, the more fundamental, and perhaps more rewarding, problems of *why* and *how* steroids are excreted through the biliary system have received little attention. In fairness to workers in this area of research, it should be stated that very little is known about the mechanisms of renal excretion of steroid hormone metabolites, and knowledge of the fundamental mechanisms of renal function is far in advance of that of the mechanisms of biliary secretion.

Some workers have put forward general hypotheses about the factors which determine whether particular steroid metabolites will be excreted by the hepatic or renal route. These hypotheses have become untenable as more information has been accumulated. Taylor (1965b) has discussed this early work and pointed out the deficiencies of the various hypotheses.

It is reasonable to assume that the fundamental mechanism of biliary secretion is common to all higher animals. Evidence to support a contrary view is lacking. However, the major stumbling block to a full understanding of biliary secretion is the technical problem of obtaining primary bile, i.e., bile present in the canaliculi. Advances in renal physiology were to a large extent consequent upon the technique of obtaining samples of glomerular filtrate from various regions of the renal tubules. But the task of obtaining primary canalicular bile by such a technique at the present time seems to be impossible. Therefore theories about the mechanism of bile secretion must be dependent for the time being on secondary information. It is generally accepted that the primary event in bile secretion is the active transport of bile salts (in the form of anions) from the hepatocytes into the bile canaliculi. The osmotic gradient resulting from this process promotes the passage of water and solutes into the canaliculi. It is also possible that water and solutes are able to pass along the intercellular spaces and so reach the canaliculi by this route. However, the net result would be the same in that primary bile would accumulate in the canaliculi and then pass down the biliary tree. There is indirect evidence that changes in bile composition occur by transfer of water and solutes across the epithelial cells of the bile ductules and larger ducts, and that it is this part of biliary secretion which is influenced by the hormone secretin.

It is also well established that many substances (particularly acids) which are excreted in bile by active transport cause an increase in bile production. This aspect of biliary secretion and the corresponding phenomenon in urine formation have been discussed by Sperber (1959, 1965).

Brauer (1959) distinguished three classes of substances which are excreted in bile, the classification being based on the ratios of their concentrations in bile and plasma. Class A substances (bile:plasma ratio = 1) included Na^+, K^+, Cl^-, and glucose; Class B substances had a bile:plasma ratio of 10–1000:1 (e.g., BSP, bilirubin glucuronide, bile salts); Class C substances had a ratio of less than 1 (sucrose, inulin, phosphate, cholesterol, and mucoproteins). Class B substances have been the most thoroughly studied, but the validity of many such studies is open to question because of the inadequacy of the analyses carried out. Usually, for technical reasons, only the amount of a substance excreted in bile was measured, and the Brauer concept of bile:plasma ratio was lost sight of. Schanker (1968) has stressed the need for rigorous experimental design in work carried out to study biliary excretion. The substances should be determined in both plasma and bile, and whenever possible the concentration of the substance in liver tissue and the volume of bile produced should also be measured. Ideally, the plasma concentration of the substance should be kept constant by administering the substance by continuous infusion, and if the substance is excreted partly in urine, the renal pedicles should be ligated. If a substance is rapidly excreted in bile then it is probable that an active transport mechanism is involved. However, if biliary excretion of a substance is low, no valid conclusions can be made. Schanker quotes the example of guanethidine. In rats only about 0.2% of the dose is excreted in bile in 2 hours. However the bile:plasma ratio is about 25:1. The low biliary excretion is due to the low plasma concentration because most of the compound is tightly bound to muscle proteins. Other examples of how erroneous conclusions can be drawn from specific examples are given by Schanker (1968).

He has also suggested that the isolated perfused liver provides a useful preparation for the study of biliary excretion. The plasma levels of a compound presented to the biliary system can be more readily controlled and the influence of extrahepatic metabolism and excretion are eliminated. The effects of metabolic inhibitors, anaerobic conditions and temperature change can be readily investigated. This preparation has been widely used for studying the mechanism of biliary secretion (e.g., Bizard, 1965; Brauer, 1965; Vanlerenberghe, 1965). However, the perfused liver preparation has been used for very few investigations of biliary excretion of steroid hormones. Berliner et al. (1962) studied the conjugation and biliary excretion of corticosteroids by isolated perfused rat liver. The results obtained were similar to those from in vivo experiments on intact animals. Perfusion pressure and temperature were kept constant and no metabolic inhibitors were added to the perfusate. In spite of the limited nature of this investigation, it does show that the isolated perfused liver could be a valuable tool for studying the secretion of steroids in bile.

A large number of a wide variety of drugs and chemicals are excreted in bile. A comprehensive survey of such investigations has been made by Smith (1966). In that review, most of the work referred to was carried out on rats. This convenient laboratory animal may have proved to be more of a bane than a boon in providing information about biliary excretion of drugs and steroids. For instance, in a review by Stowe and Plaa (1968) a list of 91 drugs which are excreted in bile is given. In 62 instances the experimental animal was the rat. Thus, many general conclusions about biliary secretion of drugs have been arrived at from results on this one species. While some of these conclusions may be valid *for the rat*, these conclusions do not apply generally to all species. It has already been stressed that the rat differs from other species, particularly man, in its metabolism and excretion of steroid hormones.

It is worthwhile to provide a specific example of investigations designed to provide a generally acceptable theory to explain the biliary excretion of metabolites of organic compounds.

Abou-El-Makarem et al. (1967a) compared the biliary and urinary excretion by rats of metabolites of benzene and 21 of its simple derivatives. The general conclusion was drawn that, in the rat, compounds with a molecular weight of less than 300 are poorly excreted in bile. When the renal pedicles were tied, biliary excretion of these metabolites increased slightly but was still less than 10% of the dose. Therefore the low biliary excretion was not due to the kidney having a greater capacity for clearing these metabolites. Millburn et al. (1967) carried out similar studies with compounds of greater molecular weight (154–495). The biliary excretion of these compounds ranged from 10 to 100% of the dose. They concluded that the extent of biliary secretion of compounds in the rat depends on its molecular weight, polarity, and metabolism. The minimum molecular weight appeared to be 325 ± 50; the rate at which substances are metabolized may also affect the extent of biliary secretion. Most of the substances were excreted as glucuronides. Millburn et al. suggested that the reason why substances with these properties are excreted in bile is that they are transported into bile by the same route as bile salts which have molecular weights of about 466–516 and pK_a values of 1.56–4.54. Bilirubin mono- and diglucuronides have molecular weights of 761 and 937, respectively. Sperber (1965) has also suggested that substances of molecular weights 200–400 are preferentially excreted by the kidney, and those with a molecular weight greater than 400 are efficiently excreted in bile. Abou-El-Makarem et al. (1967b) found that species differences exist in the ability of animals to excrete organic compounds in bile. In general, however, compounds of higher molecular weight tended to be excreted more readily in bile. Stilbestrol glucuronide (molecular weight, 445) provides an example of this species difference. The rat, dog, hen, and cat excrete 60–100% of this compound in bile, whereas the guinea pig and rabbit excrete only 20–30% by this route. When phenolphthalein glucuronide was administered, 3 grades of biliary excretion of the compound were found: rat, dog, and hen, 50–90%; cat and sheep, 30%; rabbit, guinea pig, and rhesus monkey 5–15%.

Further studies were carried out on the biliary excretion of [^{14}C]succinylsulfathiazole in rats and rabbits. In the rat 34% of an intravenous dose was excreted in bile in 3 hours, but only 1.3% in the rabbit. Ligation of the renal pedicles increased the amount in rat bile to 82%, but only to 2.5% in the rabbit. This species difference was attributed to the differences in permeability of the cells to the drug and also to a deficiency in the rabbit for transferring the drug from the liver cell to the canaliculus. It was also found that phenolphthalein glucuronide and bile salts compete with succinylsulfathiazole for biliary excretion in the rat but not in the rabbit (Abou-El-Makarem et al., 1967b).

These investigations have been quoted at some length because of their relevance to the biliary excretion of steroid metabolites. Steroid hormone metabolites have molecular weights of the order of 300–350, and conjugation with glucuronic acid would increase this value to about 500. Such glucuronides fit the criteria for substances which would be expected to be excreted in bile, i.e., a high molecular weight, a polar (glucuronide or sulfate) group and a pK of 3–4. Therefore, on the basis of the hypothesis propounded above, steroid metabolites ought to be excreted mainly in the bile. This is valid to a certain extent for the rat, but does not explain the large differences in biliary excretion of metabolites of the same steroid by different species, nor of different steroid by the same species (Table I).

If, as has been stated above, it is reasonable to suppose that the fundamental mechanism of bile formation is the same in all species, it follows that the biliary excretion of steroid metabolites is not linked to this fundamental process. It is also unlikely that the proposal of Millburn *et al.* (1967) that the substances they investigated are excreted into bile by the same mechanism for the bile salts is tenable. Indeed, J. Sjövall and Sjövall (1970) found that plasma bilirubin levels were normal in some patients with pruritis of pregnancy even though steroid sulfate and bile acid levels in plasma were elevated. There was also little or no correlation between plasma bile acid and steroid sulfate levels nor between $C_{21}O_2$ steroids and 5α-pregnane-3α,20α,21-triol. Furthermore, after parturition the plasma levels of certain steroid monosulfates decreased normally, whereas the decrease in disulfates was less rapid. There may be many explanations of these findings, but the most likely is that biliary function is impaired in these patients. However, the variable and unrelated levels of bilirubin, bile acids, some steroids and their mono- and disulfates provide strong evidence that there is a differential disturbance of biliary secretion. If this is so, then it follows that bile salts, bilirubin, and steroid conjugates are not secreted into bile by the same mechanism.

A few examples taken from experiments described in Section IV (Table I) will illustrate the complexity of the problem. The rat excretes metabolites of all steroids so far studied to a considerable extent in bile (or feces). When the bile duct of rats is ligated, the metabolites of progesterone are diverted to the urine. These findings are in agreement with the observations of R. T. Williams and his group, and also with the criteria proposed for the excretion of substances in bile. In contrast, the cat excretes metabolites of neutral and phenolic steroids almost completely into bile, and ligation of the bile duct does not divert metabolites of estradiol into the urine. Also, the cat excretes phenolphthalein glucuronide in both urine and bile (Karim and Taylor, 1970c). A possible explanation of this is that the cat kidney will not "accept" estrogen metabolites but will "accept" more phenolphthalein glucuronide when the biliary route is not available. The administered estradiol is metabolized and the plasma level of radioactivity remains virtually constant (Fig. 9) until the biliary route of excretion becomes available. Plasma bilirubin increases steadily during the period of ligation of the bile duct.

Human subjects excrete different steroid metabolites to different extents in bile and urine. In general, metabolites of the more polar steroids are excreted almost entirely in urine, while those of less polar steroids are excreted to some extent in the bile. Some work suggests that there is not an absolutely selective excretion of metabolites in bile and urine based on the structure of the steroid moiety or on the type of conjugate. Evidence for this is sparse; Wiest *et al.* (1958) isolated the same metabolites of progesterone from the glucuronide fraction of bile and urine. On the other hand, studies on endogenous steroids suggest that sulfoconjugated steroids occur in human bile in greater amounts than do glucuronides (Section VI).

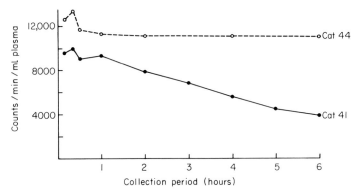

Fig. 9. Plasma radioactivity in cats with cannulated bile ducts after administration of [4-¹⁴C]estradiol. The lower (solid) line shows the values in a normal experiment; the upper (broken) line the values in a cat with the common bile duct ligated. (Karim and Taylor, 1970b).

These observations indicate that the secretion of steroid metabolites into bile involves a number of complex factors, most of which are not clearly understood. However, certain unlikely mechanisms can be eliminated. It is probable that molecular weight, polarity and pK are not major factors influencing biliary excretion of steroids; steroid metabolites (and bilirubin) are not secreted into bile by the same process as bile salts, and so are not associated with the primary mechanism of bile formation; the stereochemical conformation and nature of conjugation of the steroid molecule may be major factors in determining the route of excretion (e.g., sulfates of 5α-steroids predominate in bile and glucuronides of 5β-steroids appear to be preferentially cleared by the kidney: Section X).

Haslewood (1965, 1967) has suggested that during evolution organisms developed the ability to produce "more efficient" bile salts as they became less "primitive." He has also shown than, within limits, it is possible to assess the relationships between, and the development of, species by considering the nature of the bile salts formed. Thus, the concept of "biochemical taxonomy" was derived. It is difficult to classify the animals considered in the present review in a precise order from more "primitive" to less "primitive," either by general or "biochemical" taxonomy. However, it is reasonable to suggest that rodents are more "primitive" than man in many biochemical and physiological respects. Such a classification does not rule out the concept that the fundamental mechanism of bile secretion is common to all higher animals. If this is accepted, further proposals about bile formation may be made. It is generally accepted that different species synthesize "primary" bile acids from cholesterol, and these may be conjugated with glycine and/or taurine to yield the bile salts. Some examples relevant to the present argument are worth quoting. The "primary" bile acids produced by various species are shown in Table XIII. The "secondary" bile acids are formed from the "primary" acids by the intestinal microflora of the terminal ileum (and possibly cecum), the region of the gastrointestinal tract in which most reabsorption of bile acids occurs. The bile acids found in animal bile are, therefore, a mixture of "primary" and "secondary" acids. These acids have different structures and are conjugated with glycine and taurine to different extents in different species. This conjugation depends to some extent on diet: carnivores and omnivores produce mainly taurine conjugates, and herbivores both taurine and glycine conjugates. Thus the biliary secretory mechanism for bile salts in different animals will require the canalicular

TABLE XIII
"PRIMARY" AND "SECONDARY" BILE ACIDS OF ANIMAL AND HUMAN BILE[a]

Species	Primary acid	Secondary acid
Human Rabbit Ox	Cholic	Deoxycholic
Human Rat	Chenodeoxycholic	Ursodeoxycholic (?)
Human Rabbit Guinea pig	Chenodeoxycholic	Lithocholic

[a] From Haslewood (1967).

membrane to have the ability to "recognize" different bile salts so that active secretion of these substances into the canaliculus can occur. There is evidence that this type of specific "recognition" exists. The rat and mouse do not tolerate deoxycholic acid but convert it into cholic acid. Bile obtained by fistula from rats contains no deoxycholic acid, and if this labeled acid is injected into rats it is rapidly converted into taurocholic acid. The same occurs in the mouse. However, the rabbit does not possess the 7α-hydroxylase system for converting deoxycholic to cholic acid and so appears to "prefer" dihydroxy bile acids.

Bile salts appear to be secreted only into bile. There is no substantial evidence that any appreciable quantities of these substances appear in urine, except in human patients with severe obstructive jaundice and even then the amounts are small.

The strongly basic anion exchange resin cholestyramine is able to sequester bile salts in the intestine and so prevent the enterohepatic circulation of bile salts. This leads to a decrease in the levels of plasma bile salts and cholestyramine has been used to decrease these levels in patients with jaundice and pruritus (see Haslewood, 1967, for references).

Jensen et al. (1966) have discussed the role of specific "receptor sites" for target organs of estrogens and testosterone. The sites are highly specific for a particular hormone in particular target tissues.

Cronholm et al. (1970) found that during the jaundiced phase in patients with hepatitis total plasma bile acids were markedly elevated. Deoxycholic acid was practically absent from plasma, but returned during recovery from the disease. This strongly indicates an interrupted enterohepatic circulation of bile acids. However, the extent of the increase in steroid sulfates was not so great as that of bile acids. They quote evidence that biliary secretion of bile acids is not completely blocked in hepatitis. J. Sjövall and Sjövall (1970) observed similar changes in patients with pruritus of pregnancy, but found no correlation between the absolute levels of bile acids and steroid sulfates. When cholestyramine was administered to some of the patients, plasma bile acids were decreased 2- to 3-fold, but there was no significant change in steroid sulfates.

On the basis of the evidence quoted in the preceding paragraphs a hypothesis is now put forward to account for the secretion of steroid hormone metabolites into bile. The membrane of the bile canaliculus contains "receptor sites" which are as specific for certain steroid metabolites as are other "receptor sites" for bile salts. The "binding" of these substances at the "receptor sites" is an obligatory step prior to active transfer of the substances across the canalicular membrane. In the more "primitive" animals, such as rats and mice, the "receptor sites" have poor specificity and so are able to "bind" metabolites of most steroid hormones. In other species, particularly man, evolution has resulted in a decrease in the number, specificity and "binding capacity" of these sites. Therefore, some steroid metabolites are partially "bound" and so excreted into bile (e.g., progesterone metabolites), whereas others are less firmly, or not, bound and so return to the blood by a passive or active transport mechanism. The "binding sites" have a greater affinity (1) for conjugated, especially diconjugated, metabolites than for free steroids and (2) for sulfoconjugates than for glucuronides. The presence of these "binding sites" in the canalicular membrane would result in the removal of the "bound" metabolites from the steroid-metabolizing and conjugating enzyme systems within the cell, thus allowing the entry of more steroid into the cell by active or passive transport.

This hypothesis goes some way to explaining the differences in biliary excretion of steroid metabolites by different species, and the excretion of different steroids by the same species. If the canalicular membrane suffers damage due to toxic substances or disease these postulated "binding sites" might lose their activity more readily than the "sites" for bile acids. This would explain the different effects of disease on plasma bile acids and plasma steroids, and also the difference in the ability of the liver to retain its normal secretory capacity during recovery from disease. The hypothesis does not exclude the possibility that specific binding proteins might also be present within the hepatocyte. However, the transport of steroid metabolites into bile is a rapid process. Taylor and Wright (1970) investigated the disposition of metabolites of tritiated progesterone in the liver of mice. Figure 10 shows the heavy deposition of silver grains in a small bile duct in an autoradiograph of a sample of liver taken 10 minutes after administration of the steroid. No localization of silver grains within hepatocytes could be observed in livers taken at times ranging from 1.5 to 30 minutes after administration of the labeled progesterone. This is not highly convincing evidence for the proposed mechanism of "binding" of steroid metabolites by the canalicular membrane, but useful evidence for or against the hypothesis could be obtained by combined electron microscopy–autoradiography.

The degree of specificity of the "binding sites" for hormone (and drug) metabolites will determine the degree of inhibition produced by some substance on the biliary secretion of others. Therefore, the hypothesis could be tested by investigating the extent of competition for biliary excretion of steroids and other substances by administration of the possible competitors in differing amounts. Ideally the substances administered should not undergo further metabolism before being excreted in the liver. Doubly labeled steroid conjugates and the isolated perfused liver would provide a useful experimental system for such studies.

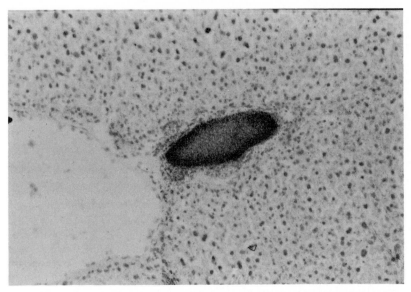

FIG. 10. Autoradiograph of mouse liver taken 10 minutes after administration of [7α-³H]progesterone. Note the heavy deposition of silver in the bile ductule and the absence of deposition in the blood vessel (×180). From Taylor and Wright (1970).

Other possible ways of disposing of this highly tentative suggestion will no doubt occur to the critical reader.

XII. CONCLUDING REMARKS

In 1889 L. S. Beale began the Introduction to his book "The Liver" with these words: "Our knowledge of the intimate structure and action of the liver still remains in many respects vague and incomplete, and as compared with what is known of the minute anatomy and physiology of many secreting organs our information concerning this large gland is still imperfect. Not only must it be admitted that the exact arrangement and precise relation to one another of the most important structural elements have not yet been conclusively determined, but we are unable at this time to give an adequate explanation of the most important changes which occur during the healthy action of the liver."

Although an enormous amount of information about the liver and biliary system has been published in the intervening 80 years, the statement of Beale is almost as true today as it was then.

The study of biliary and fecal excretion of steroid hormone metabolites has greatly extended our knowledge of steroid metabolism. However, an equally important aspect of this field of study is that the judicious use of steroid metabolites could provide valuable information about the mechanism(s) involved in bile production. It is hoped that this review will encourage those mainly involved with steroid investigations to use the new highly sensitive and precise techniques of steroid analysis to study the mechanism of biliary excretion; and also that those mainly concerned with studying bile formation in normal and pathological conditions will include steroid hormone metabolites in their investigations. Some interdisciplinary work of this kind is already in progress, but the time is now ripe for much more collaboration and a change in attitudes to particular aspects of work on the biliary system. Biomedical scientists are often accused of being specialists of a specialized aspect of a specialized field of research. The biliary system and steroid metabolism offer two specialized fields which could be united to blunt the accusation.

ACKNOWLEDGMENTS

I wish to thank Mr. B. McFarlane of the Department of Anatomy of this Medical School for the electron microscopy of cat liver (Fig. 2), and also Mrs. M. Cheek for so ably typing the manuscript. My thanks are also due to Blackwells Scientific Publications and the Editor of the *Journal of Clinical Endocrinology and Metabolism* for permission to reproduce diagrams from their publications.

ADDENDUM

After the review had been completed Despopoulos (1971) described experiments with isolated perfused rat livers, and other types of liver preparation, designed to assess the role of some natural and synthetic estrogens, progestins, and corticoids in hormone-induced cholestasis. He has proposed that steroid-induced cholestasis could be the result of interference with any steps in bile formation. The primary effect seemed to be on the conversion of cholic acid to taurocholate by most of the steroids examined. The reduction in formation of bile salts would result in a decrease in bile flow. However, this proposal does not provide a general explanation of steroid-induced cholestasis since Mestranol did not have any effect on taurocholate formation. Nor would species differences in response to steroid administration and the differential changes in plasma levels of steroids, bile acids, and bilirubin in hepatitis and pruritis of pregnancy in man be explicable on the basis of this hypothesis. However, the interesting proposals of Despopoulos are worthy of fuller investigation in man and other animals with different types of cholestasis.

REFERENCES

Aach, R. D. (1969). *Gastroenterology* **56**, 363.
Abdel-Aziz, M. T., and Williams, K. I. H. (1970). *Steroids* **15**, 695.
Abou-El-Makarem, M. M., Millburn, P., Smith, R. L., and Williams, R. T. (1967a). *Biochem. J.* **105**, 1269.
Abou-El-Makarem, M. M., Millburn, P., Smith, R. L., and Williams, R. T. (1967b). *Biochem. J.* **105**, 1289.
Adlercreutz, H. (1962). *Acta Endocrinol. (Copenhagen)*, *Suppl.* **72**.
Adlercreutz, H. (1965). *In* "The Biliary System" (W. Taylor, ed.), p. 369. Blackwell, Oxford.
Adlercreutz, H. (1970). *J. Endocrinol.* **46**, 129.

Adlercreutz, H., and Luukkainen, T. (1965a). *J. Reprod. Fert.* **9**, 137.
Adlercreutz, H., and Luukkainen, T. (1965b). *Biochim. Biophys. Acta* **97**, 134.
Adlercreutz, H., and Luukkainen, T. (1967). *Acta Endocrinol. (Copenhagen) Suppl.* **124**, 101.
Adlercreutz, H., and Luukkainen, T. (1970). *Ann. Clin. Res.* **2**, 365.
Adlercreutz, H., Diczfalusy, E., and Engstrom, L. (1960). *Endocrinology* **66**, 80.
Adlercreutz, H., Svanborg, A., and Anberg, A. (1967a). *Amer. J. Med.* **42**, 335.
Adlercreutz, H., Svanborg, A., and Anberg, A. (1967b). *Amer. J. Med.* **42**, 341.
Allan, J. S., and Tyler, E. T. (1967). *Fert. Steril.* **18**, 112.
Allen, J. G., and Thomas, G. H. (1967). *J. Endocrinol.* **37**, 477.
Allen, J. G., and Thomas, G. H. (1968). *J. Endocrinol.* **42**, 27.
Archer, S. E. H., Scratcherd, T., and Taylor, W. (1965). *Biochem. J.* **94**, 778.
Arias, I. M. (1963). *Ann. N. Y. Acad. Sci.* **104**, 1014.
Barry, M. C., Eidenoff, M. L., Dobriner, K., and Gallagher, T. F. (1952). *Endocrinology* **50**, 587.
Bercovici, J. D., and Mauvais-Jarvis, P. (1970). *Proc. Int. Congr. Horm. Steroids, 3rd, 1970* Int. Congr. Ser. No. 210, p. 136.
Berliner, D. L., Leong, G. F., Cazes, D. M., and Berliner, M. L. (1962). *Amer. J. Physiol.* **202**, 420.
Birke, G. (1954). *Acta Med. Scand., Suppl.* **291**, 53.
Bizard, G. (1965). *In* "The Biliary System" (W. Taylor, ed.), p. 315. Blackwell, Oxford.
Brauer, R. W. (1959). *J. Amer. Med. Ass.* **169**, 1462.
Brauer, R. W. (1965). *In* "The Biliary System" (W. Taylor, ed.), p. 41. Blackwell, Oxford.
Brooks, C. J. W., Brooks, R. V., Fotherby, K., Grant, J. K., Klopper, A., and Klyne, W. (1970). *J. Endocrinol.* **47**, 265.
Brown, J. B. (1955). *Biochem. J.* **60**, 185.
Burstein, S., Ungar, F., Gut, M., and Dorfman, R. I. (1955). *Endocrinology* **56**, 267.
Butt, H. R., Foulk, W. T., Baggenstoss, A. H., and Dickson, E. R. (1965). *In* "The Biliary System" (W. Taylor, ed.), p. 619. Blackwell, Oxford.
Calvin, H. I., and Lieberman, S. (1962). *Biochemistry* **1**, 639.
Calvin, H. I., Wiele, R. L. V., and Lieberman, S. (1963). *Biochemistry* **2**, 648.
Cargill, D., Steinetz, B., Gosnell, E., Beach, V., Meli, A., Fujimoto, G., and Reynolds, B. (1969). *J. Clin. Endocrinol. Metab.* **29**, 1051.
Chang, E., Slaunwhite, W. R., and Sandberg, A. A. (1960). *J. Clin. Endocrinol. Metab.* **20**, 1568.
Clifton, J. A., Ingelfinger, F. J., and Burrows, B. A. (1958). *J. Lab. Clin. Med.* **51**, 701.
Collins, D. C., and Layne, D. S. (1969). *Steroids* **13**, 783.
Collins, D. C., Williams, K. I. H., and Layne, D. S. (1967). *Endocrinology* **80**, 893.
Cooke, A. M., Rogers, A. W., and Thomas, G. H. (1963). *J. Endocrinol.* **27**, 299.
Cronholm, T., Norman, A., and Sjövall, J. (1970). *Scand. J. Gastroenterol.* **5**, 297.
Despopoulos, A. (1971). *J. Pharmacol. Exp. Ther.* **176**, 273.
Diczfalusy, E., Franksson, C., and Martinsen, B. (1961). *Acta Endocrinol. (Copenhagen)* **38**, 59.
Diczfalusy, E., Franksson, C., Lisboa, B. P., and Martinsen, B. (1962). *Acta Endocrinol. (Copenhagen)* **40**, 537.
Doisy, E. A., Jr. (1965). *In* "The Biliary System" (W. Taylor, ed.), p. 685. Blackwell, Oxford.

Elias, H. (1965). *In* "The Biliary System" (W. Taylor, ed.), p. 1. Blackwell, Oxford.

Emerman, S., Twombly, G. H., and Levitz, M. (1967). *J. Clin. Endocrinol. Metab.* **27**, 539.

Emslie-Smith, A. H. (1965). *Ernobrungsforsch.* **10**, 302.

Eneroth, P., and Gustafsson, J. A. (1969). *Acta Endocrinol. (Copenhagen) Suppl.* **138**, 69.

Engel, L. L., Carter, P., and Fielding, L. L. (1955). *J. Biol. Chem.* **213**, 99.

Ericsson, J. L. E. (1969). *In* "The Biological Basis of Medicine" (E. E. Bittar and N. Bittar, eds.), Vol. 5, p. 143. Academic Press, New York.

Eriksson, H. (1971). *Eur. J. Biochem.* **18**, 86.

Eriksson, H., and Gustafsson, J. A. (1970a). *Eur. J. Biochem.* **15**, 132.

Eriksson, H., and Gustafsson, J. A. (1970b). *Eur. J. Biochem.* **13**, 198.

Eriksson, H., and Gustafsson, J. A. (1971). *Eur. J. Biochem.* **18**, 146.

Eriksson, H., Gustafsson, J. A., and Sjövall, J. (1968). *Eur. J. Biochem.* **6**, 219.

Eriksson, H., Gustafsson, J. A., and Sjövall, J. (1970). *Eur. J. Biochem.* **12**, 520.

Erlinger, S., Dumont, M., and Benhamov, J. P. (1969). *Rev. Fr. Etud. Clin. Biol.* **14**, 1007.

Fahim, M. S., and Hall, D. G. (1970). *Amer. J. Obstet. Gynecol.* **106**, 183.

Forker, E. L. (1969). *J. Clin. Invest.* **48**, 654.

Fotherby, K., Kamyab, S., Littleton, P., and Klopper, A. (1968). *J. Reprod. Fert., Suppl.* **5**, 51.

Francis, F. E., and Kinsella, R. A. (1966). *J. Clin. Endocrinol. Metab.* **26**, 128.

Francis, F. E., Shen, N. C., and Kinsella, R. A. (1960). *J. Biol. Chem.* **235**, 1957.

Francis, F. E., Shen, N. C., and Kinsella, R. A. (1962). *Biochemistry* **1**, 1184.

Fukushima, D. K., Bradlow, H. L., Dobriner, K., and Gallagher, T. F. (1954). *J. Biol. Chem.* **206**, 863.

Gallagher, T. F., Mueller, M. N., and Kappas, A. (1966). *Medicine (Baltimore)* **45**, 471.

Goebelsmann, U., Sjoberg, K., Wiqvist, N., and Diczfalusy, E. (1965). *Acta Endocrinol. (Copenhagen)* **50**, 261.

Gustafsson, B. E., Bergstrom, S., Lindstedt, S., and Norman, A. (1957). *Proc. Soc. Exp. Biol. Med.* **94**, 467.

Gustafsson, B. E., Gustafsson, J. A., and Sjövall, J. (1968a). *Acta Chem. Scand.* **20**, 821.

Gustafsson, B. E., Gustafsson, J. A., and Sjövall, J. (1968b). *Eur. J. Biochem.* **4**, 568.

Gustafsson, J. A. (1968). *Eur. J. Biochem.* **6**, 248.

Gustafsson, J. A. (1970). *Eur. J. Biochem.* **14**, 560.

Gustafsson, J. A., and Sjövall, J. (1968a). *Eur. J. Biochem.* **6**, 227.

Gustafsson, J. A., and Sjövall, J. (1968b). *Eur. J. Biochem.* **6**, 236.

Gustafsson, J. A., Shackleton, C. H. L., and Sjövall, J. (1969). *Eur. J. Biochem.* **10**, 302.

Gustafsson, J. A., Shackleton, C. H. I., and Sjövall, J. (1970). *Acta Endocrinol. (Copenhagen)* **65**, 18.

Haemmerli, P., and Weiss, H. I. (1967). *Medicine (Baltimore)* **46**, 299.

Hargreaves, T. (1965). *Nature (London)* **206**, 154.

Haslewood, G. A. D. (1965). *In* "The Biliary System" (W. Taylor, ed.), p. 107. Blackwell, Oxford.

Haslewood, G. A. D. (1967). "Bile Salts." Methuen, London.

Heikel, T. A. J., and Lathe, G. H. (1970a). *Brit. J. Pharmacol.* **38**, 593.

Heikel, T. A. J., and Lathe, G. H. (1970b). *Biochem. J.* **118**, 187.

Hellman, L., Bradlaw, H. L., Adesman, J., Fukushima, D. K., Kulp, J. L., and Gallagher, T. F. (1954). *J. Clin. Invest.* 33, 1106.

Hellman, L., Zumoff, B., Fishman, J., and Gallagher, T. F. (1970). *J. Clin. Endocrinol. Metab.* 30, 161.

Hellström, K., Sjövall, J., and Víhko, R. (1969). *Acta Endocrinol. (Copenhagen)* 60, 501.

Hobkirk, R., and Nilsen, M. (1969a). *Steroids* 13, 679.

Hobkirk, R., and Nilsen, M. (1969b). *Steroids* 14, 533.

Hobkirk, R., Nilsen, M., and Blahey, P. R. (1969). *J. Clin. Endocrinol. Metab.* 29, 328.

Hyde, P. M., and Williams, R. H. (1957). *J. Biol. Chem.* 227, 1063.

Hyde, P. M., Elliott, W. H., Doisy, E. A., Jr., and Doisy, E. A. (1954). *J. Biol. Chem.* 207, 287.

Inoue, N., Sandberg, A. A., Graham, J. B., and Slaunwhite, W. R. (1969a). *J. Clin. Invest.* 48, 380.

Inoue, N., Sandberg, A. A., Graham, J. B., and Slaunwhite, W. R. (1969b). *J. Clin. Invest.* 48, 390.

Jensen, E. V., Jacobson, H. I., Flesher, J. W., Saha, N. N., Gupta, G. N., Smith, S., Colucci, V., Shiplacoff, D., Neuman, H. G., DeSombre, E. R., and Jungblut, P. W. (1966). *In* "Steroid Dynamics" (G. Pincus, J. Tait, and T. Nakao, eds.), p. 133. Academic Press, New York.

Jirku, H., and Levitz, M. (1969). *J. Clin. Endocrinol. Metab.* 29, 615.

Karim, M. F., and Taylor, W. (1970a). *Biochem. J.* 117, 267.

Karim, M. F., and Taylor, W. (1970b). *Proc. Int. Congr. Horm. Steroids, 3rd, 1970* Int. Congr. Ser. No. 210, p. 233.

Karim, M. F., and Taylor, W. (1970c). Unpublished observation.

Katz, R., Ducci, H., and Alessandri, H. (1957). *J. Clin. Invest.* 36, 1370.

Kirdani, R. Y., Slaunwhite, W. R., and Sandberg, A. A. (1969). *J. Steroid Biochem.* 1, 265.

Kleiner, G. J., Kresch, L., and Arias. I. M. (1965). *N. Engl. J. Med.* 273, 420.

Klopper, A., Strong, J. A., and Cook, L. R. (1957). *J. Endocrinol.* 18, 319.

Korenman, S. G., Perrin, L. E., and McCallum, T. (1969). *J. Clin. Invest.* 48, 45a.

Kreek, M. J., Sleisenger, M. H., and Jeffries, G. H. (1967a). *Amer. J. Med.* 43, 795.

Kreek, M. J., Weser, E., Sleisenger, M. H., and Jeffries, G. H. (1967b). *N. Engl. J. Med.* 277, 1391.

Kreek, M. J., Peterson, R. E., Sleisenger, M. H., and Jeffries, G. H. (1969). *Proc. Soc. Exp. Biol. Med.* 131, 646.

Kulkarni, B. D., Kammer, C. S., and Goldzieher, J. W. (1970). *Gen. Comp. Endocrinol.* 14, 68.

Laatikainen, T. (1970a). *Steroids* 15, 139.

Laatikainen, T. (1970b). *Eur. J. Biochem.* 14, 372.

Laatikainen, T. (1970c). *Ann. Clin. Res.* 2, 338.

Laatikainen, T., and Víhko, R. (1969a). *Eur. J. Biochem.* 10, 165.

Laatikainen, T., and Víhko, R. (1969b). *Steroids* 14, 119.

Laatikainen, T., and Víhko, R. (1970a). *Eur. J. Biochem.* 13, 534.

Laatikainen, T., and Víhko, R. (1970b). *Proc. Int. Congr. Horm. Steroids, 3rd, 1970* Int. Congr. Ser. No. 210, p. 124.

Laatikainen, T., and Víhko, R. (1970c). *Ann. Clin. Res.* 2, 350.

Laatikainen, T., Peltokallio, P., and Víhko, R. (1968). *Steroids* 12, 407.

Lanman, R. C., and Schanker, L. S. (1970). *Life Sci.* 9, 1003.

Lathe, G. H., and Walker, M. (1958a). *Biochem. J.* **68,** 6p.

Lathe, G. H., and Walker, M. (1958b). *Quart. J. Exp. Physiol.* **63,** 257.

Layne, D. S., Sheth, N. A., and Kirdani, R. Y. (1964). *J. Biol. Chem.* **239,** 3221.

Lehtinen, A., Nurmikko, V., and Hartiala, K. (1958a). *Acta Chem. Scand.* **12,** 1585.

Lehtinen, A., Hartiala, K., and Nurmikko, V. (1958b). *Acta Chem. Scand.* **12,** 1589.

Lester, R. (1965). *In* "The Biliary System" (W. Taylor, ed.), p. 223. Blackwell, Oxford.

Levitz, M., and Katz, J. (1968). *J. Clin. Endocrinol. Metab.* **28,** 862.

Lisboa, B. P., Drossé, I., and Breuer, H. (1965). *Hoppe-Seyler's Z. Physiol. Chem.* **342,** 106.

Longwell, B., and McKay, F. B. (1942). *J. Biol. Chem.* **142,** 757.

Lowy, J., Albepart, T., and Pasqualini, J. R. (1969). *Acta Endocrinol. (Copenhagen)* **61,** 483.

Luckey, T. D. (1965). *Ernobrungsforsch.* **10,** 302.

Luukkainen, T., Leroux, G., and Adlercreutz, H. (1970). *Proc. Int. Congr. Horm. Steroids, 3rd, 1970* Int. Congr. Ser. No. 210, p. 188.

Marti, M., Schindler, O., and Buehrer, R. (1961). *Gynaecologia* **152,** 265.

Menini, E., and Diczfalusy, E. (1960). *Endocrinology* **67,** 500.

Menini, E., and Diczfalusy, E. (1961). *Endocrinology* **68,** 492.

Migeon, C. J., Sandberg, A. A., Paul, A. C., and Samuels, L. T. (1956). *J. Clin. Endocrinol. Metab.* **16,** 1291

Millburn, P., Smith, R. L., and Williams, R. T. (1967). *Biochem. J.* **105,** 1275.

Mitchell, F. L. (1967). *Vitam. Horm. (New York)* **25,** 191.

Mueller, M. N., and Kappas, A. (1964). *J. Clin. Invest.* **43,** 1905.

Pasqualini, J. R. (1969). *J. Steroid Biochem.* **1,** 25.

Pearlman, W. H., Rakoff, A. E., and Contarow, K. C. (1947). *J. Biol. Chem.* **170,** 173.

Pearson, J. R., and Martin, R. B. (1966). *Endocrinology* **78,** 914.

Peterson, R. E. (1959). *Recent Progr. Horm. Res.* **15,** 231.

Peterson, R. E. (1965). *In* "The Biliary System" (W. Taylor, ed.), p. 385. Blackwell, Oxford.

Peterson, R. E., Pierce, C. E., Wyngaarden, J. B., Bunim, J. J., and Brodie, B. B. (1957). *J. Clin. Invest.* **36,** 1301.

Rao, L. G. S., and Taylor, W. (1964). Unpublished observation.

Rao, L. G. S., and Taylor, W. (1965). *Biochem. J.* **96,** 172.

Roberts, K. D., Bandi, L., Calvin, H. I., Drucker, W. D., and Lieberman, S. (1964). *J. Amer. Chem. Soc.* **86,** 958

Roberts, R. J., Shriver, S. L., and Plaa, G. L. (1968). *Biochem. Pharmacol.* **17,** 1261.

Rogers, J. (1956). *J. Clin. Endocrinol. Metab.* **16,** 114.

Rogers, J., and McLellan, F. (1951). *J. Clin. Endocrinol. Metab.* **11,** 246.

Romanoff, L. P., Morris, C. W., Welch, M. T., Rodriquez, R. M., and Pincus, G. (1961). *J. Clin. Endocrinol. Metab.* **21,** 1413.

Rommel, P., and Zschintzsch, A. (1965). *Acta Endocrinol. (Copenhagen)* **50,** 47.

Rouiller, C., ed. (1963). "The Liver," Vol. 1, p. 161. Academic Press, New York.

Sandberg, A. A., and Slaunwhite, W. R. (1956). *J. Clin. Invest.* **35,** 1311.

Sandberg, A. A., and Slaunwhite, W. R. (1957a). *Proc. Soc. Exp. Biol. Med.* **96,** 658.

Sandberg, A. A., and Slaunwhite, W. R. (1957b). *J. Clin. Invest.* **36,** 1266.

Sandberg, A. A., and Slaunwhite, W. R. (1958). *J. Clin. Endocrinol. Metab.* **18,** 253.

Sandberg, A. A., and Slaunwhite, W. R. (1965). *J. Clin. Invest.* **44,** 694.

Sandberg, A. A., Kirdani, R. Y., Back, N., Weyman, P., and Slaunwhite, W. R. (1967). *Amer. J. Physiol.* **213,** 1138.

Sandberg, A. A., Slaunwhite, W. R., and Kirdani, R. Y. (1970). *In* "Metabolic Conjugation and Metabolic Hydrolysis" (W. H. Fishman, ed.), Vol. 2, p. 123. Academic Press, New York.

Sandberg, E., Gurpide, E., and Lieberman, S. (1964). *Biochemistry* 3, 1256.

Schanker, L. S. (1968). *In* "Handbook of Physiology" (Amer. Physiol. Soc., J. Field. ed.), Sect. 6, Vol. V, p. 2433. Williams & Wilkins, Baltimore, Maryland.

Schedl, H. P. (1965). *J. Clin. Endocrinol. Metab.* 25, 1309.

Schedl, H. P., and Clifton, J. A. (1963). *Gastroenterology* 44, 1134.

Scherb, J., Kirschner, M., and Adrias, I. M. (1963). *J. Clin. Invest.* 42, 404.

Schmid, R., and Hammaker, L. (1959). *N. Engl. J. Med.* 260, 1310.

Schneider, J. J. (1952). *J. Biol. Chem.* 199, 235.

Schoenfield, L. J., and Foulk, W. T. (1964). *J. Clin. Invest.* 43, 1419.

Schubert, K., Schlegel, J., and Horhold, C. (1962). *Z. Naturforsch. B* 17, 84.

Schulster, D., and Kellie, A. E. (1967). *Biochem. J.* 103, 759.

Senciall, I. R., and Thomas, G. H. (1970). *J. Endocrinol.* 48, 61.

Shackleton, C. H. L., Gustafsson, J. A., and Sjövall, J. (1970). *Steroids* 15, 131.

Shaver, J. C., Roginsky, M. S., and Christy, N. P. (1963). *Lancet* 2, 335.

Shen, N.-H. C., Elliott, W. H., Doisy, E. A., Jr., and Doisy, E. A. (1954). *J. Biol. Chem.* 208, 133.

Sherlock, S. (1963). "Diseases of the Liver and Biliary System." Blackwell, Oxford.

Sherlock, S. (1965). *In* "The Biliary System" (W. Taylor, ed.), p. 585. Blackwell, Oxford.

Shirley, I. M., and Cooke, B. A. (1968). *J. Endocrinol.* 40, 477.

Sjövall, J., and Sjövall, K. (1970). *Anal. Clin. Res.* 2, 321.

Sjövall, J., and Víhko, R. (1968). *Acta Endocrinol. (Copenhagen)* 57, 247.

Sjövall, K. (1970). *Anal. Clin. Res.* 2, 393.

Slaunwhite, W. R., and Sandberg, A. A. (1961). *J. Clin. Endocrinol. Metab.* 21, 753.

Slaunwhite, W. R., Burgett, H. J., and Sandberg, A. A. (1967). *J. Clin. Endocrinol. Metab.* 27, 663.

Song, C. S., and Kappas, A. (1968). *Vita. Horm. (New York)* 26, 147.

Smith, R. L. (1966). *Progr. Drug. Res.* 9, 299.

Sperber, I. (1959). *Pharmacol. Rev.* 11, 109.

Sperber, I. (1965). *In* "The Biliary System" (W. Taylor, ed.), p. 457. Blackwell, Oxford.

Støa, K. F., and Levitz, M. (1968). *Acta Endocrinol. (Copenhagen)* 57, 657.

Stowe, C. M., and Plaa, G. L. (1968). *Annu. Rev. Pharmacol.* 8, 337.

Stupnicki, R., McCracken, J. A., and Williams, K. I. H. (1969). *J. Endocrinol.* 45, 67.

Svandborg, A., and Ohlsson, S. (1959). *Amer. J. Med.* 27, 40.

Taylor, W. (1954). *Biochem. J.* 56, 463.

Taylor, W. (1956). *Biochem. J.* 72, 442.

Taylor, W., ed. (1965a). "The Biliary System." Blackwell, Oxford.

Taylor, W., ed. (1965b). "The Biliary System," p. 399. Blackwell, Oxford.

Taylor, W. (1965c). *Biochem. J.* 97, 89.

Taylor, W. (1969). *Biochem. J.* 113, 259.

Taylor, W. (1970). *Biochem. J.* 117, 263.

Taylor, W. (1971). *Acta Endocrinol. (Copenhagen)* 67. Suppl. 155, 118.

Taylor, W., and Scratcherd, T. (1961). *Biochem. J.* 81, 398.

Taylor, W., and Scratcherd, T. (1962). *Proc. Int. Congr. Horm. Steroids, 1st, 1962.* Int. Congr. Ser. No. 51, p. 142.

Taylor, W., and Scratcherd, T. (1963). *Biochem. J.* **86**, 114.
Taylor, W., and Scratcherd, T. (1967). *Biochem. J.* **104**, 250.
Taylor, W., and Wright, D. E. (1970). *J. Endocrinol.* **48**, liii.
Twombly, G. H., and Levitz, M. (1960). *Amer. J. Obstet. Gynecol.* **80**, 889.
Vanlerenberghe, J. (1965). *In* "The Biliary System" (W. Taylor, ed.), p. 263. Blackwell, Oxford.
Velle, W. (1963). *Gen. Comp. Endocrinol.* **3**, 621.
Vermeulen, A., Slaunwhite, W. R., and Sandberg, A. A. (1961). *J. Clin. Endocrinol. Metab.* **21**, 1534.
Wheeler, H. O. (1968). *In* "Handbook of Physiology" (Amer. Physiol. Soc., J. Field, ed.), Sect. 6, Vol. V, p. 2409. Williams & Wilkins, Baltimore, Maryland.
Wiest, W. G., Fujimoto, G. I., and Sandberg, A. A. (1958). *J. Endocrinol. Metab.* **18**, 972.
Williams, K. I. H. (1969). *Steroids* **13**, 539.
Williams, R., and Billing, B. H. (1961). *Lancet* **2**, 392.
Williamson, D. G., and Layne, D. S. (1970). *Can. J. Biochem.* **48**, 523.
Willoughby, H. W., Chen, C., and Freeman, S. (1959). *Endocrinology* **65**, 539.
Wotiz, H. H. (1963). *Biochim. Biophys. Acta* **69**, 415.
Zumoff, B., Bradlow, H. L., Gallagher, T. F., and Hellman, L. (1967). *J. Clin. Invest.* **46**, 1735.
Zumoff, B., Bradlow, H. L., Cassouto, J., Gallagher, T. F., and Hellman, L. (1968). *J. Clin. Endocrinol. Metab.* **28**, 92.

The Action of Thyrotropin on Thyroid Metabolism

J. E. DUMONT

Laboratory of Nuclear Medicine and Experimental Medicine, School of Medicine, University of Brussels, and Biology Department, Euratom, Brussels, Belgium

I. Introduction

Growth and function of the thyroid are mainly controlled by the level of thyrotropin (TSH)* concentration in the plasma (for references, see Brown-Grant, 1969; Dumont et al., 1969b). The principal element of this control, the action of TSH on its target, the thyroid follicular cell, has been investigated intensively during recent years. TSH activates rapidly the steps of thyroidal iodine metabolism, i.e., the formation of thyroid hormones from iodide and tyrosines and the secretion of these hormones, and induces, after a delay, the growth of thyroid tissue.

Among the various systems available for the study of the interaction of a tropic hormone with its target cell, the thyroid and TSH present several advantages and disadvantages. The specialized metabolism of the follicular cell, the metabolism of iodine, is easily studied with the various radioisotopes of iodine. Thyroid tissue is very resistant to adverse conditions, which explains the great stability and the great variety of *in vitro* thyroid systems. This variety allows a large choice of experimental systems from the most complex and physiological, the intact animal, to the simplest and less physiological system, purified subcellular preparations, with useful intermediates such as organ perfusion *in vivo*

---

*Abbreviations: cAMP: cyclic 3′,5′-adenosine monophosphate; dATP: deoxy-adenosine triphosphate; DB-cAMP: N^6-2′-O-dibutyl cyclic 3′,5′-adenosine monophosphate; 5AI₄C: 5-aminoimidazole-4-carboxamide; DFP: diisopropylfluorophosphate; DIT: diiodotyrosine; cGMP: cyclic 3′,5′-guanosine monophosphate; GSH: reduced glutathione; GSSG: oxidized glutathione; MIT: monoiodotyrosine; NAD⁺, NADH: oxidized and reduced forms of diphosphopyridine nucleotide; NADP⁺, NADPH: oxidized and reduced forms of triphosphopyridine nucleotide; NAD = NAD⁺ + NADH; NADP = NADP⁺ + NADPH; P_i: inorganic phosphate; PBI: protein-bound iodine; PGE, PGF: prostaglandins E and F; PTU: 6-N-propylthiouracil; Synkavit: 2-methyl-1,4-naphthohydroquinonedimethylphosphoric acid; TRH: thyrotropin-releasing hormone; TSH: thyrotropin; T₃: triiodothyronine; T₄: thyroxine.

The hexose monophosphate pathway is mostly called the pentose phosphate pathway. The term iodide organification has been used in place of iodide binding to proteins or to trichloroacetic acid-precipitable material.

and *in vitro*, and incubation of slices or isolated cells. The only experimental system lacking in this field is the culture of stable, well differentiated lines of tumor cells. Such a system would be very valuable for the study of long-term hormonal effects. Among the disadvantages of the thyroid–thyrotropin system, one may mention the fragility of TSH and the fact that TSH structure was unknown until 1970 so that analogs of TSH are not yet available. Also, in most experimental animals, the thyroid is small and contains only a small population of cells. The heterogeneity of the thyroid presents problems: heterogeneity in cell composition (e.g., the high proportion of mast cells in the rat thyroid), heterogeneity in the reactivity of neighbor cells to the same stimulus. The most serious difficulty in the study of the action of TSH is, however, the variability of thyroid metabolism and of its reactions to various agents, between different species and, within the same species, between animals submitted to various diets or experimental conditions.

The literature on the action of TSH on thyroid is often hard to assess. The great variability of thyroid metabolism and responses to TSH makes it difficult to compare data obtained in different experimental systems. Each laboratory uses its own experimental protocol and provides little correlative information (e.g., relation of concentration of TSH to one of its well defined effects). Moreover, there is little common ground between morphological studies and physiological or biochemical investigations. The action of TSH on thyroid structure or ultrastructure is generally studied *in vivo* without any evaluation of thyroid metabolism. On the other hand, most metabolic investigations, *in vivo* or *in vitro*, lack controls of the ultrastructure of the investigated system. Therefore, in the absence of correlative evidence, one should be cautious about using data from one study (e.g., on ultrastructure *in vivo*) to interpret results in another system (e.g., on metabolism *in vitro*).

In this review, we have tried to analyze the available evidence on the action of TSH on thyroid function and growth, on the metabolic and morphological patterns of resting and activated tissue. Other problems, among which the binding of TSH to the thyroid cell, the possible action of TSH on thyroid differentiation, and the action of other hormones on the thyroid, have not been considered. The literature since 1960 has been covered as completely as possible. We have tried to present a comprehensive picture of current concepts of the mechanism of action of TSH, and also to differentiate what has been proved from what remains only possible, plausible, speculative, or entirely unknown. The astonishing outpouring of data and literature on the mechanism of action of TSH during the last few years has made it necessary to examine very closely the validity of experimental evidence. We have first considered the evidence that the cyclic 3',5'-AMP (cAMP) model of Sutherland applies to thyroid and TSH. The actions of TSH on thyroid morphology and on the principal metabolic pathways have then been analyzed successively. In each section, we tried to consider *in vivo* and *in vitro* effects, acute and chronic stimulation, the mechanism of each TSH effect as related to other hormonal effects, and the role of cAMP in the mediation of specific effects. Finally, the action of activators and inhibitors of the cAMP system on the various TSH effects has been analyzed.

The early literature on thyroid morphology, metabolism and regulation has been analyzed in Pitt-Rivers and Trotter (1964), while TSH action, mainly on thyroid morphology, was reviewed in articles on the bioassay of TSH (Sonenberg, 1958; J. R. Brown, 1959; McKenzie, 1960). Some aspects of TSH action were considered in reviews on more general or different subjects (Söderberg, 1959; Ingbar and Galton, 1963; Maloof and Soodak, 1963; Freinkel, 1964; Rosenberg and Bastomsky, 1965; Pastan, 1966a; McKenzie, 1967, 1968; Werner and Nauman, 1968). The mechanism of action of TSH on the thyroid (Dumont, 1968; Field, 1968) and the relation of TSH with its postulated thyroid receptor and the thyroid adenyl cyclase system (Schell-Frederick and Dumont, 1970) have been reviewed more recently. The general role of cAMP in hormone action has been considered several times during recent years (Sutherland *et al.*, 1965; Robison *et al.*, 1968; Sutherland and Robison, 1966, 1969).

II. Thyrotropin (TSH) and Thyroid Adenyl Cyclase

A. The Sutherland Model of Hormone Action

During the last decade, a large body of evidence has been presented which favors the hypothesis that the effects of many hormones are mediated by intracellular cAMP (Robison *et al.*, 1968). We shall analyze the evidence which has been presented in favor of or against the applicability of the Sutherland model of hormone action to thyroid and thyrotropin. The principal features of the model are schematized in Fig. 1. As applied to thyrotropin and thyroid, this model postulates that TSH binds to a specific receptor on the outer side of the follicular cell plasma membrane. This binding activates adenyl cyclase at the inner side of the membrane. Adenyl cyclase catalyzes ATP transformation to cAMP. Intracellular cAMP activates various enzymes and thus elicits, more or less directly, the hormonal effects. In all the tissues in which this system has been demonstrated, NaF greatly enhances adenyl cyclase activity in disrupted cell preparations, homogenates, or particulate fractions. cAMP is hydrolyzed to 5'-AMP by a specific phosphodiesterase. cAMP

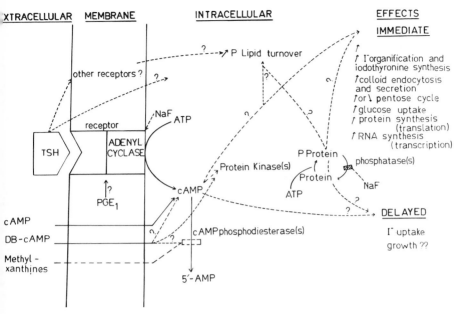

FIG. 1. Mechanism of action of thyrotropin on the thyroid cell: application of the cyclic 3′,5′-adenosine monophosphate (cAMP) concept of Sutherland to the thyroid and thyrotropin (TSH). *P-Protein,* phosphorylated protein.

phosphodiesterase is inhibited by methylxanthines (theophylline, caffeine, etc.). It is now known that 2 or several specific cAMP phosphodiesterases with different K_m may coexist in the cell.

The evidence on the action of TSH on a plasma membrane receptor of the follicular cell has been discussed previously (Schell-Frederick and Dumont, 1970). Both direct and indirect experiments indicate that TSH binds at the cell surface, but other intracellular binding sites have not been ruled out. The nature of the binding site(s) is completely unknown. Insofar as the activation of thyroid adenyl cyclase accounts for many intracellular effects of TSH, evidence on the subcellular location of this enzyme is very relevant. In all mammalian cells so far tested, the enzyme has been shown to be located in the plasma membrane (Robison *et al.,* 1968; Rodbell *et al.,* 1968). The specific activity of the thyroid enzyme is increased by a factor of 10 in a purified preparation of plasma membrane (Yamashita and Field, 1970). It is therefore probable that thyroid adenyl cyclase and its/a TSH receptor are located on the plasma membrane of the follicular cell.

The validity of the Sutherland model of hormone action for a tissue and a hormone can be tested in several ways. Four criteria should be satisfied: (1) TSH should increase the level of cAMP in intact thyroid cells. (2) TSH should activate thyroid adenyl cyclase in acellular systems (homogenates or particulate). (3) Agents which enhance the cAMP content of thyroid cells should mimic the action of TSH. (4) Agents which decrease the cAMP content of thyroid cells should inhibit the action of TSH. To fulfill the first two criteria, specificity of hormone and of tissue, the concentration-effect relationship and the time-effect relationship should be consistent with the model.

We shall analyze first the evidence that cAMP acts as an intracellular "messenger" for TSH (criteria 1 and 2). The evidence on the applicability of the model to the various effects of TSH will be reviewed separately in the sections concerning these specific effects.

B. Criterion 1: TSH Enhances cAMP Accumulation in
    Thyroid Tissue

TSH *in vitro* causes an increase in the cAMP content of bovine thyroid slices (Fig. 2) (Gilman and Rall, 1968a). This effect is potentiated by addition of 1 mM theophylline to the incubation medium. It is present at the first measurement, i.e., 3 minutes after the beginning of the incubation, and is maximal after 3–6 minutes. The cAMP content of the slices returns slowly toward control values after this early peak. The maximum cellular cAMP level is observed at about the same time or earlier than the earliest *in vivo* and *in vitro* effects of TSH (Dumont and Rocmans, 1965). In beef thyroid slices, depression of glucose carbon-1 oxidation by TSH begins 15 minutes after the beginning of the incu-

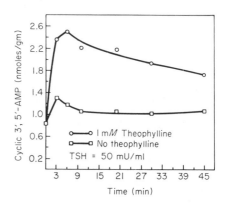

Fig. 2. Time course of cyclic 3',5'-adenosine monophosphate (cAMP) content of bovine thyroid slices after addition of 50 mU/ml of thyrotropin (TSH). Incubations were performed in the presence or the absence of 1 mM theophylline as indicated. From Gilman and Rall (1968a), with permission of the authors and publisher.

bation (Gilman and Rall, 1968b). So far as it has been tested, the increased cAMP content in the thyroid is specific for TSH. It is obtained with TSH preparations of various purities, and is not caused by other polypeptide hormones (ACTH, LH, FSH, GH, human chorionic gonadotropin, prolactin). Epinephrine is the only compound tested which has a similar although weaker and shorter effect in beef thyroid slices (Gilman and Rall, 1968a). The effect of TSH on the thyroid slices is tissue specific (Zor et al., 1969b). Increased cAMP content after 10 minutes of incubation in the presence of TSH has also been observed in dog thyroid slices (F. R. Butcher and Serif, 1969; Zor et al., 1969a; Van Sande and Dumont, 1970), in rat thyroid lobes (Tonoue et al., 1970), and in isolated calf thyroid cells (Knopp et al., 1970); this effect is still observed after 120 minutes; it is potentiated by 1 mM theophylline (Zor et al., 1969b). Increased cAMP formation from adenine-^{14}C has also been observed in stimulated dog thyroid slices (Ahn and Rosenberg, 1970a). The effect of TSH on cAMP formation in intact cells is obtained for hormone concentrations (0.25–10 mU/ml) not far from the range of concentrations which elicit other effects (Gilman and Rall, 1968a,b; Dekker and Field, 1970; Kaneko et al., 1970). It is surprising, however, that in the only study in which the TSH concentration-effect relationship for cAMP accumulation and for another TSH effect was investigated in the same system, the action of TSH on cAMP accumulation was only barely detectable at or above 0.2 mU/ml while the inhibition of glucose oxidation was nearly maximal at this concentration (Gilman and Rall, 1968a,b). Systematic studies of such relationships will have to be provided before the first criterion of Sutherland for the thyroid and thyrotropin can be considered as completely satisfied.

C. CRITERION 2: ACTIVATION OF THYROID ADENYL CYCLASE BY TSH

TSH could increase the cAMP content of thyroid tissue by increasing its synthesis or by decreasing its hydrolysis. The experiments of Klainer et al. (1962) already suggested the possibility of an activation of thyroid adenyl cyclase by TSH. They showed that TSH stimulated the formation of cAMP by a sheep particulate preparation. However, in this preliminary study, the TSH concentration was very high (500–1000 mU/ml), only crude hormone was used, the effect was weak (25% increase), and no attempt was made to confirm the identity of the product cAMP. Pastan and Katzen (1967) and Zor et al. (1969b) have shown that TSH enhances the accumulation of cAMP in beef and dog thyroid homogenates within 30 seconds (Fig. 3). This effect is obtained with purified TSH, but not with other polypeptide hormones. Although the cAMP formed has not been biologically characterized, it has been identified

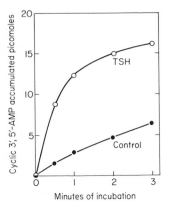

Minutes of incubation

Fig. 3. Time course of the effect of thyrotropin (TSH) on the accumulation of cyclic 3',5'-adenosine monophosphate (cAMP) in beef thyroid homogenate. Each 0.06 ml reaction mixture contained 0.67 mg of thyroid homogenate protein, 1.3 mM ATP, 2×10^6 cpm of α-labeled ATP-^{32}P, 8 mM theophylline; 2 mM MgCl$_2$; 21 mM tris·Cl, 0.08% albumin, and, where indicated, 20 mU of TSH. From Pastan and Katzen (1967), with permission of the authors and publisher.

by paper chromatography in several systems. The TSH effect is tissue specific. Confirmatory results have been reported for ovine particulate preparations (Burke, 1970b), and for dog thyroid homogenates (Ahn and Rosenberg, 1970a). Adenyl cyclase activity in dog thyroid homogenate is increased within 3 minutes after the injection of TSH *in vivo* (Zor *et al.*, 1969b). Low concentrations of TSH (1 mU/ml) activate adenyl cyclase in dog thyroid homogenate (Zor *et al.*, 1969b). However, until now, no systematic study has been made to show that the TSH concentration effect relationships for adenyl cyclase activation in acellular systems and for other hormones effects in intact cells are compatible with the postulated model of TSH mechanism of action.

On the basis of his data on the inhibitory action of various nucleotide triphosphates on cAMP formation in acellular systems, Burke (1970e) concluded that sheep thyroid adenyl cyclase was base specific, utilizing only ATP and dATP. Purification of thyroid plasma membrane is accompanied by an increase in the specific activity of TSH and NaF-stimulated adenyl cyclase (Yamashita and Field, 1970; Wolff *et al.*, 1970). This suggests that, in the thyroid as in other tissues, this enzyme is located in the plasma membrane.

In beef thyroid homogenates, TSH does not decrease the hydrolysis of cAMP to 5'-AMP (Pastan and Katzen, 1967), i.e., phosphodiesterase activity. An objection has been raised that the latter experiments would not demonstrate any ATP-dependent destruction of the cyclic nucleotide (Gilman and Rall, 1968a). However, such a process would have been demonstrated in the confirmatory experiments of Zor et al. (1969b). Therefore, there is no evidence of an action of TSH on cAMP catabolism. In conclusion, the second criterion of Sutherland is satisfied to a large extent for the thyroid and TSH: TSH activates the thyroid adenyl cyclase, and this reaction may account for TSH effects.

D. CRITERIA FOR THE DEMONSTRATION THAT cAMP MEDIATES
   A PARTICULAR EFFECT OF TSH

Three types of experiments have been proposed to test the hypothesis that a given effect of TSH is secondary to increased formation of cAMP in thyroid cells: (1) The effect is mimicked by cAMP itself in intact cells. (2) The effect is mimicked by DB-cAMP, a less polar derivative of cAMP. (3) The effect is reproduced or enhanced by inhibitors of cAMP phosphodiesterase, the methylxanthines, theophylline, and caffeine.

In experiments on whole animals, one should always take into account the possibility that factors affecting cAMP metabolism may modify thyroid function by acting at other levels than the thyroid. For instance, cAMP has been implicated in the stimulation of pituitary hormone secretion and more particularly in TSH secretion (Steiner et al., 1970). Effects on TSH secretion would be difficult to demonstrate because of the very short half-life of the hormone in blood (± 35 minutes) (Bakke et al., 1962). To prove the absence of TSH secretion under a given set of experimental conditions, one would have to provide serial measurements of plasma TSH beginning within minutes after the injection of active compounds, or control experiments showing that TRH does not induce secretion under these conditions.

Besides the general drawback of in vivo experiments, each of the proposed tests may give false negative and false positive results.

1. Reproduction of the Effect by cAMP

The reproduction by extracellular cAMP of a hormone effect mediated by intracellular cAMP obviously depends on the penetration and rate of intracellular degradation of the nucleotide, and on the sensitivity of the target system, i.e., in part on the basal level of cAMP intracellular concentration and of organ metabolic activity. These factors may vary with the species and with the pretreatment of the animal as well as with the nature of the experimental system. For instance, whereas cAMP and DB-cAMP, as well as TSH, enhance the organic binding of iodide in the thyroids of rats pretreated with thyroxine and low doses of TSH, only TSH does so in untreated animals (Ahn and Rosenberg, 1968). In tissues with high phosphodiesterase activity, the small amounts of cAMP penetrating the cells would be rapidly hydrolyzed, and thus hormonelike activity would not be expected to be observed unless cAMP phosphodiesterase is inhibited. Optimal conditions for reproducing TSH effects with extracellular cAMP would therefore seem to be the use of relatively high concentrations of the nucleotide, effective concentrations of methylxanthines and resting thyroids from pretreated animals (Rodesch et al., 1969).

If the effect of cAMP on the thyroid has any specificity, one should not expect other nucleotides to mimic this effect. However, the addition of adenine nucleotides or adenosine to the incubation medium of brain slices results in an increased intracellular concentration of cAMP (Kakiuchi et al., 1969). Reproduction in the thyroid of cAMP effects by other adenine nucleotides or adenosine could be caused by increase of the cellular cAMP content and therefore does not necessarily bear against the significance of hormone mimicry by cAMP.

Recent reports of divergent biological effects of cAMP and DB-cAMP on glucose metabolism in the fat cell (S. S. Solomon et al., 1970) and on glycogen level in HeLa cells (Hilz and Tarnowski, 1970) cast some doubt on the validity of the use of these nucleotides in the extracellular medium as analogs of the intracellular active secondary messengers. The simplest explanation of such discrepancies may be that cAMP might exert an action at the cell surface, possibly by inhibiting adenyl cyclase (Hilz and Tarnowski, 1970). Therefore, the actions of extracellular cAMP and DB-cAMP should always be compared with each other.

2. Reproduction of the Effect by DB-cAMP

In many systems, acyl derivatives of cyclic 3',5'-AMP, such as DB-cAMP, mimic the effects of the hormones on intact cells while cAMP itself is inactive. The effectiveness of DB-cAMP has been attributed to two of its characteristics: (1) Acyl derivatives of cAMP are more resistant to the action of phosphodiesterase than the parent compound. (2) These derivatives were synthesized with the hope that, being more lipophilic, they would penetrate more rapidly into intact cells (Posternak et al., 1962; Robison et al., 1968); this assumption has not yet been verified experimentally. An effect of DB-cAMP on a system of an intact cell depends on the penetration and the intracellular degradation of the nucleotide, like cAMP, and on the activity of its intracellular derivatives. Intracellular activity probably requires the removal of at least one (2'-0) of the butyryl moieties (Gilman and Rall, 1968b; Robison et al., 1968), although this may not apply to all systems (Blecher et al., 1970). Failure of DB-cAMP to reproduce qualitatively or quantitatively TSH effects in intact cells may therefore be due to low rates of penetration or of spontaneous or enzymatic deacylation, to high phosphodiesterase activity or to low intrinsic activity of the acyl derivatives on the target enzymes systems. Acyl derivatives of the cAMP might even compete in the cell with cAMP itself for allosteric sites of enzymes and therefore, when used with the hormone, partially inhibit the hormonal effects. This hypothesis would explain the partial inhibition of TSH stimulation of glucose oxidation by DB-cAMP reported by Burke (1968a).

The reports of a biphasic effect of DB-cAMP, but not of TSH, on ^{32}P incorporation into phospholipids in sheep and dog thyroid slices (Burke, 1968a), and on phospholipid metabolism and glucose oxidation in pig thyroid slices (Macchia et al., 1970), suggests that at high concentrations this nucleotide may exert unspecific inhibitory effects. In some animals not pretreated with TSH and/or thyroxine and in all hypophysectomized animals, DB-cAMP, injected by carotid infusion, failed to stimulate thyroid secretion in the dog (Ahn et al., 1969). Penetration of the nucleotide or reactivity of the target system could be involved. Simultaneous measurements of other cAMP-sensitive parameters, or of reactivity to TSH might have explained these results.

It has been reported (Murad et al., 1969) that an inhibitor of cAMP action, very similar in structure to cAMP, could be formed in acellular systems in parallel to cAMP and perhaps from cAMP. ^{6}N-monobutyryl cAMP blocks the formation of this inhibitor. This could explain why in some cases DB-cAMP, which would not give rise to this antagonist, could have higher stimulatory effect, than the native hormone. If the effect of DB-cAMP on the intact tissue is by the same mechanism as the action of cAMP, one would expect this effect not to be produced by butyrate. This should be controlled as it is known that fatty acids alter profoundly the metabolism of thyroid tissue (Freinkel, 1965). Mimicry by adenine nucleotides of DB-cAMP effects does not necessarily bear against the significance of these effects, as these nucleotides may also, as discussed previously (Section II,D,1), raise the intracellular concentration of cAMP.

3. Reproduction and Enhancement of the Effect by Methylxanthines

The third way of attempting to increase the intracellular cAMP concentration has been to block its catabolism by phosphodiesterase. The mimicry or potentiation by methylxanthines of hormonal effects mediated by cAMP has the following requirements:

a. The methylxanthines penetrate the cell in sufficient concentrations.

b. Basal phosphodiesterase activity is relatively high.

c. Most of cAMP catabolism occurs by way of the methylxanthine-inhibited cAMP phosphodiesterase; the existence in toad bladder of another catabolic pathway has been suggested (Gulyassi, 1968).

d. Further increases in intracellular cAMP levels can enhance the effect; no potentiation by methylxanthines would be expected at hormone concentrations at which the effect is already maximal.

e. Methylxanthines do not inhibit cAMP formation as theophylline does in brain slices (Kakiuchi et al., 1969).

f. The action of cAMP is not interfered with by other unrelated effects of the methylxanthines on cellular metabolism, such as the probable stimulation by theophylline of phosphorylase A phosphatase activity (Hess et al., 1963), the inhibition of glucose oxidation in fat cells (Zor et al., 1969a), the inhibition of glucose oxidation and ^{32}P incorporation into phospholipids in dog thyroid slices (Zor et al., 1969a), or the activation of a glycogen synthetase phosphatase activating enzyme (De Wulf et al., 1970). For instance, the activation by caffeine of phosphatases, (e.g., phosphorylase phosphatase) (Stalmans et al., 1970) could antagonize the effects of cAMP which are secondary to an activation of kinases.

Failure to meet any one of these requirements may bring about a false negative result, i.e., a negative finding that does not invalidate the model. The fact that methylxanthines may have other effects in intact cells than inhibition of phosphodiesterase raises the alternative possibility that observed positive, i.e., hormonelike or hormone-potentiating effects, may be unrelated to cyclic 3',5'-AMP.

In evaluating evidence on methylxanthines, it is important to distinguish between hormone mimicry and hormone potentiation: the first suggests that intracellular cAMP can reproduce a hormonal effect, and the second is the only evidence suggesting that cAMP actually mediates the hormonal effect.

Some information is available on the inhibition of thyroid cAMP phosphodiesterase by theophylline. In beef thyroid homogenates, 1 mM theophylline inhibits phosphodiesterase activity 80–85% (Pastan and Katzen, 1967). A similar concentration considerably increases the effect of TSH on intracellular cAMP accumulation in beef thyroid slices (Gilman and Rall, 1968a). In fact, in the absence of theophylline, the effect of TSH is small. In this system, one would therefore also expect theophylline to potentiate very markedly the subsequent effects of TSH. However, the true potentiation by theophylline of the stimulation of cAMP formation may have been overevaluated in these experiments. In the absence of methylxanthine in the cells, rapid hydrolysis of cAMP between the end of the incubation and the chemical inactivation of phosphodiesterase may considerably decrease the observed values of cAMP content in the slices.

4. Negative Evidence

The best evidence that a given effect of TSH is not mediated by cAMP would be that agents which mimic other TSH effects by way of the cAMP system do not reproduce the effect in question. However, such a refutation of the model must include compatible data on the concentration-response and time-effect relationships for all the effects, both with TSH and the other agents. There are a few data available on such concentration-response relationships.

Even high concentrations of cAMP and DB-cAMP may correspond only to very small concentrations of TSH. For instance, as evaluated from their respective effects on glucose C-1 oxidation by thyroid slices of pretreated dogs, concentrations of 5 mM cAMP (in the presence of caffeine), and of 0.075 mM DB-cAMP would be less active than concentrations of 1 mU of bovine TSH per milliliter (Willems and Dumont, 1969). On the same material, concentrations of TSH, 0.25 mU/ml, 3.5 mM cAMP + 1 mM caffeine, and 0.075 mM DB-cAMP are equally effective in stimulating secretion (Willems et al., 1970). With dog thyroid slices, Zor et al. (1968) obtained lower effects with 0.75 mM DB-cAMP than with TSH 1 mU/ml on glucose oxidation, and Ahn and Rosenberg (1970a) got similar stimulation of iodide organification with 0.3 mM DB-cAMP and TSH, 0.15 mU/ml. In beef thyroid slices, 1 mM DB-cAMP has a similar or slightly lower effect than 2 mU of TSH per milliliter on glucose carbon-1 oxidation and glycolysis (Gilman and Rall, 1968b). In mouse thyroids in vitro (Ensor and Munro, 1969), 10 mM cAMP and human TSH, 0.66 mU/ml (MRC Human Thyrotrophin Research Standard A) have similar effects on ^{131}I release. In the same system, DB-cAMP is approximately 50 times more potent than cAMP on a basis of molarity (Kendall-Taylor and Munro, 1970). In all systems, therefore, it appears almost impossible to use concentrations of cAMP or DB-cAMP corresponding to more than 2 mU of TSH per milliliter.

In most negative experiments on hormone mimicry, cAMP, DB-cAMP, and methylxanthines have been compared to concentrations of TSH much higher than their "equipotent" concentration. It is of course hardly possible to increase further the concentrations of cAMP, DB-cAMP, and methylxanthines used, for fear of introducing new artifacts, but the effects of lower TSH concentrations should be explored. Time-effect relationships should also be checked, since Gross and Gafni (1968) have shown that for the TSH-induced secretion this relation varies greatly with the concentration of the hormone. Even with compatible data on concentration-response and time-effect relationships, in the evaluation of negative evidence for one TSH effect, one should take into account the possibilities that DB-cAMP and its derivatives may not act like cAMP on some target enzyme systems, that methylxanthines may inhibit some effects of cAMP, and perhaps that exogenous substances may not get equal access to all intracellular sites.

In conclusion, positive evidence that cAMP, DB-cAMP, or methylxanthines mimic an effect of TSH thus suggests that intracellular cAMP could account for a TSH effect and therefore that cAMP is involved in this effect. Potentiation of a TSH effect by a methylxanthine further suggests that the effect of TSH is mediated by cAMP. On the contrary, negative evidence, i.e., the failure to mimic or potentiate a TSH effect, should not be considered to bear against this hypothesis unless other obvious alternative explanations have been ruled out.

III. Action of TSH on the Structure and Biochemical Composition of the Thyroid Gland

A. Introduction—Heterogeneity of Cell Response

Different aspects of the action of TSH on the morphology and the biochemistry of the thyroid gland have been studied in several species. Most of the studies do not provide physiological data on thyroid stimulation or correlations between the results of biochemical analysis, histology, and electron microscopy of the stimulated tissue. However, when comparable, the results of these studies are, in general, qualitatively similar. Our data (Dumont and Rocmans, 1964; Nève and Dumont, 1970a) on the kinetics of TSH stimulation in dog thyroid will be used as the framework of this section (Fig. 4), but we shall rely heavily on previous results obtained in other species to explain these data. The mechanisms of thyroid secretion and its morphological counterparts have been excellently reviewed by Wollman (1969).

The first ultrastructural changes may be observed in a resting thyroid within a few minutes after the injection of TSH into the animal. In the rat, different changes appear successively, showing a sequence of morphological reactions to the stimulation: images of colloid engulfment, appearance of intracellular colloid droplets at the apex, then deeper in the cells (Nadler et al., 1962; Wollman et al., 1964; Wetzel et al., 1965; Ekholm and Smeds, 1966; Seljelid, 1967a,c,d). In the dog, similar changes become progressively apparent followed by alterations suggestive of increased synthetic activity. The latter changes are seen only in cells in which colloid droplets are already observed. One can therefore describe a sequence of morphological stages in thyroid cell stimulation. In the

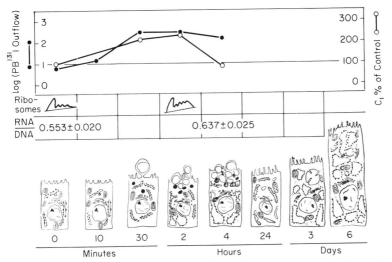

FIG. 4. Effect of thyrotropin (TSH) on dog thyroid *in vivo:* secretion, glucose oxidation, RNA concentration, ultrastructure. ●, Log (PBI-^{131}I outflow): log of the radioactivity of protein-bound iodine secreted in the venous outflow from prelabeled dog thyroid. +, C-1: oxidation of glucose carbon-1 *in vitro* by slices of thyroids removed at various times after TSH administration. Data from Dumont and Rocmans (1964a) and Nève and Dumont (1970a).

dog, the same stages are observed in neighbouring cells at different times after the administration of TSH, but only 3 hours after this injection do all cells show signs of stimulation. This suggests that if the sequence of events in each cell follows the same pattern, the beginning of this sequence in different cells is more or less delayed. In the rat thyroid, such different latencies are more (Wetzel *et al.*, 1965) or less (Nadler *et al.*, 1962) evident between cells of different follicles. This interfollicular heterogeneity can perhaps be explained by local variations of blood flow and therefore of TSH delivery to the follicles (Nadler *et al.*, 1962). Intrafollicular heterogeneity of response in dog thyroid cannot be accounted for in this way. This phenomenon suggests that the response of the thyroid cell to a first part of the chain of reactions following the interaction of TSH with a thyroid cell is more or less delayed, depending on the functional state of this cell. One wonders then whether with lower doses of TSH only the cells or the follicles which are at the moment of the injection in a responsive state would react to the hormone. In thyroid slices of dogs pretreated with thyroid extract, TSH *in vitro*, at very low concentrations (0.01 mU/ml), induces the formation of several colloid droplets in scarce cells dispersed in all follicles, while having apparently no effect on all the other cells (Willems *et al.*, 1970). A quantitative difference in reactivity to TSH between adjacent thyroid cells has been observed by Seljelid (1967a).

These morphological data have two important general consequences: (a) The various delays between the injection of TSH and the onset of the sequence of effects in different thyroid cells will tend to blur any differences in time relationship between the different actions of TSH as evaluated on the whole gland. (b) They emphasize the importance in the stimulation of any thyroid cell of the reactivity of this cell at the time of the injection.

When increasing the amount of TSH, one may wonder how much of the increase in TSH effect is due to the activation of a greater number of cells and how much to an increased activation of each cell.

B. EFFECTS OF ACUTE ADMINISTRATION OF TSH

1. Colloid Resorption

The effects of TSH on the thyroid have generally been studied in animals deprived of endogenous TSH secretion by hypophysectomy or thyroid hormone administration. In our dogs, suppression of TSH secretion was obtained by pretreatment for 3 days with thyroid extract. Such "resting thyroids" (Freinkel, 1964) are characterized by a low epithelium, with flattened ergastoplasmic vesicles but no colloid droplets (Fig. 5).

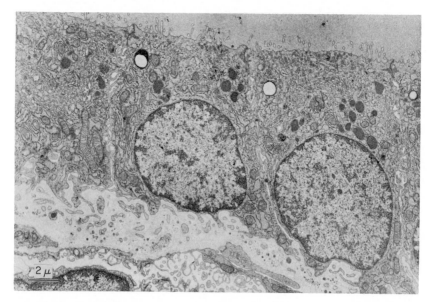

FIG. 5. Electron micrograph of a normal dog thyroid: part of a follicle with cubic follicular cells. ×6,600. Courtesy of Dr. P. Nève.

Within 5–10 minutes after injection of TSH, intense apical cell surface activity may be observed; this consists of the formation of large bulbous pseudopods which project into the follicular lumen and apparently engulf the luminal colloid, by phagocytosis. Intracellular colloid droplets are formed in this way (Nadler et al., 1962; Wetzel et al., 1965; Ekholm and Smeds, 1966; Seljelid, 1967a,b,c), which may be identified by their PAS+ staining in light microscopy. Masses of colloid droplets rapidly fill the apices of the follicular cells, which therefore increase in height and bulge in the follicular lumen (Dumont and Rocmans, 1964; Nève and Dumont, 1970a) (Fig. 6). Several arguments strongly support the concept that at least the majority of the colloid droplets which appear in the cells originate from the luminal colloid. The droplets appear first in the pseudopods, then in the apex, then in the body of the cell (Nadler et al., 1962; Wollman et al., 1964; Wetzel et al., 1965); their occurrence is remarkably reduced when the lumen is depleted of colloid (Wollman et al., 1964). Colloid droplets are labeled with leucine-^{3}H (Nadler et al., 1962) or with iodine-^{125}I (Stein and Gross, 1964; Sheldon et al., 1964; Bauer and Meyer, 1965; Ekholm and Smeds, 1966) when, and only when, the delay between the injection of the tracer and the administration of TSH has been sufficient to allow the labeling of luminal colloid. Finally, follicular cells ingest intraluminally injected ferritin (and serum), along with the colloid (Seljelid, 1967b). This last finding also suggests that the phagocytotic process itself is not selective for colloid or its main protein component thyroglobulin. The ingestion by isolated horse thyroid cells of latex beads in vitro supports this hypothesis (Rodesch et al., 1970).

The phagocytosis of colloid proceeds in parallel with a general mobilization of dense bodies. These seem to migrate from the base of the cell (Wollman et al., 1964; Wetzel et al., 1965) or from the whole cell (Seljelid, 1967a,c,d,e; Ekholm and Elmqvist, 1967; Nève and Dumont, 1970a) to the apex, where they mix with droplets. These dense bodies have been identified as primary lysosomes by their structure and by their acid phosphatase and esterase activity (Wetzel et al., 1965; Ekholm and Smeds, 1966; Seljelid, 1967a,d). The mobilization of lysosomes does not appear to be secondary to phagocytosis, since it occurs also when phagocytosis has been inhibited by intraluminal injection of cysteine (Seljelid, 1967b) or by prior treatment of the animal with actinomycin (Ekholm and Elmqvist, 1967). However, we know of no argument for the converse hypothesis (Onaya et al., 1969) that phagocytosis is secondary to lysosomal labilization.

There is strong evidence that lysosomes which have moved to the apex of the follicular cells fuse with colloid droplets. This allows contact between acid hydrolases and ingested colloid, and leads to progressive thyroglobulin hydrolysis and thyroid hormone release. Acid phosphatase and thyro-

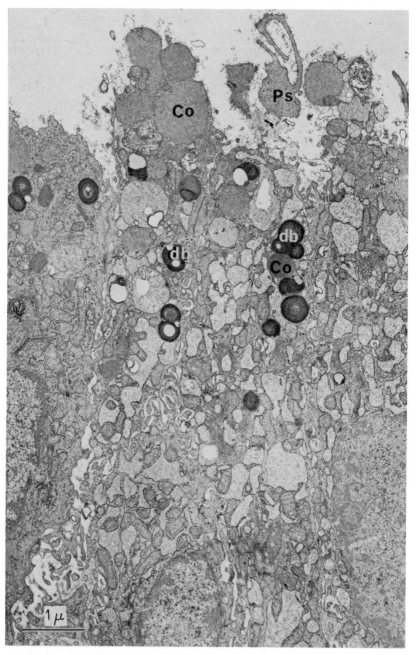

FIG. 6. Electron micrograph of dog thyroid cells 2 hours after thyrotropin (TSH) administration. Pseudopods (*Ps*) engulfing colloid droplets (*Co*) are found at the top of some follicular cells. The cytoplasm contains dilated granular reticulum. Dense bodies (*db*) are often in contact with colloid droplets. ×17,000. From Nève and Dumont (1970a) with the permission of the publisher.

globulin hydrolyzing activities have a similar subcellular distribution and structure-linked latency, which would suggest that the two enzymatic activities are localized in the same population of particles (Ekholm et al., 1966). Transfer of these activities from the lysosomes to the droplets has been suggested by different morphological data. Structures suggestive of fusion of dense bodies and droplets have been observed by electron microscopy (Wetzel et al., 1965; Ekholm and Smeds, 1966; Seljelid, 1967d; Nève and Dumont, 1970a). Immediately after stimulation, droplets are unstained by histochemical procedures for acid phosphatase, but at later stages, they are often stained (Wetzel et al., 1965). Similarly, droplets without phosphatase activity are usually located near the apex, while those displaying activity are located more basally (Seljelid, 1967d). The positive staining of many colloid droplets is concomitant with a decreased number of primary lysosomes, the total acid phosphatase and thyroglobulin hydrolyzing activity remaining constant. This also suggests a redistribution of enzymatic activity (Seljelid, 1967d; Kosanovic et al., 1968). As they progress toward the base of the cell, the colloid droplets decrease in size, while their density and acid phosphatase activity increase (Wetzel et al., 1965). These changes appear to indicate a progressive degradation of colloid in the droplets. The lifetime of the colloid droplet in the cell has been estimated at more than 20 minutes (Seljelid, 1967b) and less than 2 hours (Wollman et al., 1964).

The heterogeneous appearance of colloid droplets and their unequal labeling has been interpreted by Ekholm and Smeds (1966) to suggest that some of the droplets represent other processes than thyroglobulin resorption and degradation, presumably synthetic processes. For Wetzel et al. (1965), on the contrary, the heterogeneity of the droplets reflects the different stages in the resorption and degradation of follicular colloid. Quantitative analysis of the kinetics of labeling of droplets after the injection of labeled amino acids could determine whether or not some of the droplets are batches of newly synthesized thyroglobulin on their way to the lumen.

Evidence on the transfer of colloid from the lumen to a particulate fraction containing the droplets and of the hydrolysis of colloid in the droplets by lysosomal enzymes has been provided by Deiss and his group. They prepared the fraction of the thyroid homogenate which sediments at 15,000 g but not at 800 g; this fraction contains various organelles including colloid droplets (Balasubramaniam et al., 1965) and lysosomes with a characteristic cathepsin (Balasubramaniam and Deiss, 1965). After administration of TSH to dogs previously labeled with radioiodine and treated with methimazole, the radioactive iodoprotein increased in the colloid droplets fraction. When this fraction was suspended in $0.45\,M$ sucrose, the iodoprotein remained largely particle bound over a pH range of 3.6–8.5. The particles showed lysis of the iodoprotein into butanol-extractable iodine (BEI-^{131}I), during the *in vitro* incubation. That this hydrolysis took place in the intact particulate and not in the medium was suggested by the inhibition of proteolysis by Triton X100 which presumably disrupts colloid droplets and lysosomes. Particles from TSH-treated animals hydrolyzed a greater fraction of their iodoproteins than particles from control dogs (Balasubramaniam and Deiss, 1965). However, the interpretation of these experiments is not clear cut: (a) The identification and even more so the proportion of colloid droplets in the "15,000 g" fraction of cellular organelles is uncertain. (b) The possibility that bound iodoproteins are in fact adsorbed on membranes or subcellular particles has not been ruled out (Wollman, 1969).

The early morphological effects of TSH on thyroid tissue therefore disclose the process of thyroid secretion. This process may be schematized as follows: stimulated thyroid cells phagocytize colloid from the lumen, thus forming intracellular colloid droplets; primary lysosomes migrate to the apex of these cells and fuse with the droplets in secondary lysosomes; digestion of thyroglobulin in the secondary lysosomes results in the release of thyroid hormone (Wollman, 1969). This scheme is well in keeping with present concepts on lysosome function and phagocytosis (de Duve and Wattiaux, 1966). However, quantitative data on the amount of colloid taken up by the cells, on the life time of colloid droplets and on thyroid secretion would be needed to prove that this process fully accounts for thyroid secretion. The presence in stimulated thyroid cells of "bristle-coated pits" in the apical plasma membranes and of small vesicles containing intraluminally ingested ferritin in the apical cytoplasm has suggested to Seljelid (1967b,c) that micropinocytosis could also contribute to colloid ingestion by these follicular cells.

The biochemical consequence of colloid uptake and digestion is an important loss of colloid in the stimulated gland: total thyroglobulin, as estimated by iodine and sialic acid decreases (Rawson, 1949; Sonenberg, 1958; Bates and Warren, 1963); colloid concentration in the follicle lumen, as evaluated by interference microscopy, is also reduced (Sage and Robins, 1970); the Na$^+$ content of the gland decreases (D. H. Solomon, 1961). The gland becomes more hydrated as evidenced by an increased wet weight to dry weight ratio (Dumont and Rocmans, 1964; Creek, 1965).

After TSH injection, the number of colloid droplets in the stimulated thyroid increases steadily to a peak, after which it decreases progressively to a baseline level. The duration of the cycle varies with the dose of TSH (Wollman *et al.*, 1964).

2. Signs and Consequences of Increased Synthetic Activity

Beginning 2 hours after the injection of TSH to dogs, new ultrastructural changes are observed in the follicular cells in which colloid droplets indicate previous stimulation: membrane-free clustered ribosomes seem to be more numerous; the cisternae of the endoplasmic reticulum become dilated, mainly at the basal pole of the cell, and the Golgi apparatus seems more developed. This last observation (Wissig, 1963; Wetzel et al., 1965; Nève and Dumont, 1970a) has not been confirmed by Seljelid (1967a). At any rate such observations are only qualitative impressions. In the rat, increased numbers of 0.1 μ vesicles are observed near the Golgi zone and beneath the apical plasma membrane (Wetzel et al., 1965). It has been suggested that these vesicles carry the newly synthesized colloid to the follicular lumen (Nadler et al., 1962; Wetzel et al., 1965). Four hours after stimulation, it has been reported that microvilli increase in length in dogs as well as in rats (Wissig, 1963; Seljelid, 1967b) and in the guinea pig (Kosanovic et al., 1968). Such an effect is difficult to prove (Wissig, 1963) and its physiological meaning is unknown. All these changes could be interpreted as signs of hypertrophy and increased synthetic activity in the stimulated follicular cells.

Increased cell height (Olin-Lamberg and Lamberg, 1953; Wahlberg, 1955; Gedda, 1960; Nève and Dumont, 1970a) and increased nuclear volume (Lamberg and Olin-Lamberg, 1955) observed by light microscopy 2–4 hours after stimulation also suggest cell hypertrophy. The results of biochemical analysis of stimulated thyroids are not always statistically significant, but taken together they give some evidence of hypertrophy at this time. These include increases in RNA content in the dog (Nève and Dumont, 1970a), the chick (Creek, 1965), the guinea pig (Kerkof and Tata, 1967), and the rat (Fiala et al., 1957); increases in phospholipid content in the guinea pig (Kerkof and Tata, 1967), increases in K^+ content in the guinea pig (Gedda, 1960) and the chick (D. H. Solomon, 1961), and increase in succinic dehydrogenase activity in the rat (Kytomaki and Rinne, 1963). Cellular RNA is mainly ribosomal RNA; most of the cell phospholipids constitute membranes (plasma, mitochondrial, rough and smooth membranes) (Ansell and Hawthorne, 1964); tissue K^+ reflects the cell mass (D. H. Solomon, 1961). Therefore, a few hours after TSH injection, the cell mass, the membrane, and the ribosome contents appear to be increased in the stimulated thyroid.

The delay between TSH injection and significant histological (Rawson, 1949) or biochemical (Degroot and Dunn, 1968) evidence of cellular hypertrophy is in some cases longer than a few hours and certainly depends on the experimental conditions (species, dose of TSH, etc.). The fact that the increases in acid phosphatase and thyroglobulin hydrolyzing activities and in the number of lysosomes are apparent when no sign of secretory activity is any longer observed (Kosanovic et al., 1968) suggests that the growth response of TSH outlasts the secretory effect.

Cell hypertrophy and colloid digestion both contribute to increase the relative proportion of epithelium to colloid in thyroid tissue, an effect which has been the most used histological index of TSH stimulation (Sonenberg, 1958; J. R. Brown, 1959; Kirkham, 1966).

The last morphological effect of TSH is the onset of mitoses in some thyroid cells. In the guinea pig, this effect does not appear until 12 hours after TSH injection. These mitoses are scanty and do not become numerous until after 2 or 3 daily injections (Borell, 1945; Gedda, 1960). Thus TSH induces cell hypertrophy, but also cellular hyperplasia.

C. EFFECTS OF PROLONGED ADMINISTRATION OF TSH

Repeated daily injections of TSH, prolonged goitrogen administration, and cold exposure induce qualitatively similar morphological and biochemical changes in the thyroid (Matovinovic and Vickery, 1959; Maloof and Soodak, 1963; Chow and Woodbury, 1965; Panda and Turner, 1966; Graig, 1967; Lupulescu and Petrovici, 1968). That the effects of goitrogens and cold are entirely mediated by TSH is questionable. Therefore, we shall use data obtained on animals injected with TSH for several days to describe the chronically stimulated thyroid.

1. Morphology

The thyroid of dogs stimulated for 6 days by TSH is characterized by increased weight, high proportion of cell mass to colloid mass, and cellular hypertrophy. Light microscopy shows, as in other animals (Rawson, 1949; Lamberg and Olin-Lamberg, 1955; Sonenberg, 1958; Gyllenstein et al., 1959; Matovinovic and Vickery, 1959; Gedda, 1960; Sobel and Geller, 1965; Kirkham, 1966; Lupulescu and Petrovici, 1968), a much reduced follicular lumen containing scant colloid, a high epithelium with many infoldings, and some dilation of the intercellular and interfollicular space. The proliferation of capillaries as estimated by histology (Wissig, 1964) or by indices of vascular volume such as hemoglobin or total iron content (Gyllensten et al., 1959; Gedda, 1960) seems to proceed pari passu with the proliferation of the parenchyma. Similar histological observations have been quantitated in guinea pig thyroids after 7 days of stimulation (Matovinovic and Vickery, 1959). The thyroid weight is multiplied by 2.3; the follicular lumen space is decreased from 0.51 of the total to 0.25 (i.e., the relative proportion of this space is decreased, but the absolute value is slightly increased); the cell space increases from 0.29 of the total to 0.55 (i.e., the relative proportion of this space was multiplied by 1.9 while the absolute value was multiplied by 4.3), and the stromal space remains constant at 0.2 of the total, i.e., its absolute value increases in proportion to thyroid weight. Similar changes are observed by histology and by evaluation of the stromal and luminal volumes with inulin-^{14}C and $^{35}SO_4^{2-}$ in chronically stimulated rat thyroids (Chow and Woodbury, 1965). Converse results are obtained in hypophysectomized animals.

Various data suggest that, in addition to decreasing the luminal volume, TSH also decreases the concentration of thyroglobulin in luminal fluid: it decreases guinea pig luminal fluid concentration, as evaluated by microscopic ultraviolet absorption (Gersh and Casperson, 1940); it decreases the viscosity of the colloid removed directly from the lumen of rat thyroid follicles (De Robertis, 1941); it increases the SO_4^{2-} and Cl^- spaces while decreasing the luminal space in guinea pig thyroid (Chow and Woodbury, 1965); it decreases the voltage between the lumen and interstitial fluid (Gorbman and Ueda, 1963), a finding that suggests a decreased Donnan distribution ratio of nondiffusible anions between lumen and stroma, i.e., a decreased concentration of protein in the lumen.

Cellular hypertrophy is best shown by electron microscopy. The very high epithelial cells appear vacuolated because of the great increase in volume of the dilated ergastoplasmic cisternae, which nearly fill the cytoplasm (Fig. 7). The development of the ergastoplasm and the numerous membrane-free polysomes indicate a great increase in the number of ribosomes per cell. The Golgi apparatus is more complex and more dispersed throughout the cytoplasm and appears larger. Similar observations have been made in the thyroids of various animals treated by TSH, cold exposure or goitrogen administration (Dempsey and Peterson, 1955; Wissig, 1964; Hajos et al., 1964; Sobel and Geller, 1965; McKenzie, 1967; Pantic, 1967; Lupulescu and Petrovici, 1968). TSH-stimulated rat thyroids also show a greater complexity of the basal membrane, which forms deep invaginations and whose processes become longer and more tortuous (Wissig, 1964). An increase in the concentration of mitochondrial elements in follicular cells is suggested by electron microscope observations (Wissig, 1964; Sobel and Geller, 1965) and by the histochemical demonstration of increased activity of a mitochondrial enzyme, succinic dehydrogenase (Tellkä and Kuusisto, 1955). However, measurement of mitochondrial enzymes (succinic cytochrome c reductase and cytochrome oxidase) in homogenates of stimulated rat thyroids showed that increments of the activity of these enzymes are similar to increases in RNA content. This finding suggests that mitochondrial elements increase in parallel with cellular growth (Degroot and Dunn, 1968). Histology

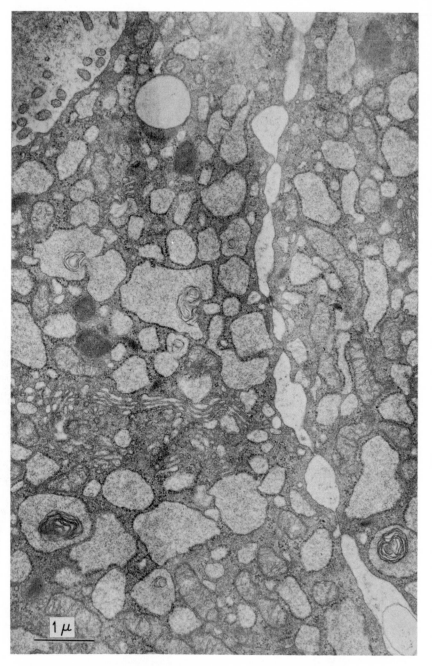

Fig. 7. Electron micrograph of dog thyroid cells after 3 days of stimulation by thyrotropin (TSH); the granular reticulum is very dilated and the Golgi apparatus is well developed. ×17,500. From Nève and Dumont (1970a), with the permission of the publisher.

has shown long ago that prolonged TSH administration also increases the nuclear volume (Sonenberg, 1958; J. R. Brown, 1959; Kirkham, 1966).

2. Biochemical Analysis

Qualitative morphological changes observed in chronically stimulated thyroids have been confirmed by quantitative biochemical analysis (Matovinovic and Vickery, 1959). These authors assume that the slight increase in DNA concentration concomitant with a slightly decreased cell population density in TSH-stimulated thyroid reflects an increase in the number of cells with polyploid nuclei, i.e., of cells preparing for mitosis. From this assumption, they infer that the DNA content of the thyroid cells is constant, and is not modified by TSH. Analyzing their data on the DNA content of hyperplastic mouse and rat thyroids, Wollman and Breitman (1970) arrive at a similar conclusion. The DNA content of the gland would therefore measure the number of cells. The total cell mass of a gland is evaluated by the product of the weight of the gland by the fraction of the gland occupied by cells; this fraction is measured by histometry. By use of these parameters, it is possible to calculate that in the chronically stimulated guinea pig thyroid the number of cells is multiplied by 2.5, the mean cell mass is multiplied by 2.2, and the mean RNA content per cell is multiplied by 3.3. Therefore, this gland is characterized by cellular hypertrophy and hyperplasia. Comparable results have been presented by Ekholm and Pantic (1963). Qualitatively similar changes have been observed in chronically stimulated rat thyroids, i.e., the number of cells is multiplied by a factor of 3, the mean follicular cell volume by 1.5, while the RNA content per cell (RNA:DNA ratio) only slightly increases (Greig et al., 1969; Philp et al., 1969).

Numerous enzyme activities are enhanced in chronically stimulated thyroids: ATPase (S. Lindsay, 1963), oxidative enzymes (S. Lindsay and Jenks, 1961) and lysosomal enzymes (Sobel, 1962), as demonstrated by histochemical methods, creatine phosphokinase, lactic dehydrogenase (Graig, 1967), isocitric dehydrogenase, glucose-6-phosphate dehydrogenase, TPNH cytochrome c reductase, and DPNH-TPNH dichlorophenol indophenol reductase (Degroot and Dunn, 1968) by assay in thyroid homogenates. Although these increases certainly reflect the increment in cell mass in the stimulated tissue, marked differences in the kinetics and in the degree of stimulation between the various enzymes suggest some selectivity in TSH action (Degroot and Dunn, 1968). Thyroid citrate content, which is normally high, is very much decreased in tissue chronically stimulated by TSH or by thiouracil (Belotti and Ravera, 1954; Kaellis and Goldsmith, 1965). It has been suggested that this decrease reflects the decrease in colloid content of the thyroid (Kaellis and Goldsmith, 1965).

In the chronically stimulated dog thyroid, few intracellular colloid droplets are observed. Therefore, there is little morphological evidence of the intense secretion which is going on. This could be explained by a very fast turnover of thyroglobulin in the lumen and in the cell or by the operation of secretory mechanisms which would not involve colloid secretion into and resorption from the follicular lumen. The observation of intracellular colloid droplets in chronically stimulated mouse thyroid, the follicular lumen of which still contains colloid (McKenzie, 1967), suggests that resorption from the lumen is taking place in such thyroid, but that it is apparent only when the colloid is ingested in bulk.

3. Hyperplasia

Therefore, a great part of thyroid enlargement induced by chronic stimulation is due to cellular hyperplasia. The development of this hyperplasia has been studied under various conditions in vivo. Within days after the beginning of chronic stimulation, thymidine-^{3}H incorporation in thyroid DNA increases (Al-Indawi and Wilson, 1965; Greig et al., 1969; Wollman et al., 1969). The labeling index, i.e., the proportion of cells labeled with thymidine-^{3}H, increases in parallel with the specific activity of DNA, which indicates a large increase in the fraction of cells participating in DNA synthesis (Al-Indawi and Wilson, 1965; Greig et al., 1969). The labeling index also parallels the rate of cellular multiplication and of thyroid growth (Philp et al., 1969; Sheline, 1969); it therefore reflects both the rates of DNA synthesis and of cellular multiplication. TSH enhances thymidine-^{3}H incorporation into DNA (Speight et al., 1968) and growth (Bengmark et al., 1963) in thyroid cultures. The cellular multiplication in chronically stimulated thyroids in vivo, may therefore result from a direct action of TSH.

Under chronic stimulation of rat and mouse thyroids, the labeling index is higher in the stromal cells, i.e., endothelial cells and fibroblasts, than in follicle cells (Wollman et al., 1969). Moreover, the proportion of stromal cells in the population increases (Greig et al., 1969). Apparently, all thyroid cells respond to the stimulation. In the mouse, thymidine labeling of stromal cells begins several days before the labeling of follicle cells (Wollman et al., 1969). Therefore, the increase in stromal cell population is not a consequence of follicle cell hyperplasia. Stromal cell hyperplasia raises the question whether these cells respond directly to TSH or to the follicle cell hyperactivity caused by TSH.

In chronically stimulated rat thyroids, the duration of S and G_2 phases of the generation cycle of epithelial cells have been evaluated at 7 to 10 hours and around 7 hours (Wollman et al., 1969; Sheline, 1969). The duration of G_2 appears to be very variable. As mitoses could not be obtained before the wave of cell labeling with thymidine, Wollman et al. (1969) concluded that in the cell population of resting thyroids, few cells were in the G_2 stage. Most of the cells must therefore be in the G_1 phase of the cycle, i.e., in the phase preceding DNA synthesis.

Deriving from the curve of labeled mitoses an evaluation of follicle cell generating time (45 hours) in stimulated rat thyroids, and using the data in the literature on follicle cell population doubling time, Sheline (1969) estimated that in stimulated rat thyroids more than 20% of these cells participate in the proliferation. In fact, the exponential growth curve of cell population (Philp et al., 1969) in such thyroids, is compatible with the hypothesis that the whole cell population participates in this process.

Under chronic stimulation, thyroid cell population often increases to a new plateau, suggesting either that a new steady state level in thyroid pituitary feedback has been reached, or that the thyroid cell population is unable to increase further. In culture, TSH increases thymidine-^{3}H incorporation into DNA, but also accelerates labeled DNA degradation (Speight et al., 1968). In rats treated with PTU, the persistence of DNA-^{3}H is reduced (Al-Hindawi and Wilson, 1965; Speight et al., 1968). These results suggest that TSH not only stimulates DNA synthesis, but also increases the rate of cell death. TSH would therefore induce cell multiplication and increase cell turnover in the thyroid. Other mechanisms must, however, play a role in the plateauing of cell population in rats submitted to a constant stimulation by a diet enriched in PTU. Indeed, both the fractional increase in the number of cells per day and the thymidine-^{3}H labeling index decrease after an early peak indicating a slackening in the rate of cell multiplication. It is possible that the tissue gets less sensitive to TSH stimulation or that the TSH secretion in response to PTU decreases after a certain time (Wollman and Breitman, 1970).

Involution of the thyroid caused by an iodine-rich diet decreases the thyroid DNA content to a new plateau, which suggests the death of a class of unstable cells (Wollman and Breitman, 1970). The decrease begins within a few days after the change in diet.

It seems probable that cellular hyperplasia in the chronically stimulated thyroid is accompanied by follicle hypertrophy and hyperplasia (Goss, 1967). Follicle hyperplasia might result from production of new microfollicles by fragmentation of larger units or by development of aggregates of interfollicular cells, as described by Gibadulin (1962).

IV. The Physiology and Iodine Metabolism of the Thyroid Gland

Like the morphological effects, the *in vivo* effects of TSH on thyroid metabolism are characterized by a very definite time action relationship. The order of appearance of the effects is generally identical in different species, but the time scale of the sequence may vary. Within this time scale, one may distinguish early and delayed effects: the early effects, for instance secretion of thyroid hormone, begin during the first hour after the injection of TSH, the delayed effects, for instance increased iodide trapping, become apparent only several hours after the administration of the hormone.

A. Thyroid Blood Flow

TSH administration enhances thyroid blood flow. This effect is observed within a few minutes after hormone injection in the guinea pig (Söderberg, 1958) and the rat (Clayton and Szego, 1967), but is delayed until 2 hours in the chick (D. H. Solomon *et al.*, 1963), and is not detected even after 3 hours in the dog (Rosenberg *et al.*, 1960; Dumont and Rocmans, 1964). The early effect observed in the rat is presumably not due to nonspecific protein as it is also obtained with purified preparations of TSH. The increase in thyroid blood flow following TSH administration cannot be the cause of the early *in vivo* TSH effects observed in the chick and dog thyroid. Neither can it be the cause of the many TSH effects which are measurable *in vitro*, either after *in vivo* or *in vitro* administration of hormone (Taurog *et al.*, 1958b). On the contrary, increased blood flow might be secondary to earlier metabolic activation. However, increased blood flow could contribute to the delayed effects of TSH, such as the stimulation of iodide uptake. Indeed, in the dog, large variations of the thyroid blood flow take place without any change in the iodide extraction coefficient (Rocmans and Dumont, 1968), i.e., the total uptake of iodide is proportional to the blood flow. Increased perfusion of the thyroid, by increasing the availability of substrates, could also allow or facilitate the metabolic action of TSH.

Perfusion of DB-cAMP in the carotid artery rapidly tends to increase dog thyroid venous outflow (Ahn *et al.*, 1969). Since in this species TSH has no such rapid effect, it is probable that in this case DB-cAMP rather mimics the activation of β-adrenergic vascular receptors (Robison *et al.*, 1968).

B. Iodide Trapping

The first step in the iodine metabolism of the thyroid gland is the trapping of iodide. It is believed that this uptake is achieved by a mechanism of active transport located at the basal plasma membrane of the follicular cell (Wolff, 1964; Tyler et al., 1968). In the intact thyroid, most of the trapped iodide is located in the follicle lumen, where it may "flow downhill" with the electrical gradient across the apical membrane (Wolff, 1964). TSH decreases iodide trapping by the thyroid in the early phase of its action, and increases it afterward.

Iodide trapping in the thyroid is usually studied, both in vivo and in vitro, in tissues in which iodide organification has been blocked by inhibitors such as methimazole or propylthiouracil; it is evaluated by the ratios T/S, T/M, or C/M, where T, C, S, and M are the radioactivities per unit volume of iodide in the tissue, isolated cells, the serum, and the incubation medium, respectively.

1. Early Decrease

In the rat, TSH in vivo decreases iodide trapping for several hours and enhances it thereafter (Halmi et al., 1960). This initial decrease is not due to contaminants in the TSH as it has been obtained with purified preparations of TSH. The decrease in iodide trapping is a general effect: thyrotropin also induces a release of recently trapped iodide from blocked dog and human thyroid glands and a release of pertechnetate from dog thyroids (Isaacs et al., 1966; Isaacs and Rosenberg, 1967). In short-term incubations it also lowers the C:M in isolated beef thyroid cells (Wilson et al., 1968) and in dog thyroid slices (Ahn and Rosenberg, 1970a).

The fact that TSH decreases the T:S ratio while not modifying the unidirectional clearance of plasma radioiodide suggests that it enhances the exit rate constant for thyroidal radioiodide (Halmi et al., 1960). The observations of TSH-induced release of recently trapped iodide and of pertechnetate from blocked and unblocked dog thyroids in which the unidirectional glandular clearance of plasma iodide is unchanged also supports the hypothesis of a TSH stimulation of glandular efflux of iodide (Isaacs et al., 1966; Isaacs and Rosenberg, 1967). The effect of TSH is not mainly due to a washout of trapped iodide by iodide produced in the gland as has been previously suggested (Rosenberg et al., 1961). Indeed, TSH also lowers the C:M in isolated thyroid cells which are deprived of colloid (Wilson et al., 1968). Moreover, increased iodide efflux has been observed in rats chronically treated with PTU, to render the thyroids devoid of thyroglobulin (Halmi et al., 1960). Increased efflux is also observed in animals in which elevated plasma iodide levels are maintained and glandular content of trapped iodide is thus increased many fold (Isaacs et al., 1966; Isaacs and Rosenberg, 1967). The influence on iodide efflux of a constant amount of iodide released from the iodotyrosines of thyroglobulin should be much decreased when the pool of trapped iodide is greatly increased by elevating the plasma iodide level. The fact that this is not observed (Rosenberg *et al.*, 1965) bears against the hypothesis that the increase of iodide efflux is secondary to iodide release from thyroglobulin. Halmi *et al.* (1960) have suggested that the TSH enhancement of iodide efflux reflects an increased permeability of the stimulated cell plasma membrane.

The early decrease of iodide trapping in isolated beef thyroid cells is mimicked by DB-cAMP, but not by ATP or AMP (Wilson *et al.*, 1968). The absence of a cAMP effect in these experiments is probably explained by the concentrations used: TSH, 100 mU/ml; DB-cAMP, 3 mM; cAMP, 3 mM (see Section II,D,4). DB-cAMP, like TSH, decreases the T:M in dog thyroid slices (Ahn and Rosenberg, 1970a), but in these experiments, the possibility that the effect is caused by iodide release from thyroglobulin has not been ruled out. Therefore, the available evidence is compatible with the hypothesis that the TSH enhancement of thyroid iodide efflux is mediated by cAMP.

2. *Delayed Enhancement*

The delayed stimulation of iodide trapping by TSH is due to an increase in the rate of unidirectional clearance of radioiodide (Wollman and Reed, 1959). This effect has not been reproduced *in vitro* except in isolated cells (Wilson *et al.*, 1968; Knopp *et al.*, 1970), where the possibility that it may reflect other phenomena has not been ruled out (Nève *et al.*, 1968).

The iodide transport system and the Na$^+$/K$^+$ activated, ouabain-sensitive ATPase in thyroid have many common properties suggesting that iodide transport may be linked to the fundamental cation transport system of the cell (Wolff, 1964). TSH *in vivo* enhances the T:S ratio and ouabain-sensitive ATPase activity in a parallel fashion (Wolff and Halmi, 1963). This parallelism is also observed during goitrogen treatment (Brunberg and Halmi, 1966). These observations could be interpreted as indicating that TSH affects thyroidal iodide transport as a result of a prior action on ouabain-sensitive ATPase. However, treatment with triiodothyronine or hypophysectomy markedly decreases the T:S ratio in rats without inducing consistent changes in ouabain-sensitive ATPase activity; treatment of rats for a few days with PTU, or treatment of hypophysectomized rats with TSH and PTU much enhances the T:S ratios without increasing ouabain-sensitive ATPase activity (Brunberg and Halmi, 1966). An active ouabain-sensitive ATPase is probably required for sustained iodide transport in the thyroid, but stimulation of the iodide pump by TSH is not secondary to an overall increase of ouabain-sensitive ATPase activity in the gland. Neither is the stimulation of the iodide pump by TSH merely a consequence of thyroid growth. T:S ratios are much more sensitive to TSH than thyroid growth (Greer, 1959; Halmi, 1961), and decrease much faster after hypophysectomy (Vanderlaan and Greer, 1950). Present evidence is compatible with the hypothesis that TSH stimulates the transport of iodide in the thyroid by enhancing the activity or the synthesis of a carrier specific for iodide and similar anions. This hypothesis is supported by the finding that in isolated thyroid cells TSH increases iodide influx, more specifically the V_{max} of iodide influx, and that this effect is inhibited by incubation in the presence of inhibitors of protein and RNA synthesis (Knopp et al., 1970). However, the latter evidence will not be conclusive as long as the possibility of other phenomena (cell reaggregation, reformation of closed luminal spaces, etc.) (Nève et al., 1968) has not been ruled out.

In rats, the delayed stimulation by TSH of iodide trapping by the thyroid has also been observed with doses of TSH and theophyliine, which are inactive when administered separately (Bastomsky and McKenzie, 1967). In isolated beef thyroid cells, enhancement of iodide trapping is induced by DB-cAMP as well as by TSH, but not by other adenine nucleotides or by cAMP itself (Wilson et al., 1968). Some reservations are necessary in the interpretation of both types of experiments: in vivo experiments do not demonstrate a direct effect of theophylline on the thyroid, and the increased iodide uptake in isolated cells might be related to a structural reorganization of the cells rather than to an activation of iodide transport (Nève et al., 1968). Nevertheless the combination of these two types of results suggests the involvement of cAMP in the TSH stimulation of iodide transport in the thyroid.

C. SYNTHESIS OF THYROID HORMONES

The synthesis of thyroid hormones (thyroxine $= T_4$, triiodothyronine $= T_3$) involves at least 2 steps: the binding of iodide to tyrosyl groups of thyroglobulin and the oxidative coupling of iodotyrosines into iodothyronines in the thyroglobulin molecule. It is not known whether the latter reaction involves 2 or 1 iodotyrosyl group from thyroglobulin. These processes could be catalyzed by at least 2 enzymatic systems: an H_2O_2 generating system with NADPH as coenzyme and a peroxidase catalyzing the oxidation of iodide; the iodination itself does not require a specialized enzyme in reconstituted systems, which does not rule out the existence of an iodinase in the thyroid. It has been suggested that iodination would take place at the interface of cell and follicular lumen, perhaps on the microvilli. However, the possibility of intracellular iodination has not yet been ruled out (Degroot, 1965).

1. *Iodide Binding to Protein*

The *in vivo* estimation of organic binding of radioiodide by Nagataki *et al.* (1961) was based on the difference between the calculated total radioiodide release from thyroglobulin in unblocked stimulated dog thyroids and radioiodine venous output. The value they calculated can be considered only as an approximation (Dumont and Rocmans, 1964). Using this method, Nagataki *et al.* (1961) showed that, within minutes after its injection, TSH accelerates the organic binding of iodide in dog thyroids. This effect roughly parallels the secretory effect of the hormone. Subsequent studies using more refined methods have confirmed this action of TSH. If TSH does stimulate organic binding of iodide promptly, it should, as a result, increase the clearance of iodide under conditions in which transport is not rate limiting. Since the iodide transport capacity of the gland greatly exceeds its organic binding capacity, raising plasma iodide concentration creates such conditions. When radioiodide is administered with carrier to dog, subsequent TSH injection exerts a prompt stimulating effect on the thyroid clearance of iodide (Rosenberg *et al.*, 1965; Rosenfeld and Rosenberg, 1966). The increment of radioiodide taken up is almost entirely organically bound (Rosenberg *et al.*, 1965). A similar effect is observed within minutes in dogs in which increased efflux of recently trapped iodide is demonstrated by pertechnetate release (Isaacs *et al.*, 1966). These experiments suggest that the stimulation of organic binding of iodide is not due to an enhanced trapping. A similar conclusion can be drawn from experiments on rats *in vivo*. TSH increases the uptake and binding of radioiodide when it is injected with carrier, i.e., under conditions in which binding is limiting, but it decreases the trapping of carrier-free iodide; it renders glandular organification resistant to the inhibitory effects of high plasma iodide concentration. This effect is not abolished by $NaClO_4$ (Rosenfeld and Rosenberg, 1966; Ahn and Rosenberg, 1970a).

A prompt stimulation of the binding of iodide to proteins has been observed in *in vitro* incubated pig (Kondo, 1961a,b; Kerkof and Tata, 1969), calf, sheep, and dog (Rodesch *et al.*, 1969; Ahn and Rosenberg, 1970a) thyroid slices, and in fetal rat thyroids (Nataf and Chaikoff, 1964). In experiments with slices, as *in vivo*, the effect is best observed in the presence of carrier iodide (Rodesch *et al.*, 1969). TSH also rapidly enhances iodide organification in isolated calf (Pastan, 1961), bovine (Tong, 1964a), sheep (Rodesch and Fontaine, 1968), and horse (Rodesch *et al.*, 1969) thyroid cells and in cultured sheep thyroid cells (Dickson, 1966). The effect is observed when iodide trapping is not increased

(Kondo, 1961b; Nataf and Chaikoff, 1964; Tong, 1964b; Dickson, 1966) do not trap iodide, because of deterioration (Pastan, 1961) or inhibition and when iodide uptake is decreased (Rodesch *et al.*, 1969; Ahn and Rosenberg, 1970a) in the tissue preparations; it is obtained in cells which with perchlorate (Tong, 1964c; Rodesch *et al.*, 1968). The effect of TSH is observed for low concentrations of hormone [in our dog thyroid slices: 0.1 to 1 mU/ml (Fig. 8)] (Rodesch *et al.*, 1969). TSH specifically enhances the iodination of thyroglobulin (Kondo, 1961b; Raghupathy *et al.*, 1965; Wilson *et al.*, 1968).

The effect of TSH on iodide trapping (increased efflux) and on iodide binding to proteins are independent and opposite. This explains the conflicting results obtained in studies of the early action of TSH on total iodide uptake *in vivo* and *in vitro* (Rosenberg *et al.*, 1965; Dumont, 1965).

2. Iodothyronine Formation

Under conditions in which tissue preparations contain little colloid, i.e., in rat fetal thyroids in culture (Nataf *et al.*, 1965), in thyroids of newborn rats incubated *in vitro* after *in vivo* TSH administration (Nataf and Chaikoff, 1964), in isolated cells (Tong, 1964a) or in cells in culture (Dickson, 1966), the TSH induced increase in iodide organification is accompanied by a marked enhancement of iodothyronine synthesis. Ahn and Rosenberg (1970a) have also reported a stimulation by TSH of ^{131}I incorporation into thyroxine in dog thyroid slices. However, the proportion of ^{131}I recovered in thyroxine was extremely small in both control and stimulated slices. Increased iodothyronine synthesis has also been observed *in vivo*. In PTU-treated rats subsequently injected with TSH, the iodotyrosines and iodothyromines disappear from the gland in proportion to their concentration, whereas in animals not given PTU, TSH induces a relatively greater depletion of iodotyrosines than iodothyronines. Determination of the specific activities of iodotyrosines and iodothyronines further suggests an acceleration of the conversion of iodotyrosines to iodothyronines (Sasson and Rosenberg, 1963). A marked stimulation of ^{131}I-labeled iodide incorporation into iodothyronines is observed within 30 minutes after TSH injection in Purina fed and in hypophysectomized rats (S. I. Shimoda *et al.*, 1966). In the *in vivo* experiments, no stimulation of overall iodide organification was observed. This was to be expected since these experiments were carried out in the absence of carrier iodide. The data establish that increased iodothyronine formation is not a consequence of the enhanced iodide organification.

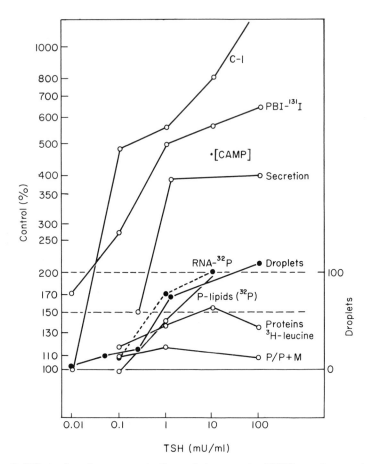

FIG. 8. Effect of various concentrations of thyrotropin (TSH) on the metabolism of dog thyroid slices *in vitro*. Results obtained in different experiments on similarly pretreated dogs (300 mg thyroid extract per day for 3 days) with one brand of TSH (Thytropar Armour). *C-1:* glucose carbon-1 oxidation; *PBI-^{131}I:* binding of iodide-^{131}I (10 μM) to proteins; *cAMP:* accumulation of ^{14}C AMP 10 minutes after TSH in slices prelabeled with adenine-^{14}C; *secretion:* release of butanol-extractable iodine-^{131}I from prelabeled slices; *RNA-^{32}P:* incorporation of ^{32}P$_i$ into RNA; *droplets:* number of intracellular colloid droplets per 20 nuclei; *Plipids(^{32}P):* incorporation of ^{32}P$_i$ into phospholipids; *proteins leucine-^{3}H:* incorporation of leucine-^{3}H into proteins; *P/P+M:* ratio of ribosomes in the polysome fraction (P) and in the total ribosome pellet (P + M) of incubated slices. Data from the author's laboratory: Dumont *et al.* (1939a); Rodesch *et al.* (1969); Willems *et al.* (1970); Lamy *et al.*, 1969, Lecocq and Dumont, 1970).

3. Thyroglobulin Maturation

Within 2 hours after its injection into the rat, TSH induces a shift of recently synthesized thyroglobulin from a sedimentation constant of 15 S to 19 S, i.e., it induces an acceleration of thyroglobulin maturation (Cavalieri and Searle, 1967). If maturation of thyroglobulin is dependent upon iodination reactions (Seed and Goldberg, 1965), the effect of TSH on maturation may be secondary to the stimulation of these iodination reactions.

4. Mechanisms—Role of cAMP

The parallel stimulation of protein iodination and of iodotyrosines coupling suggests the activation of one or more of the common enzyme systems, i.e., of the hydrogen peroxide generating system or the peroxidase (Degroot, 1965). This hypothesis would explain why TSH still stimulates the coupling reaction when iodination is limited by iodide supply. Exogenous H_2O_2 mimics the action of TSH; maximal effects of TSH and H_2O_2 are similar and not additive (Ahn and Rosenberg, 1970a). TSH *in vitro* enhances the formation of H_2O_2 in calf, hog (Bénard and Brault, 1970), and dog (Ahn and Rosenberg, 1970c) thyroid slices. There is therefore strong support for the concept that the stimulation by TSH of iodide binding to proteins and of iodothyronine synthesis takes place at the level of the H_2O_2 generating system.

The very fast effect of TSH on iodination in intact thyroid cells contrasts with the very sluggish response (of the order of days) of thyroid iodinating activity, as measured in acellular particulate preparations, to PTU or thyroxine treatment, to thyroxine withdrawal or to hypophysectomy (Zimmerman and Yip, 1968). This suggests that the rapid effect of TSH on iodination is not due to increased enzyme synthesis. A similar conclusion may be reached from the facts that, *in vitro*, the stimulation by TSH of iodide binding to proteins and thyroxine formation are not inhibited by actinomycin and puromycin (Tong, 1965; Nataf, 1968).

A direct stimulatory effect of TSH on iodination of thyroglobulin by a cell-free particulate system from pig thyroid has been reported (Kondo, 1961c). However, the TSH used was impure, and this finding has never been confirmed.

DB-cAMP, as well as cAMP, other adenine nucleotides, and theophylline stimulate iodide organification in rat thyroid *in vivo* (Ahn and Rosenberg, 1968). For cyclic 3',5'-AMP, this effect has been reproduced in hypophysectomized animals, suggesting that it is direct. This conclusion is supported by the observation that DB-cAMP as well as TSH stimulates iodide organification in various *in vitro* preparations: thyroid slices from pig (Kerkof and Tata, 1969) and dog (Rodesch *et al.*, 1969; Ahn and Rosenberg, 1970a), and isolated cells from beef (Wilson *et al.*, 1968), and sheep (Rodesch *et al.*, 1969) (Fig. 9). No similar effects were obtained with adenine nucleotides or with butyrate (Rodesch *et al.*, 1969). Under suitable conditions, i.e., in thyroid slices from animals pretreated with thyroid extract, and in the presence of 1 mM caffeine, cAMP also stimulates iodide organification. In these slices, the effect of low concentration of TSH is potentiated by 1 mM caffeine, which by itself has no effect (Rodesch *et al.*, 1969). In isolated beef thyroid cells, TSH, like DB-cAMP, enhances the incorporation of iodide preferentially into thyroglobulin (Wilson *et al.*, 1968). In guinea pig thyroid tissue incubated for 40 hours in a culture medium, TSH and theophylline enhance the binding of iodide to proteins, and the effects are additive at less than maximal concentrations (Desbarats-Schönbaum *et al.*, 1970). In this case, the length of the incubation is such that several different mechanisms may be involved. These data therefore strongly support the hypothesis that the stimulation of iodide organification by TSH is mediated by cAMP.

TSH injection increases the ratio of DIT-^{131}I to MIT-^{131}I and the radioiodine labeling of iodothyronines in rat thyroid *in vivo*. This effect

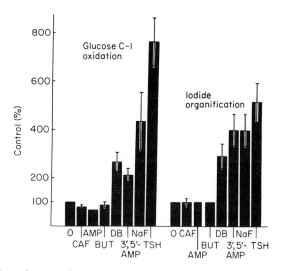

Fig. 9. Action of agents interfering with the cAMP system on glucose oxidation, iodide binding to proteins, and intracellular colloid droplet formation in dog thyroid slices. *CAF:* caffeine 1 mM; AMP, 5′-AMP 7 mM + caffeine 1 mM. *BUT:* butyrate 0.6 mM. *DB:* DB-cAMP 0.3 mM. *3′,5′-AMP:* cAMP 7 mM + caffeine 1 mM. NaF: 3 mM. TSH: 100 mU/ml. Incubation times: 45 minutes and 1 hour. Intracellular colloid droplets: TSH, +++; NaF, 0; 3′,5′-AMP, ++; DB, +++; BUT, 0; CAF, 0; control, 0. Data from Rodesch *et al.* (1969).

is mimicked by cAMP, other adenine nucleotides, and theophylline (Ahn and Rosenberg, 1968). In mice, doses of TSH and theophylline, which by themselves are ineffective, increase the ratio DIT:MIT and enhance the synthesis of iodothyronines (Bastomsky and McKenzie, 1967). The action of effective doses of TSH is increased by theophylline (Bastomsky and McKenzie, 1968). These effects appear to be direct since they are also obtained *in vitro*, with DB-cAMP in isolated beef thyroid cells (Wilson *et al.*, 1968), and in the case of iodothyronine synthesis, with cAMP, DB-cAMP, caffeine, and theophylline but not with other adenine nucleotides, also in mouse thyroids prelabeled *in vivo* (Ensor and Munro, 1969; Kendall-Taylor and Munro, 1970). In the latter experiments cAMP, unlike TSH, appeared to stimulate the formation of iodothyronines less than it stimulated iodine secretion. However, in the absence of kinetic data, one could not conclude that there is an important discrepancy between the effects of cAMP and TSH; TSH may have a more sustained effect than the rapidly hydrolyzed cAMP, and iodothyronine formation may depend more closely than secretion on a continuous increase of intracellular cAMP level. DB-cAMP has also been reported to stimulate thyroxine formation in dog thyroid slices (Ahn and Rosenberg, 1970a). Since there is evidence that the activation by TSH of iodide organification and of iodothyronine synthesis may be secondary to enhanced H_2O_2 formation, it is of great interest that DB-cAMP is reported to mimic the action of TSH in stimulating this formation (Bénard and Brault, 1970; Ahn and Rosenberg, 1970b). Therefore, the effect of TSH on thyroid DIT/MIT ratio and on iodothyronine synthesis, like the stimulation of iodide organification, seems to be mediated by cAMP.

D. THYROID SECRETION

The thyroid secretes, mainly in the venous outflow, thyroid hormones and some iodide. The secretion of thyroid hormones involves at least two consecutive processes: the endocytosis of colloid by phagocytosis resulting in the formation of intracellular colloid droplets, and the digestion of colloid thyroglobulin by lysosomal enzymes with the release of thyroid hormone (Nadler *et al.*, 1962; Wetzel *et al.*, 1965) (Fig. 10). The digestion of thyroglobulin also releases iodotyrosines which are deiodinated by a NADPH requiring desiodase; part of the iodide derived from the iodotyrosines is reorganified while another part "spills out" of the cell (Rosenberg *et al.*, 1965).

1. *In Vivo Nature of Secretion*

TSH increases the secretion of PBI and induces the release of inorganic iodide into the venous blood within a few minutes after its injection. In the dog, for example, the venous concentrations of PBI may

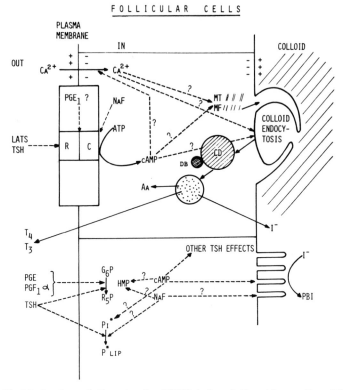

FIG. 10. Mechanism of thyrotropin (TSH)-induced thyroid secretion. Model exemplifying various hypotheses on this mechanism: role of cAMP, role of microtubules and/or microfilaments, stimulation secretion coupling by way of Ca^{2+} penetration in the cell, etc. *p*lip:* incorporation of $^{32}P_i$ into thyroid phospholipids; LATS: long-acting thyroid stimulator; MT: microtubule; MF: microfilament; CD; colloid droplet; DB: dense body; R: receptor; C: adenyl cyclase.

reach a peak of 9 $\mu g/100$ ml (control 2.9 $\mu g/100$ ml), 1–2 hours after TSH (Rosenberg *et al.*, 1961). There is a parallelism between the kinetics of the formation of intracellular colloid droplets, of the appearance of PBI in isolated droplets, and of the release of PBI and iodide in venous blood, i.e., between the kinetics of three aspects of the secretory process (Dumont and Rocmans, 1965; Balasubramaniam *et al.*, 1965; Rosenberg *et al.*, 1965). The PBI released by the stimulated thyroid represents thyroxine and some triiodothyronine (Taurog *et al.*, 1964; Dumont and Rocmans, 1964; Rosenberg *et al.*, 1965). *In situ* perfusion of the rat thyroid has shown that TSH does not markedly change the $T_3:T_4$ ratio in the effluent (Inoue *et al.*, 1967). Previous observations *in vivo* (Matsuda and Greer, 1965), suggesting a very marked increase in this ratio in the secreted PBI were probably due to the high basal level of thyroxine in the thyroid arterial blood. It has been shown that the iodide secreted by the stimulated thyroid originates essentially from the iodotyrosines of the thyroid proteins (see review of Rosenberg *et al.*, 1965; Isaacs *et al.*, 1966).

Iodotyrosines are not usually secreted by the thyroid after TSH injection although they constitute a major part of the total thyroid iodine (Taurog *et al.*, 1964; Rosenberg *et al.*, 1965). Traces (Dumont and Rocmans, 1964; Inoue *et al.*, 1967) or small amounts (Matsuda *et al.*, 1964) of iodotyrosines have been detected in the effluent of intensely stimulated glands. This presumably results from saturation of the deiodinating system. Overloading with exogenous iodotyrosines *in vivo* also induces iodotyrosine release by the thyroid (Serafimov and Sestakov, 1967).

Concomitant with the release of thyroid hormone and iodide into the blood, TSH stimulates the release of iodide, thyroxine, and mainly iodoprotein into the lymphatics of cat and monkey thyroids. In the absence of precise data on lymphatic flow, it is impossible to quantitate this secretion, but the available information suggest that of the total thyroid output, secretion into the lymphatic system accounts for all of the secretion of iodoprotein, part of the thyroxine secretion and a minor fraction of iodide release (Daniel *et al.*, 1967a). Outflow of iodoproteins in the lymphatics consists at least partly of thyroglobulin: thyroglobulin has been identified by radioimmunoassay in the lymph from resting and activated glands. Since no radioisotopes had been administered to the experimental animals, this release is physiological and is not secondary to radiation damage (Daniel *et al.*, 1967b; Kotani *et al.*, 1968).

2. *Endocytosis of Colloid*

The endocytosis of colloid, its mechanism and its ultrastructural counterparts, have been described in Section III,B,1. *In vitro*, as the endocytosis of colloid or other material by thyroid cells has not yet been studied directly, the information available on endocytosis is mainly derived from studies on the formation of apical pseudopods or intracellular colloid droplets in stimulated thyroid tissue. Pseudopod formation is difficult to quantitate, and therefore the frequency of intracellular colloid droplets (number of droplets per cell) has been taken as a measure of the activity of the endocytic process. In interpreting these experiments, one must keep in mind that (1) light microscope examination may fail to reveal small or less-colored droplets; (2) the frequency of droplets does not necessarily reflect the amount of colloid present in the cells as the size and density of the droplets varies; (3) the amount of colloid present in a cell at a given time is a function not only of the rate of endocytosis, but of the equilibrium between the processes of endocytosis and colloid digestion.

TSH *in vitro* causes the formation of colloid droplets in follicular cells of thyroid slices from guinea pig (Junqueira, 1947), dog (Dumont, 1965; Pastan and Wollman, 1967; Onaya *et al.*, 1969), rat (Pastan and Macchia, 1967) and sheep (Burke, 1969d, 1970c).

The effect of TSH on colloid droplet formation is mimicked in dog thyroid slices by DB-cAMP (Pastan and Wollman, 1967; Rodesch *et al.*, 1969), and by 10 times higher concentrations of cAMP in the presence of caffeine (Rodesch *et al.*, 1969), but not with concentrations of cAMP equivalent to those of DB-cAMP in the absence of caffeine (Pastan and Wollman, 1967); these observations have been confirmed by electron microscopy (Nève and Dumont, 1970b). The effect is not mimicked by other adenine nucleotides (Pastan and Wollman, 1967; Rodesch *et al.*, 1969), by caffeine, or by butyrate (Rodesch *et al.*, 1969). Onaya *et al.* (1969) have confirmed that DB-cAMP induces the formation of colloid droplets in dog thyroid slices. In rat thyroid slices, DB-cAMP did not mimic this effect of TSH (Pastan and Macchia, 1967); however, in these experiments, DB-cAMP also failed to reproduce the TSH stimulation of glucose oxidation. As discussed earlier, there are many possible explanations for such a discrepancy, the most obvious one being that 0.38 mM DB-cAMP is too low a concentration to mimic TSH 50 mU/ml. Burke (1969d) has reported that DB-cAMP enhances intracellular colloid droplet formation in sheep thyroid slices. The available evidence is therefore very suggestive of an involvement of cAMP in the induction of colloid phagocytosis in thyroid cells. It would be of great interest to investigate the possible role of cAMP on phagocytosis in other cells.

3. *Thyroglobulinolysis in vitro—Iodotyrosine deiodination*

The release of nonprotein-bound ^{131}I iodine by slices of prelabeled rat thyroids has been studied by Ahn and Rosenberg (1967). In their system, the release could be induced only by prior *in vivo* administration of TSH; the rate of accumulation of ^{131}I in the medium rapidly tapered off and no further release was observed after 2 hours of incubation. In these experiments, at the time of thyroid removal (2 hours after TSH injection), the follicular cells must have been already filled with colloid droplets. These observations suggest that in this system only proteolysis of already ingested colloid took place, i.e., that the experiments explored the second step of thyroid secretion. Proteolysis in prelabeled rat thyroid was enhanced by cysteine, mercaptoethanol, and GSH, and was not inhibited by DFP. These characteristics correspond to those of the acid protease(s) of the lysosomal fraction of thyroid homogenates (Ahn and Rosenberg, 1967). The particulate alkaline protease which had been identified in rat thyroid homogenate (Pastan and Almqvist, 1965) has been shown to belong to mast cells rather than thyroid follicular cells (Pastan and Almqvist, 1966) ; in addition, its characteristics (sensitivity to DFP, reduction of the activity by *in vivo* treatment with compound 48/80) do not correspond to those of the proteolytic system involved in thyroglobulin hydrolysis in intact cells (Ahn and Rosenberg, 1967). These authors have suggested that the stimulation of intracellular proteolysis by GSH and cysteine is due to reduction of disulfide bonds in substrate thyroglobulin; this reduction would render the molecule more susceptible to the action of intracellular proteinases. Inhibitors of energy metabolism do not inhibit proteolysis in acellular systems (Ahn and Rosenberg, 1967), which suggests that once secondary lysosomes are formed, thyroglobulinolysis does not require any more energy. The data obtained *in vitro* therefore support the concept of the digestion of thyroglobulin in secondary lysosomes of thyroid cells. The morphological observations which led to this hypothesis have been discussed in Section III,B,1.

Enhanced thyroidal deiodinating activity has been observed in rat thyroid homogenates 3 hours after *in vivo* TSH administration. This observation suggested that increased deiodination was a factor in accelerating glandular iodine depletion after TSH administration (Maayan and Rosenberg, 1963). However, deiodination of exogenous iodothyrosines by beef slices is dependent on the quantity of iodotyrosine substrates and is not enhanced by TSH (Powell et al., 1964). Moreover, increased deiodinating activity in rat thyroids is not observed 1 hour after the injection of TSH, i.e., at a time when iodine release by the thyroid should be near its peak. No change in activity is observed in dog thyroid slices 1 hour after stimulation (Bastomsky and Rosenberg, 1966). Changes in deiodinating capacity of the thyroid cell therefore seem to play little part in the acute stimulation of thyroid iodide release by TSH.

4. Secretion in Vitro

The effect of TSH on the overall process of thyroid secretion has been studied *in vitro* by a variety of methods: by the release of butanol-soluble ^{131}I from prelabeled rat thyroid glands; by the release of free α-aminonitrogen, tyrosine, and inorganic [127]I in beef and sheep thyroid slices (Poffenbarger et al., 1963; Powell et al., 1964; Tonoue et al., 1970) ; by the release of non-TCA precipitable iodine-^{131}I from prelabeled dog thyroids (Dumont, 1966) ; by the release of iodine-^{131}I from prelabeled rat (Botkin et al., 1954), dog (Ahn and Rosenberg, 1970b), or mouse thyroid (W. Brown and Munro, 1967); and by the release of butanol-extractable ^{131}I from prelabeled and preincubated dog thyroid slices (Willems et al., 1970). Although all these systems give results of a similar nature, the two latter procedures give a much lower signal-to-noise ratio, and a lower spontaneous release of ^{131}I in the controls. Several facts suggest that the BEI release from dog thyroid slices results from the uptake of colloid by phagocytosis and its digestion by lysosomal enzymes: the absence of intracellular colloid droplets and of basal release in control slices, the kinetic data showing that droplet formation largely precedes BEI release, the parallel TSH concentration-effect relationships (Fig. 11). Other arguments also strongly support the hypothesis that the in vitro release corresponds to the in vivo secretion: the specificity of the activating agent TSH, the nature of the release (T₄, T₃, and iodide), the linear kinetics of release (Willems et al., 1970), and the similarity of the ultrastructural aspects of secretion in vivo and in vitro (Nève and Dumont, 1970b). Secretion in vitro takes place in the same range of TSH concentrations that cause other hormonal effects (Fig. 8) (Willems et al., 1970).

In dog thyroid slices, secretion is inhibited by inhibitors of glycolysis (NaF, oxamate). For NaF, the inhibition is total in the absence of glucose in the medium, but it is partly relieved when glucose is added to the medium, i.e., when the Embden-Meyerhof pathway is reactivated. NaF and oxamate also inhibit intracellular colloid droplet formation (Willems et al., 1970). Anaerobiosis suppresses iodide release from beef thyroid slices (Powell et al., 1964), and antimycin blocks colloid droplet formation in dog thyroid slices (Willems and Dumont, 1968). These results suggest that both glycolytic and mitochondrial ATP are required

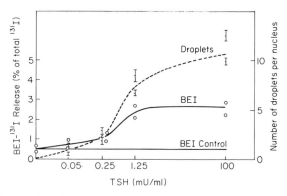

Fig. 11. Effects of various TSH concentrations on intracellular colloid droplet formation and secretion in dog thyroid slices in vitro. BEI-^{131}I release: release of butanol-extractable ^{131}I iodine (iodine and iodothyronines) from prelabeled slices. From Willems et al. (1970), with permission of the publisher.

for the secretory process and that depletion of cellular ATP stores blocks secretion at the level of colloid endocytosis.

5. Mechanism of TSH Secretory Effect—Role of cAMP

The stimulation of radioiodine release from mice thyroids *in vivo* is mimicked by theophylline, by cAMP and adenine nucleotides, but not by other nucleotides. Doses of TSH and theophylline, which are inactive by themselves, considerably enhance the secretion when they are combined. The latter phenomenon is also observed in the rat *in vivo* (Bastomsky and McKenzie, 1967). Similar results were obtained with DB-cAMP (Burke, 1968a) and with DB-cAMP, cAMP, and other adenine nucleotides (Ochi and Degroot, 1969a) in mice. These *in vivo* effects might be at least partly secondary to an effect at the level of the pituitary. However, DB-cAMP, but not cAMP or 5'-AMP, injected by carotid arterial infusion enhances the secretion of the ipsilateral thyroid lobe without affecting the contralateral lobe (Ahn *et al.*, 1969).

The stimulation of thyroid iodine secretion by TSH has been reproduced *in vitro* with prelabeled intact mouse thyroids. The effect of TSH is mimicked by theophylline, caffeine, and cAMP, but not by other adenine nucleotides. However, in the case of methylxanthines, a large part of the radioiodine release is represented by proteins (Ensor and Munro, 1969). This peculiarity may suggest that this effect of methylxanthines does not correspond to the physiological secretion, or that methylxanthines inhibit the hydrolysis of thyroglobulin. Combinations of maximally effective concentrations of TSH and theophylline, TSH and cAMP, or of cAMP and theophylline produce no increase over the plateau effect of each of these compounds acting separately. The levels of these plateaus differ only slightly. These observations are compatible with the hypothesis of a final common pathway in the mechanism of action of these agents. Concentrations of theophylline which give minimal responses potentiate the effects of lower than maximal concentrations of cAMP and of TSH (Ensor and Munro, 1969). Ochi and Degroot (1969a) reported that neither cAMP nor DB-cAMP stimulated iodine ^{125}I release *in vitro* from prelabeled mouse thyroids. However, no effect of TSH was observed either, which indicates that this system was unsatisfactory. DB-cAMP mimics the TSH induced release of iodide and iodothyronines *in vitro* from prelabeled mouse (Kendall-Taylor and Munro, 1970) and rat (Tonoue *et al.*, 1970) thyroids and from dog thyroid slices (Ahn and Rosenberg, 1970b). In the latter system, the stimulating effects of maximally effective concentrations of TSH and DB-cAMP were not additive, suggesting a common pathway of their actions. In our dog thyroid slices system, not only DB-cAMP but also cAMP and caffeine (but not ATP,

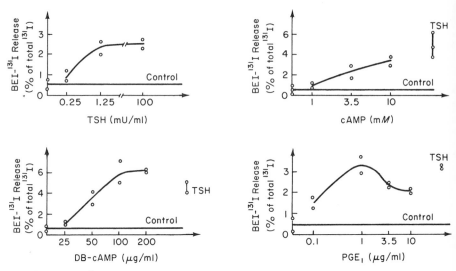

Fig. 12. Effects of various concentrations of thyrotropin (TSH), cyclic 3′,5′-adenosine monophosphate (cAMP) (in the presence of 1 mM caffeine), (DB-cAMP), and prostaglandin E₁ (PGE₁) on secretion by dog thyroid slices *in vitro*. In the experiments with cAMP, DB-cAMP, and PGE₁, the action of TSH 1.25 mU/ml in the same experiment is shown for comparison. From Willems *et al.* (1970), with permission of the publisher.

ADP, or AMP) mimic the TSH action on secretion and its ultrastructural counterparts (Fig. 12) (Willems *et al.*, 1970; Nève and Dumont, 1971). There is therefore very good evidence that the secretory effect of TSH is mediated by cAMP.

Microtubules and microtubular proteins which have been identified in the thyroid as in other tissues may have a role in cell movement. Therefore, the hypothesis was proposed that the stimulation by TSH of colloid endocytosis and thyroid secretion might result from an action of cAMP on microtubules (Fig. 10). Intracellular colloid droplet formation and secretion in activated dog thyroid slices are inhibited by colchicine, vincristine, vinblastine, ethanol, and D₂O, i.e., by agents that share the common property of interfering with the normal functioning of microtubules. These data suggest that the microtubular system is involved (Fig. 13) in colloid endocytosis (Nève *et al.*, 1970). Therefore, it is of interest that it has recently been shown that cAMP activates the phosphorylation of microtubular proteins in nervous tissue (Goodman *et al.*, 1970). The inhibition of secretion by cytocholasin, a inhibitor of the microfilament system, in dog thyroid slices *in vitro* suggests that this system also plays a role in thyroid secretion (Nève *et al.*, 1971).

Douglas (1968) has demonstrated that many secretory phenomena are secondary to a burst of Ca²⁺ concentration inside cells. He has called this

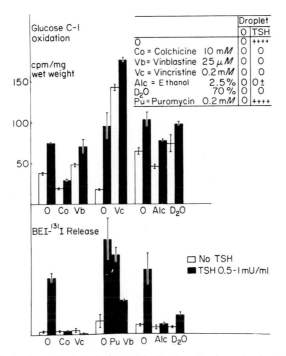

FIG. 13. Effect of agents interfering with the functioning of microtubules on the action of thyrotropin (TSH) on secretion and glucose oxidation. Droplet: intracellular colloid droplet formation. From Nève et al. (1970), with permission of the publisher.

phenomenon the stimulation-secretion coupling. Seljelid and Nakken (1969) have hypothesized that this scheme may apply to thyroid and that thyroid secretion may be triggered by an increased penetration of Ca^{2+} into the follicular cell (Fig. 10). Thyroid secretion and intracellular colloid droplet formation in resting or stimulated dog thyroid slices *in vitro* are not enhanced by Ca^{2+} or Ba^{2+}. They are not inhibited in slices preincubated in the absence of Ca^{2+} and in the presence of Mg^{2+} EDTA and incubated without Ca^{2+}. Under such conditions, other TSH effects (the activations of glucose C-1 oxidation, and of iodide organification) are abolished (Willems and Dumont, 1971). Thus, we have found no evidence in favor of the hypothesis that the classical stimulus-secretion coupling applies to TSH-induced thyroid secretion.

E. CHRONIC EFFECTS

Thyroids stimulated for several days exhibit both the early and delayed effects of TSH: increases of thyroid blood flow (as measured by ^{86}Rb uptake) (Kapitola et al., 1970), of iodide trapping (Taurog *et al.,* 1959; Wolff and Halmi, 1963), of iodotyrosine and particularly of iodothyronine formation (Taurog *et al.,* 1958b; Katakai *et al.,* 1966; Bastomsky and McKenzie, 1968), of thyroid hormone secretion (Bates and Condliffe, 1960), and of iodotyrosine deiodinating capacity (Maayan, 1964). It is interesting to note that in these chronically stimulated glands, iodide trapping may increase less than thyroid weight, lowering the T/S ratio in comparison with controls (Taurog *et al.,* 1959). A general consequence of these effects is that the turnover of iodine in the chronically stimulated thyroid is accelerated. Qualitatively similar effects are obtained in thyroid tissue culture (Kerkof *et al.,* 1964; Nataf *et al.,* 1965; Raghupathy *et al.,* 1965; Nataf, 1968), but it is difficult to evaluate to what extent these effects are specific or are secondary to a general tropic action of TSH.

In hypophysectomized animals, a converse picture is obtained; iodide trapping is much decreased, but the binding of iodide decreases even more, as shown by the decreased organification of the small amount of iodide which is taken up by the gland; iodothyronine formation (Taurog *et al.,* 1958a) and thyroid secretion (Brown-Grant *et al.,* 1954) are almost completely suppressed; iodotyrosine deiodinating capacity is much decreased (Maayan, 1964). Therefore, the rate of turnover of thyroid iodine is greatly diminished (Brown-Grant *et al.,* 1954). It is apparent that TSH controls to a variable extent all the steps of iodine metabolism in the thyroid.

F. Interrelations between the Effects of TSH on Iodine
   Metabolism

The hypothesis that TSH stimulation of one step of iodine metabolism in the thyroid causes the other effects of the hormone (Rawson, 1949) is no longer tenable. The growth effect of TSH and the early stimulation of iodination and of thyroid secretion are observed in animals or tissue preparations in which iodide trapping has been blocked by perchlorate (Taurog *et al.,* 1958b; Tong, 1964c; Rosenberg *et al.,* 1965; Rosenfeld and Rosenberg, 1966; Nataf, 1968; Ahn and Rosenberg, 1970a). These effects are therefore independent of the early increased iodide efflux and the delayed increased iodide influx caused by the hormone. Blocking of iodination by antithyroid drugs does not inhibit the action of TSH on iodide trapping, thyroid secretion or thyroid growth (Taurog *et al.,* 1958b; Bates and Condliffe, 1960; Halmi *et al.,* 1960; Rosenberg *et al.,* 1965). TSH stimulates growth and iodide trapping in thyroids deprived of iodine by long treatment with PTU (Taurog *et al.,* 1958b). TSH also enhances iodide trapping and iodination in isolated cells which contain little or no colloid (Tong, 1964a; Wilson *et al.,* 1968). Therefore, these effects are not secondary to a stimulation of the release of iodide or thyroid hormone. It can be concluded that TSH affects the various phases of iodine metabolism coordinately but independently.

Increased iodide trapping and iodide organification probably account for the higher uptake of iodide by thyroids of mice treated with TSH for 3 days (Bastomsky and McKenzie, 1967). Increased iodide uptake was also demonstrated with theophylline, and with doses of TSH and theophylline that were ineffective by themselves. Therefore, there is some support for the hypothesis that chronic as well as acute effects of TSH on iodine metabolism in the thyroid are mediated by cAMP.

V. Action of TSH on Carbohydrate and Energy Metabolism

A. General Pattern of Glucose and Oxidative Metabolism

The energy metabolism of the dog thyroid *in vitro* is characterized by an oxygen uptake which mainly reflects tightly coupled mitochondrial respiration and a very active aerobic glycosis (Table I). The two pathways account for approximately 80% and 20% of the ATP formed from ADP. The metabolism of glucose is characterized by a high aerobic glycolysis (80% of the glucose taken up), a high incorporation of glucose into proteins (6%), and a relatively low activity of the hexose monophosphate pathway (Dumont and Tondeur-Montenez, 1965).

TSH *in vitro* greatly modifies the pattern of glucose and energy metabolism in dog thyroid tissue. It enhances the uptake of oxygen and glucose, and the formation of lactate. It greatly increases the oxidation

TABLE I
Action of Thyrotropin on the Energy Metabolism of Dog
Thyroid Slices[a,b]

Action	Control	TSH
Glucose uptake	406	552
Lactate accumulation	537	775
Estimate of ATP phosphorylated by aerobic glycolysis	537	775
Oxygen uptake	637	840
Respiration inhibited by oligomycin	447	605
Estimate of ADP phosphorylated by oxidative phosphorylation	$447 \times 6 = 2682$	$605 \times 6 = 3630$
ADP phosphorylation: estimate of ratio mitochondrial:glycolytic phosphorylation	$\dfrac{2682}{537} = 5.0$	$\dfrac{3630}{775} = 4.7$

[a] Data from Dumont and Tondeur-Montenez (1965) and Lamy *et al.* (1967).

[b] Results are expressed as milliμmoles per milligram dry weight of tissue for an incubation of 4 hours in Krebs-Ringer phosphate buffer, TSH 256 mU/ml.

of glucose-1-^{14}C to $^{14}CO_2$ and to a smaller extent the oxidation of 6-^{14}C and U-^{14}C-labeled glucose. It activates the oxidation of pyruvate carbons 1, 2, and 3. In the stimulated tissue, the incorporation of glucose, labeled in the C-1 or C-6 position, into lipids is increased, while the incorporation into the fatty acids of these lipids, and into glycogenlike material and proteins is decreased (Table II) (Dumont and Tondeur-Montenez, 1965). Some aspects of this general picture of the effects of TSH on dog thyroid metabolism had been described in previous publications (Field et al., 1961; Dumont, 1964). The effects of TSH in vitro on glucose and energy metabolism in dog thyroid tissue have also been observed in vitro after an in vivo stimulation (Dumont and Rocmans, 1964) and in perfused glands (Hershman, 1967). In general, TSH has similar in vitro effects on thyroid tissue from other species (Field et al., 1960; Freinkel, 1960, 1965; Dumont, 1961a, 1962, 1964; Schussler and Ingbar, 1961; Mulvey et al., 1962; Merlevede et al., 1963; Gilman and Rall, 1968b). However, in beef tissue, glucose carbon-1 oxidation is decreased at low concentrations of TSH but is increased at high hormone concentrations (Merlevede et al., 1963; Pastan and Macchia, 1967; Gilman and Rall, 1968b). A similar situation exists in human thyroid tissue (Otten and Dumont, 1970).

The great enhancement of glucose C-1 oxidation as compared to the smaller increase of glucose C-6 oxidation, has generally been taken as indicating an activation of the pentose pathway in the TSH-stimulated

TABLE II

EFFECT OF TSH ON THE METABOLISM OF GLUCOSE BY DOG THYROID SLICES in Vitro[a,b]

Variable	Unit	Control	TSH
Glucose uptake	Nanomoles/4hr/mg	406	552
Lactate formation	Dry weight of tissue	537	775
G_1CO_2	Fraction	0.117	0.234
G_6CO_2	Fraction	0.050	0.043
G_1 lactate	Fraction	0.72	0.62
G_6 lactate	Fraction	0.90	0.79
G_6 TCA soluble	Fraction	0.130	0.115
G_6 Hot TCA soluble	Fraction	0.012	0.009
G_6 Lipids	Fraction	0.009	0.007
G_6 Fatty acids of lipids	Fraction	0.002	0.001
G_6 Proteins	Fraction	0.058	0.038

[a] Data from Dumont and Tondeur-Montenez (1965).

[b] G_1, and G_6 indicate the fraction of the ^{14}C of 1-^{14}C- and 6-^{14}C-labeled glucose taken up by the slices which can be found in the metabolic compartment, TSH 256 mU/ml.

thyroid tissue (Field *et al.*, 1960, 1961; Dumont, 1961a; Schussler and Ingbar, 1961). This interpretation has been shown to be qualitatively correct by studies using agents known to stimulate the pentose pathway (electron acceptors) or to stimulate or inhibit the tricarboxylic acid cycle (Dumont, 1961b). Quantitative evaluation of the pentose pathway has subsequently demonstrated the stimulation of this pathway by TSH *in vitro* in beef (Merlevede *et al.*, 1963) and in dog thyroid tissue (Dumont and Tondeur-Montenez, 1965). Conversely, the decrease of glucose C-1 oxidation observed in beef thyroid tissue stimulated by low concentrations of TSH (Merlevede *et al.*, 1963) probably reflects the diminished activity of the pentose pathway. Indeed, it was not accompanied by a decreased oxidation of glucose-6-^{14}C or by a dilution of the specific activity of the thyroid hexose phosphate pool (Gilman and Rall, 1968b). The mechanism of the inhibition of the pentose phosphate pathway is unknown.

The stimulation by TSH of pyruvate oxidation, as well as the stimulation of acetate oxidation (Field *et al.*, 1961; Dumont, 1962), suggests an activation of the tricarboxylic acid cycle in the thyroid. This interpretation is supported by the fact that TSH enhances the oxidation of the carbons of pyruvate C-3 > C-2 > C-1 (Dumont and Tondeur-Montenez, 1965). Increased activity of the tricarboxylic acid cycle implies an enhanced mitochondrial respiration. The stimulation by TSH of oxygen uptake in thyroid slices, which is a reflection of mitochondrial energy metabolism, also suggests an activation of the TCA cycle. Glucose C-6 oxidation also reflects the activity of the tricarboxylic acid cycle in thyroid tissue (Dumont, 1962; Field *et al.*, 1965). However, this variable is more complex, as it measures the number of glucose molecules which are first catabolized to triose phosphates by the Embden-Meyerhof pathway and the pentose pathway, and then are completely oxidized by the oxidative decarboxylation of pyruvate and the TCA cycle (Katz and Wood, 1963; Dumont and Tondeur-Montenez, 1965).

Increased overall incorporation of glucose into lipids with concomitant decreased incorporation into the fatty acids of lipids in the stimulated tissue, suggests that TSH enhances the incorporation of α-glycerophosphate, derived from glucose, into thyroid lipids.

In summary, TSH rapidly modifies several aspects of glucose and energy metabolism in thyriod tissue: it stimulates the uptake of glucose and its metabolism through the pentose phosphate pathway and the Embden-Meyerhof pathway, it enhances the incorporation of glucose, presumably as α-glycerophosphate into lipids, it decreases the incorporation of glucose into glycogen and into proteins; it increases the activity of the tricarboxylic acid cycle, i.e., of mitochondrial oxidative metabolism.

Little information is available on the metabolism of glucose in chronically stimulated thyroid tissue.

B. Glucose Uptake and Incorporation into Proteins, Lipids, and Glycogenlike Material

1. *Glucose Uptake*

TSH *in vitro* stimulates the uptake of glucose by sheep (Freinkel, 1960, 1963; Dumont, 1964), calf (Field *et al.*, 1960; Gilman and Rall, 1968b), and dog (Dumont, 1964) thyroid slices and by sheep thyroid cells in culture (Dickson, 1966). The increases observed are of the order of 25% to 45%. No significant stimulation of glucose uptake was observed in perfused stimulated dog thyroids (Hershman, 1967). However, the data suggest that the effect was present and might have been proved by increasing the number of experiments. Moreover, *in vivo* administration of TSH enhances the uptake of glucose in dog thyroid slices *in vitro* (Dumont and Rocmans, 1964). In all these experiments, the effect was obtained with large doses or concentrations of TSH. When the concentration of TSH is decreased, the enhancement of glucose uptake in dog thyroid slices apparently decreases in parallel with other effects of the hormone on glucose metabolism (Dumont, 1964). In beef thyroid slices, on the contrary, other effects of TSH on glucose metabolism are still apparent for concentrations of TSH which do not increase glucose uptake (Gilman and Rall, 1968b). Glucose uptake is stimulated *in vitro* by insulin in calf (Field *et al.*, 1960) and sheep (Dumont, 1961b) thyroid slices.

Two mechanisms could account for the stimulation by TSH of glucose uptake in thyroid tissue: an enhancement of glucose transport into the cell or an increase in its subsequent intracellular metabolism. It may well be that both mechanisms play a role in the TSH effect. Sheep thyroid cells contain a low K_m hexokinase but no high K_m glucokinase (Abraham *et al.*, 1965). The low K_m hexokinase should be saturated at concentrations well below the physiologically prevailing plasma concentrations of glucose. This suggests that glucose phosphorylation is not the rate-limiting step in glucose utilization in thyroid. Increasing glucose concentration in the incubation medium enhances the uptake of glucose and its metabolism in sheep thyroid slices (Dumont and Eloy, 1966). In the absence of high K_m glucokinase, such an effect suggests the existence in the thyroid cell of a permeability barrier to glucose. The existence of such a barrier and of a hormone-sensitive carrier system for glucose is also suggested by the stimulation by insulin of glucose uptake in thyroid slices, during relatively short incubations (2 and 4 hours), and by the inhibition by O-methylglucose but not by 1-glucose of stimulated glucose oxidation in dog thyroid slices (Macchia and Pastan, 1968). The specific increases in the distribution spaces of xylose and 1-arabinose in TSH-stimulated calf thyroid slices strongly support the hypothesis that TSH activates the glucose transport system in the thyroid cell (Tarui and Nonaka, 1963). However, there are indications that increased intra-cellular metabolism of glucose may also enhance the uptake of this sub-strate. Cyanide, dinitrophenol, and Synkavit enhance moderately the uptake of glucose in sheep thyroid slices (Dumont, 1966). These agents activate specific pathways of glucose catabolism (glycolysis, glycolysis and the tricarboxylic acid cycle, and the pentose phosphate pathway), and presumably do not act on the cell membrane. The enhancement by TSH of glucose uptake in the thyroid may therefore be due both to a direct activation of glucose transport in the cell and to the stimulation of pathways of glucose metabolism.

The relative weakness of the insulin action on glucose uptake in the thyroid and of the glucose concentration effect on glucose metabolism (Dumont, 1961b, 1964; Gilman and Rall, 1968b) suggests that the per-meability barrier of the membrane for glucose may not be very tight and in consequence that the stimulation of glucose uptake by TSH may play only a minor, complementary role in TSH action. This hypothesis is supported by the facts that insulin, which also stimulates glucose uptake, does not mimic the action of TSH on glucose metabolism (Field et al., 1960; Dumont, 1961b), and that TSH enhances several aspects of thy-roid metabolism (phospholipid turnover, oxygen uptake, phosphate re-lease in the cell, pyruvate oxidation, endogenous glucose oxidation, etc.) (Freinkel, 1957, 1963; Dumont, 1962; Dumont and Eloy, 1966) in slices incubated in the absence of glucose in the medium.

TSH has been reported to increase the distribution space of some stereospecific sugars in calf thyroid slices. This effect was mimicked by cAMP but not by 5'-AMP (Tarui et al., 1963). These observations have suggested that TSH activates stereospecific sugar transport and that this effect may be mediated by cAMP. In beef thyroid slices, the stimulation by TSH of glucose uptake is obtained only for large concentrations of TSH and is not mimicked by DB-cAMP (Gilman and Rall, 1968b). However, the concentration of nucleotide used (1 mM) corresponds to low concentrations of TSH (≤ 2 mU/ml) when the relative potency of the two compounds on other aspects of glucose metabolism is compared. Therefore, it is possible that the effect of TSH on glucose and sugar up-take is mediated by cAMP, but the physiological meaning of this effect can be questioned.

2. Glucose Incorporation into Proteins and Glycogenlike Material

TSH decreases the incorporation of exogenous glucose into the proteins of dog thyroid slices (Dumont and Tondeur-Montenez, 1965). The hormone induced phagocytosis and digestion of colloid releases amino acids (Poffenbarger et al., 1963), sialic acid (Wollman and Warren, 1961), and other carbohydrate derivatives into the tissue, thus presumably increasing and diluting the precursors pools of thyroglobulin. Therefore, it has been suggested that this dilution of precursors pools is the cause of the decreased incorporation of glucose into the proteins of the stimulated tissue (Dumont and Tondeur-Montenez, 1965).

TSH decreases the incorporation of exogenous glucose into glycogenlike material in beef (Merlevede et al., 1963) and dog (Dumont and Tondeur-Montenez, 1965) thyroid slices. This effect requires very small concentrations of TSH (Merlevede et al., 1963). The method used in these experiments allowed contamination of the glucose-^{14}C isolated from glycogen with other carbohydrates derived from glycoproteins (Merlevede et al., 1963; Freinkel, 1965). However, Merlevede et al. (1963) showed that, in beef thyroid slices at least, glucose accounted for the largest part of the isolated radioactivity. The TSH effect on glucose incorporation into glycogen has been ascribed in part to a dilution of the precursors pools (Dumont and Tondeur-Montenez, 1965). This mechanism must play a small role, if any. Gilman and Rall (1968b) have observed no increase in the glucose 6-phosphate pool, or decrease in the specific activity of this pool in stimulated thyroid slices. Decreased incorporation of glucose into glycogen has also been explained by a stimulation by TSH of glycogenolysis in the thyroid cell (Merlevede et al., 1963; Dumont and Tondeur-Montenez, 1965). In favor of this hypothesis, F. R. Butcher and Serif (1968) showed that TSH enhances phosphorylase activity in dog thyroid slices. This effect was mimicked by DB-cAMP. However, Gilman and Rall (1968b) explained these data by the formation in stimulated tissue of increased concentrations of 5'-AMP and consequent activation of thyroid phosphorylase; they found no evidence of stimulated glycogenolysis in TSH-treated beef thyroid slices. The absence of an effect of TSH on the size and specific activity of the glucose 6-phosphate pool in thyroid suggests that the decreased incorporation of glucose-^{14}C into thyroid glycogen is due to a decreased synthesis of glycogen. Cyclic 3',5'-AMP could well mediate such an effect of TSH, as in muscle it activates the conversion of glycogen synthetase from I form (independent of glucose 6-phosphate) to the less active D form (dependent upon glucose 6-phosphate) (Larner, 1966). The action of TSH on glycogen metabolism in thyroid has probably little physiological importance. Glycogen accounts for only a small part of the metabolism of glucose (Dumont and Tondeur-Montenez, 1965), and glycogen concentration in thyroid tissue has been reported to be low (Freinkel, 1965; Field et al., 1961).

Glucose is incorporated into the lipids of resting thyroid tissue mainly as glycerol (Freinkel, 1963, 1965; Dumont and Tondeur-Montenez, 1965). In the absence of free fatty acids in the medium, this incorporation is about equally divided between neutral lipids and phospholipids. The incorporation into neutral lipids of either exogenous glucose or exogenous fatty acids is enhanced in the presence of the other substrate indicating that the synthesis of neutral lipids may be limited by the supply of both substrates (Freinkel, 1965). TSH enhances the incorporation of exogenous glucose into thyroid lipids but decreases incorporation of glucose into the fatty acids of these lipids. Therefore, it is presumably the incorporation of glycerol derived from α-glycerophosphate of glycolysis which is stimulated (Dumont and Tondeur-Montenez, 1965). In the absence of free fatty acids in the medium, the stimulated incorporation of glucose takes place essentially into the phospholipids, i.e., in the cytostructural lipids. Similarly, in the absence of glucose in the medium, TSH enhances the incorporation of exogenous free fatty acids into thyroid phospholipids but decreases the incorporation into the neutral lipids (Freinkel, 1965). These effects mainly reflect the stimulation of phospholipid turnover and synthesis induced by TSH in thyroid tissue. They are discussed in Section VIII. In the presence of free fatty acids and glucose in the medium, TSH also enhances the incorporation of both substrates into the neutral lipids of thyroid (Freinkel, 1965). This effect may be caused by the increased availability of α-glycerophosphate derived from glycolysis. Its consequence is to increase the stores of neural lipids in the cell, and it may therefore play an additive role in the delayed effects of TSH. The decreased incorporation of exogenous glucose into the fatty acids of lipids in the stimulated thyroid cell has been ascribed to a dilution of the precursor pools (Dumont and Tondeur-Montenez, 1965). TSH induces the release of large amounts of amino acids by colloid proteolysis, and could through cAMP stimulate lipolysis in thyroid as it does in adipose tissue (Freinkel, 1961; Robison et al., 1968); both effects could increase and dilute the acetyl-CoA pools. However, the fact that TSH enhances more pyruvate oxidation and glucose C-6 oxidation than oxygen uptake (Dumont, 1962) bears against the hypothesis of an increased and diluted pool of acetyl-CoA. Therefore, other hypotheses concerning the mechanism of the decreased incorporation of glucose into the fatty acids of lipids in the stimulated thyroid cell should be explored—for example, the intracellular compartmentation of acetyl-CoA pools and the inhibition by TSH of fatty acid synthesis in the thyroid cell.

No direct information is available at the present time on the role of cAMP in the metabolism of glycogen, neutral lipids, or of the glycosidic part of glycoproteins in thyroid tissue.

C. GLYCOLYSIS

TSH administered *in vivo* or *in vitro* stimulates lactate formation by rat (Irie and Slingerland, 1963), sheep, dog (Dumont, 1964; Dumont and Rocmans, 1964; Hershman, 1967) and calf (Gilman and Rall, 1968b) thyroid slices *in vitro*. The increases vary from 20% to 60%. Two mechanisms have been proposed to explain the simulation of glycolysis: stimulation secondary to increased glucose uptake (Dumont and Eloy, 1966) or activation of the Embden-Meyerhof pathway by cAMP (Gilman and Rall, 1968b). It must be kept in mind that the regulation of glycolysis is certainly complex and other factors, such as the oxidation of extramitochondrial NADH, the ratio of intracellular ADP and ATP, and the supply of fatty acids as metabolic fuel (Freinkel, 1965) must also play a role. Increasing the concentration of glucose in the medium enhances in parallel glucose uptake and lactate formation by sheep thyroid slices (Dumont and Eloy, 1966). TSH also increases in parallel glucose uptake and lactate formation in sheep (Dumont, 1964), dog (Dumont and Tondeur-Montenez, 1965), and rat (Irie and Slingerland, 1963) thyroid slices and in perfused dog thyroids (Hershman, 1967). Therefore, in these stimulated tissues the enhancement of glucose uptake could account for the increased glycolysis. However, in calf thyroids low concentrations of TSH increase the formation of lactate, but not the uptake of glucose (Gilman and Rall, 1968b), thus indicating that the two effects may be independent. A stimulation of glycolysis through activation of fructose 6-phosphate kinase by cAMP is a well known phenomenon in several tissues (Robison *et al.*, 1968). Conversion of fructose 6-phosphate to fructose 1,6-phosphate by phosphofructokinase is a rate-limiting step of glycolysis in many types of cells (Scrutton and Utter, 1968) and probably in the rat thyroid (Farnararo *et al.*, 1968). In thyroid slices DB-cAMP stimulates lactate formation (Gilman and Rall, 1968b). This suggests that in the thyroid also cAMP may activate the Embden-Meyerhof pathway directly. It is possible, as suggested by Gilman and Rall (1968b), that both increased glucose uptake and direct activation of the Embden-Meyerhof pathway by cAMP play a role in the stimulation of glycolysis in thyroid, and that only the latter mechanisms would operate at low concentrations of TSH and perhaps therefore *in vivo*.

Enhanced glycolysis is not a primary effect of TSH. Indeed, many effects of TSH occur in glucose-free media, i.e., when no lactate is formed by thyroid tissue (Dumont and Tondeur-Montenez, 1965). Moreover, inhibition of glycolysis by fluoride and iodoacetate does not suppress the stimulation by TSH of the pentose phosphate pathway (Dumont, 1966) and of iodide binding to proteins (Rodesch *et al.*, 1969).

D. Pentose Phosphate Pathway and NADP

1. *Inhibition of the Pentose Phosphate Pathway*

At low concentrations (≤ 1 mU/ml), TSH decreases the oxidation of glucose carbon 1 in beef (Merlevede *et al.*, 1963; Gilman and Rall, 1968b) and human (Otten and Dumont, 1970) thyroid slices (Fig. 14). This effect reflects a decrease of the activity of the pentose phosphate pathway; it occurs in the same range of TSH concentration as the stimulation of cAMP accumulation; it is mimicked by DB-cAMP and theophylline (Gilman and Rall, 1968b), but not by relatively high concentrations of cAMP (Gilman and Rall, 1968b; Merlevede *et al.*, 1963). Contrary to previous observations (Merlevede *et al.*, 1963), 5′-AMP has been reported to decrease glucose C-1 oxidation by beef thyroid slices (Gilman and Rall, 1968b). However, the effect of 5′-AMP appears to be of a different nature than the effect of DB-cAMP since it involves both glucose C-1 and C-6 oxidation whereas TSH and DB-cAMP decrease only C-1 oxidation. The inhibition of the pentose phosphate pathway by low concentrations of TSH is potentiated by theophylline (Gilman and

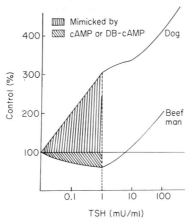

Fig. 14. Effect of various concentrations of thyrotropin (TSH) on glucose oxidation by dog, human, and beef thyroid slices. Reproduction of TSH effects by N^6-2′-O-dibutyl cyclic 3′,5′-adenosine monophosphate (DB-cAMP). Scheme from data of Merlevede *et al.* (1963), Gilman and Rall (1968b), Rodesch *et al.* (1969); and Otten and Dumont (1970).

Rall, 1968b). Therefore, there is good evidence that this effect of TSH is mediated by cAMP.

2. Activation of the Pentose Phosphate Pathway

a. Effect in Vivo and in Vitro. TSH in vitro markedly enhances the oxidation of glucose C-1 in comparison to glucose C-6 in thyroid tissue. This effect has been shown to reflect an activation of the pentose phosphate pathway (Dumont, 1961b; Merlevede et al., 1963; Dumont and Tondeur-Montenez, 1965). In dog thyroid slices, TSH increases the fraction of the glucose taken up which is oxidized to CO_2 and triose phosphate by the pentose cycle from 2 to 7.6%; i.e., it enhances the fraction of glucose which is decarboxylated in the cycle from 6 to 22.8% (Dumont and Tondeur-Montenez, 1965) (Table III).

Preferential stimulation of glucose C-1 oxidation by TSH has been observed in calf (Field et al., 1960; Stanbury, 1964), beef (Merlevede et al., 1963; Dumont, 1964), dog, human, pig (Field et al., 1961; Dumont, 1964), rat (Field et al., 1961; Mulvey et al., 1962), and sheep (Dumont, 1961a; Field et al., 1961; Schussler and Ingbar, 1961) thyroid slices and in isolated beef thyroid cells (Tong, 1964b). It is a very early effect of the hormone: its latency of less than 10 minutes decreases when TSH concentration increases (Shishiba et al., 1970). A similar effect has been observed in dog (Field et al., 1963; Dumont and Rocmans, 1964) thyroid slices after in vivo administration of TSH. TSH enhances glucose C-1 oxidation by dog thyroid slices within 20 minutes after its administration in vitro (Field et al., 1960) or in vivo (Dumont and Rocmans, 1965). However, it has been reported that 1 and 2.5 hours after TSH intraperitoneal injection in vivo, glucose C-1 oxidation in vitro was not increased in guinea pig thyroid slices (Field et al., 1961). "Attempts to explain the negative findings on the basis of route of administration or species insensitivity, are hard to reconcile with the multiple other changes that have been elicited in the guinea pig thyroid within 2 hours after intraperitoneal administration of TSH" (Freinkel, 1963). Although this report has not been confirmed, it would be interesting to investigate by available perfusion techniques the action of TSH on glucose metabolism in the thyroid in vivo.

b. Mechanism. The search for the point of action of TSH on the pentose cycle in thyroid has been based on the postulate that the hormone must act on the rate-limiting step of this pathway.

Under physiological conditions, the activity of the pentose cycle in thyroid slices is not limited by the uptake of glucose by the tissue. Indeed, the pentose cycle accounts for a relatively small part of the metabolism of glucose, and it can be greatly enhanced by factors which

TABLE III
TURNOVER OF NADP IN THE NADP OXIDATION-REDUCTION CYCLE IN
DOG THYROID SLICES[a]

	Units	Control	TSH 256 mU/ml
Glucose uptake	Micromoles/4 hours/gram wet weight	67.7	92.0
Pentose cycle (PC)	Fraction of glucose oxidized through the PC	0.020	0.076
Glucose oxidized through the PC	Micromoles/4 hours/gram wet weight	1.35	6.99
NADP$^+$ reduced per μmole of glucose oxidized through the PC	Micromoles	6	6
NADP$^+$ reduced by PC	Micromoles/4 hours/gram wet weight	8.12	41.9
(NADP$^+$ + NADPH) concentration in slices[b]	Nanomoles/gram wet weight	35.8	51.7
Minimal turnover of NADP in slices during the incubation[c]	—	8.12/0.0358 = 226	41.9/0.0517 = 809

[a] From Dumont and Tondeur-Montenez (1965).

[b] Results obtained in incubations without glucose, i.e., under conditions where TSH increases the NADP$^+$ content of the slices (TSH 128 mU/ml).

[c] Minimal turnover, because any compartmentation of the cellular NADP would increase the real turnover rate of the NADP oxidation reduction cycle.

decrease (e.g., K$^+$ enriched medium; Dumont and Van Sande, 1965) or increase only slightly (e.g., Synkavit; Dumont, 1966) the uptake of glucose.

The stimulation by TSH of the pentose cycle in thyroid is not secondary to the stimulation of glucose uptake. Despite a washing of thyroid slices preincubated in the presence of ^{14}C-labeled glucose, TSH still enhances the oxidation of tissue ^{14}C-hexoses in a second incubation (Dumont and Eloy, 1966). This suggests that the TSH effect on glucose oxidation is not caused by the stimulation of glucose uptake. Moreover, the action of TSH on glucose C-1 oxidation in thyroid slices cannot be accounted for by increased glucose uptake. Insulin, which enhances glucose uptake approximately to the same extent as TSH, does not

modify significantly the oxidation of glucose C-1 and C-6 (Field et al.,
1960; Dumont, 1961b). However, this argument is open to criticism
because insulin may affect steps of glucose metabolism other than the
uptake. In sheep thyroid slices, an increase of glucose concentration in
the medium from 3.2 mM to 6.7 mM determines an increase of 35% of
the uptake of glucose and an increase of 20% of glucose C-1 oxidation.
TSH stimulates glucose uptake by 34% and glucose C-1 oxidation by
85% in such slices (Dumont and Eloy, 1966). Therefore, the TSH-
induced increment of glucose uptake per se cannot account for the enhancement of the pentose cycle in thyroid.

The activity of the pentose cycle in incubated thyroid slices does not
appear to be limited by the cellular concentration in enzymes of this
pathway. The maximal velocity of the two dehydrogenases of this pathway, glucose 6-phosphate dehydrogenase and 6-phosphogluconate dehydrogenase, is largely superior to the activity of the pathway in intact
and stimulated dog thyroid slices (Dumont and Eloy, 1966); it is not
increased in stimulated slices (Field et al., 1960; Dumont and Eloy,
1966). The activity of the whole pentose cycle is multiplied by a factor
of 5–10 in the presence of electron acceptors such as Synkavit or methylene blue. It is 5 times higher in homogenates reinforced with coenzymes
than in intact slices, but not higher in homogenates from stimulated
slices than in homogenates from resting slices (Dumont and Eloy, 1966).
The activity of the pentose cycle in thyroid slices is therefore not limited
by the concentration of its constitutive enzymes. The stimulation of this
pathway by TSH does not require any enhancement in cell concentration
or in activity of the enzymes and there is no indication that TSH induces
such increases.

The catabolism of glucose 6-phosphate through the pentose cycle is
coupled to the reduction of NADP$^+$ (Fig. 15). If neither substrate level,
nor enzymatic concentration is the limiting factor of this pathway in
the thyroid cell, it is probable that NADP$^+$ supply is rate limiting. If
TSH does not activate the pathway by increasing the uptake of glucose
or the concentration of enzymes, it should enhance the supply of NADP$^+$.
Several lines of evidence show that NADP$^+$ supply is limiting the activity of the pentose cycle in thyroid: (1) As suggested by the data of
Field et al. (1961) and Schussler and Ingbar (1961), the activity of the
pentose cycle in thyroid homogenate essentially depends on the concentration of NADP$^+$ in this homogenate (Dumont and Eloy, 1966). This
activity greatly increases when electron acceptors are added to catalyze
the oxidation of NADPH. (2) In thyroid slices, any agent which stimulates the oxidation of NADPH, thus increasing the supply of NADP$^+$,
considerably enhances the activity of the pentose cycle. This has been

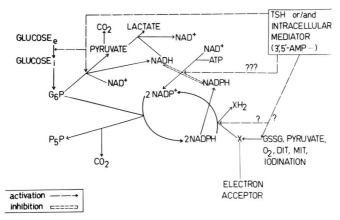

Fig. 15. Regulation of NADP metabolism in thyroid. *GLUCOSE$_e$, GLUCOSE$_i$:* glucose outside and inside the cell. *P$_5$P:* pentose 5-phosphate; *X:* any hydrogen acceptor.

shown for Synkavit, methylene blue, iodotyrosines, epinephrine, acetylcholine, and serotonin (Dumont, 1961b; Field *et al.*, 1961; Pastan *et al.*, 1961, 1962; Pastan and Field, 1962; Hupka and Dumont, 1963; Bastomsky and Rosenberg, 1966). (3) In dog thyroid slices, incubated under various conditions, there is a very good correlation between glucose C-1 oxidation and NADP+ concentration (Field *et al.*, 1963).

The NADP+ supply is therefore the limiting factor of the pentose cycle in thyroid slices. To stimulate the cycle TSH should increase this supply. This conclusion was suggested simultaneously but independently by two groups (Dumont, 1961b; Field *et al.*, 1961).

c. Effects on Pyridine Nucleotides. TSH *in vitro* increases the NADP+ content and decreases the NAD+ content in dog thyroid slices incubated in the absence of glucose in the medium (Table IV) (Pastan *et al.*, 1963; Dumont and Eloy, 1966; F. R. Butcher and Serif, 1967). Pastan and his group pointed out the increased total NADP content of the stimulated slices; the decreased NAD+ content of these slices suggested a stimulation by TSH of NADP+ synthesis from NAD+. It was later shown that such results indicate two changes in the activated tissue: a rise in the total NADP level, and a shift in the oxidation reduction equilibrium of NADP (Dumont and Rocmans, 1965; Dumont and Eloy, 1966). The rise of the NADP+ level in dog thyroid slices is very rapid; it is already observed 10 minutes after the beginning of the incubation (Oka and Field, 1967). Most of this NADP was found in the cell sap (Field *et al.*, 1966).

Pastan *et al.* (1961, 1963) and Field (1965) reasoned that, the NADP+

TABLE IV

EFFECT OF TSH *in Vitro* ON PYRIDINE NUCLEOTIDES IN DOG
THYROID SLICES[a]

	Control	TSH, 128 mU/ml
NAD⁺	81	71.5
NADH	22.5	17.3
NADP⁺	10.4	25.4
NADPH	25.4	26.3
NAD⁺ + NADH	103.5	88.8
NADP⁺ + NADPH	35.8	51.7
NAD⁺/NAD⁺ + NADH	0.76	0.80
NADP⁺/NADP⁺ + NADPH	0.29	0.49

[a] Incubation of 1 hour in the absence of glucose. Concentrations are expressed as millimicromoles per gram of tissue, wet weight. From Dumont and Eloy (1966).

level being the limiting factor of the pentose phosphate pathway in thyroid, an increase of this level by synthesis would explain the activation of the pathway. No hypothesis about the mechanism of the activation of the pentose phosphate pathway by the rise in NADP⁺ concentration (e.g., stochiometric effect of NADP⁺, or increased shuttle of NADP between oxidation and reduction sites) was proposed (Pastan *et al.*, 1961, 1963; Field, 1965). The increased NADP level in the stimulated thyroid slices cannot account for the early activation of the pentose phosphate pathway (Dumont and Rocmans, 1965; Dumont and Eloy, 1966). This increase is much less apparent when the slices are incubated in the presence of glucose, i.e., under the very conditions in which the effect of TSH on the pentose phosphate pathway is evaluated (Pastan *et al.*, 1963). It is not observed in *in vitro* stimulated sheep and beef thyroid slices (Jarrett and Field, 1964; Gilman and Rall, 1968), in calf thyroid slices stimulated *in vitro* in the presence of fluoride, dicoumarol, and iodoacetate (O'Malley and Field, 1964) or after a pretreatment with carzinophilin (Field *et al.*, 1965), in dog thyroid slices stimulated *in vivo* (Rocmans and Dumont, 1969a). In all these cases, TSH still stimulates the pentose phosphate pathway in the slices.

The evaluation of the activity of the pentose phosphate pathway and of the total NADP content of dog thyroid slices makes it possible to estimate the number of times the cellular NADP⁺ is reduced, and therefore the number of times NADPH is oxidized, during an incubation (Table III). This estimate would be too small if compartmentation reduced the pool of NADP involved in the oxidation-reduction cycle. Nevertheless, it shows that the oxidation-reduction cycle of cellular NADP is very fast in resting as well as in stimulated dog thyroid slices.

This is in contrast with what is known about the slower turnover of pyridine nucleotides by synthesis and degradation: for instance the half-life of NAD in the liver is of the order of a few hours (Gholson, 1966). Therefore, the relative concentrations of $NADP^+$ and NADPH result from the equilibrium existing between the oxidation and reduction of NADP (Dumont and Eloy, 1966). Measurements of the cellular concentrations of NAD^+ and $NADP^+$ in the absence of data on the reduced forms (Oka and Field, 1967; F. R. Butcher and Serif, 1967) may be very misleading.

In thyroid tissue, any agent which activates the oxidation of NADPH also stimulates the pentose phosphate pathway, i.e., the oxidation reduction cycle of NADP (Dumont, 1961b, 1966). The rate-limiting step of the cycle is the oxidation of NADPH, not the reduction of $NADP^+$, i.e., the pentose phosphate pathway. The fact that the ratio $NADP^+/NADPH$ is less than 1 in resting tissue supports this conclusion. The most likely explanation of the stimulation by TSH of the pentose phosphate pathway in thyroid is therefore that the hormone activates NADPH oxidation. An activation of NADPH oxidation need not increase very much the relative proportion of $NADP^+$, since any increase in the rate of NADPH oxidation will be followed by a corresponding acceleration of $NADP^+$ reduction through the pentose phosphate pathway. In the absence of exogenous glucose, i.e., under conditions of relative glucose 6-phosphate depletion, increases in the $(NADP^+)/(NADP^+) + (NADPH)$ ratio should become more apparent. This has indeed been observed in dog thyroid slices (Dumont and Eloy, 1966) (Table IV). Moreover, looking back to previously published results, one finds that, in the absence of glucose, TSH induces a shift of NADP toward the oxidized form in beef (Jarrett and Field, 1964; Gilman and Rall, 1968b), and sheep (Jarrett and Field, 1964) thyroid slices in which no change in the total NADP level is observed. A trend in the same direction can be observed in the data reported by Burke (1969b) on the action of TSH on pyridine nucleotides in sheep thyroid slices. Further indication of an increased NADPH oxidation in stimulated dog thyroid slices is provided by the data of Oka and Field (1967). In slices incubated with nicotinic acid-^{14}C, the specific activity of NAD^+ is much higher than the specific activity of $NADP^+$, the specific activity of NADPH is presumably lower than the specific activity of $NADP^+$. In the first 20 minutes after the beginning of the incubation, the specific activity of $NADP^+$ is lower in TSH-treated slices than in control slices; this suggests an increased oxidation of NADPH but no increase in $NADP^+$ synthesis. In these slices, the ratio $(NADP^+)/(NADP^+) + (NADPH)$ is already increased 10 minutes after the beginning of the incubation (Oka and Field, 1967). Therefore, these data strongly suggest that TSH activates the oxidation of NADPH in the thyroid and that this activation causes the stimulation of the pentose phosphate pathway. However, the alternative hypothesis, that TSH decreases the activity of another NADP+ reducing system (e.g., isocitric dehydrogenase) and that the pentose phosphate pathway fills in the gap could also explain these observations. An increase in cellular NADP level could accelerate the turnover of the NADP oxidation reduction cycle, but simulation studies have shown that such an increase would not change markedly the NADP+/NADPH ratio, as seen in the stimulated thyroid slices (Delcroix and Dumont, 1969).

The existing data on the effect of TSH *in vivo* on the oxidation-reduction equilibrium of thyroid pyridine nucleotides would rather support the conclusion that TSH activates NADPH oxidation. Since the supply of plasma glucose *in vivo* would tend to mask any effect on NADPH oxidation, negative evidence on this subject would have little meaning. In our dogs, no effect of TSH on pyridine nucleotides was observed 1 hour after the injection of TSH (Rocmans and Dumont, 1969a). In both normal and hypophysectomized rats, the NAD+/NADH ratio was increased 3 hours after TSH. The NADP+/NADPH ratio also was increased by TSH in hypophysectomized rats, but in normal rats TSH decreased this ratio somewhat (Maayan and Rosenberg, 1966). However, more recent data of Zakarija et al. (1969) clearly establish that 3 hours after administration in normal rats the only significant effect of TSH on thyroid pyridine nucleotides is a marked increase in the NADP+/NADPH ratio.

   d. *NADPH Oxidation.* The activation of any metabolism requiring NADPH as a reducing coenzyme could enhance the rate of glucose metabolism through the pentose cycle, and could therefore explain the stimulation of this metabolism in TSH-treated thyroid slices (Fig. 15). Several mechanisms of NADPH oxidation have been studied in this regard, but, so far, no one has been proved to account for the whole effect of TSH on the pentose phosphate pathway in thyroid.

   The reduction of pyruvate to lactate partially requires NADPH in some tissues (Futterman and Kinoshita, 1959; Wenner, 1959; Karnovsky, 1962). In such tissues, the pentose cycle is activated by pyruvate and inhibited by inhibitors of glycolysis. Exogenous pyruvate does not activate the pentose phosphate pathway in thyroid, and large concentrations of glucose, which increase glycolysis as much as TSH, induce a much smaller effect than TSH on this pathway. Moreover, fluoride and iodoacetate inhibit glycolysis but do not suppress the TSH effect on the pentose cycle. This effect is therefore not caused solely by an increase of the pyruvate supply in thyroid cell (Dumont, 1966).

   The coenzyme of iodotyrosine deiodinase is NADPH (Stanbury, 1960).

The release in stimulated thyroids of iodotyrosines from thyroglobulin could induce NADPH oxidation. Indeed, exogenous iodotyrosines activate the pentose phosphate pathway in thyroid (Dumont, 1961b,c). However, it can be calculated that the quantities of iodotyrosines released in stimulated thyroids could account for only a very small part of the effect of TSH on the pentose cycle. Moreover, the effect of exogenous iodotyrosines are rather small in comparison with those of TSH, and even a maximal effect of iodotyrosines is still further enhanced by TSH (Dumont, 1966; Burke, 1968b). The release of iodide from iodotyrosines in stimulated thyroids could also induce the activation of the pentose cycle. Indeed, iodide stimulates this pathway in sheep thyroid slices (Dumont, 1961c; Green and Ingbar, 1963; Jarrett and Field, 1964). However, the action of TSH is not inhibited by methimazole (Dumont, 1966; Green, 1970) which blocks the iodide effect (Dumont, 1961c), and it is observed in thyroids in which iodide does not stimulate the pentose cycle (Jarrett and Field, 1964).

The induction of phagocytosis causes a stimulation of the pentose phosphate pathway in various types of cells (Karnovsky, 1962). This effect is ascribed to an activation of NADPH oxidation, the mechanism of which is still doubtful. Since TSH induces the phagocytosis of colloid by thyroid cells, it was hypothesized that the stimulation of the pentose cycle in these cells could be secondary to the phagocytotic process itself (Dumont and Rocmans, 1965; Dumont, 1966; Pastan, 1966a). Several facts cast doubt on this hypothesis: (1) Stimulation of glucose C-1 oxidation by TSH, cAMP, DB-cAMP, and PGE$_1$, was observed in dog thyroid slices with no evidence of intracellular colloid droplets (Rodesch et al., 1969). (2) Chlorpramazine, 0.1 mM, blocks the formation of colloid droplets in dog thyroid slices while not inhibiting completely the activation of glucose oxidation (Onaya et al., 1969). Moreover, activation of the hexose monophosphate pathway does not seem to be required for the induction of phagocytosis. (3) PGF$_1\alpha$ and PGF$_1\beta$ have been reported to induce intracellular colloid droplet formation without stimulating glucose C-1 oxidation in sheep thyroid slices (Burke, 1970a). (4) Iodide, 1 mM, has been reported to inhibit the TSH, PGE$_1$, and DB-cAMP action on glucose C-1 oxidation, but not the induction of colloid droplets in sheep thyroid slices (Burke, 1970d). (5) EDTA and the absence of Ca^{2+} in the medium abolish the action of TSH on glucose C$_1$ oxidation (Dumont and Van Sande, 1965; Zor et al., 1968), but not on colloid endocytosis (Dekker and Field, 1970) or thyroid secretion in dog thyroid slices in vitro (Willems et al., 1970). However, GSH oxidation in the hydrolysis of thyroglobulin (Peake et al., 1967) could be followed by NADPH oxidation and activation of the pentose phosphate pathway. Iodide binding to proteins may require NADPH as coenzyme (Degroot,

1965). The stimulation of this reaction by TSH could induce NADPH oxidation. Indeed, propylthiouracil, an inhibitor of iodination has been reported to inhibit partially the stimulation of the pentose cycle (Field et al., 1960), and methimazole would inhibit the stimulation of glucose-U-^{14}C in cultured thyroid cells (Dickson, 1966). However, the effect of TSH on the pentose phosphate pathway in sheep thyroid cells is obtained in the absence of iodide in the medium and despite complete suppression of iodide binding by methimazole (Dumont, 1966). Therefore, it is not caused by an activation of iodide binding.

In acellular microsomal–mitochondrial systems, iodide binding to proteins is limited by the supply of H_2O_2. NADPH, which activates the binding, is presumed to be the coenzyme of the H_2O_2 generating system (Degroot, 1965). H_2O_2, like TSH, enhances the organification of iodide by dog thyroid slices (Ahn and Rosenberg, 1970a), which suggests that H_2O_2 supply also is limiting this process in the intact cell. The effects are not additive. TSH enhances the formation of H_2O_2 by thyroid slices (Ahn and Rosenberg, 1970c; Bénard and Brault, 1970). This activation of the H_2O_2 generating system could account for the stimulation by TSH of iodide organification, of iodotyrosine oxidative coupling, of NADPH oxidation and consequently of the pentose phosphate pathway (Fig. 16).

Evidence has been presented that calf thyroid homogenate contains a GSH peroxidase and a NADPH-GSSG reductase (Bénard and Degroot, 1969). Therefore, the reduction of part of the H_2O_2 formed in the activated thyroid could, through the successive oxidation of GSH and NADPH, also activate the pentose phosphate pathway in a sort of intracellular "detoxifying mechanism" (Fig. 16). The fact that catalase partially inhibits the activation by TSH of the pentose phosphate pathway in calf thyroid slices (Bénard and Degroot, 1969) may support this hypothesis.

In conclusion, NADPH oxidation may be enhanced by several biochemical mechanisms. It is quite possible that the activation of this oxidation in stimulated thyroid tissue may result from several effects of TSH, not only one; the activation of the H_2O_2 generating system and the consequent "detoxification" of H_2O_2 is a likely hypothesis. The stimulation of the pentose phosphate pathway itself may be the end result of the activation of several NADPH-requiring metabolisms, of an inhibition of other pathways of NADP$^+$ reduction, and of the enhancement of glucose uptake in the stimulated thyroid.

e. Role of cAMP. The stimulation by TSH of glucose carbon-1 oxidation by dog thyroid slices is qualitatively reproduced by DB-cAMP but not by noncyclic adenine nucleotides (Burke, 1968c; Pastan, 1966b; Pastan and Macchia, 1967; Rodesch et al., 1969; Zor et al., 1968),

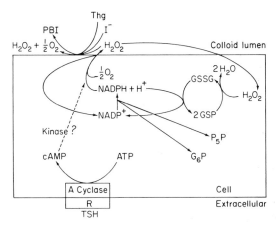

Fig. 16. Oxidation of NADPH in the thyroid. A tentative scheme to explain the activation by TSH and cAMP of NADPH oxidation and the consequent stimulation of the pentose phosphate pathway. Cyclic 3′,5′-adenosine monophosphate (cAMP) would activate the H_2O_2 generating system and thus oxidize NADPH. Some of the H_2O_2 formed would flow in the cell, where it would be reduced by glutathione peroxidase and NADPH glutathionine reductase, thus also oxidizing NADPH. Increased NADP supply would in its turn activate the pentose phosphate pathway and NADP reduction. $R = $ TSH receptor.

butyrate, caffeine (Rodesch et al., 1969), or theophylline (Zor et al., 1969a). In the dog the highest concentrations of DB-cAMP used (1 mM) give responses lower than TSH at 5 mU/ml (Willems and Dumont, 1969). This effect is also mimicked by cAMP (3–7 mM) itself in the presence of caffeine (1 mM) (Rodesch et al., 1969). The absence of an effect of cAMP reported by other authors (Burke, 1968a; Pastan, 1966b; Zor et al., 1969a) can probably be explained by lack of pretreatment of the animals, absence of methylxanthine protection, and the low concentration of nucleotide (<1.5 mM) used. Caffeine 1 mM, although inactive by itself, enhances the stimulation of glucose carbon-1 oxidation by low, but not by high, concentrations of TSH (>2 mU/ml) (Rodesch et al., 1969). Thus, there is good evidence that this effect is mediated by cAMP. In pig thyroid slices, theophylline (50 μM) failed to enhance the activation of glucose carbon-1 oxidation by low concentrations of TSH (0.5–10 mU/ ml). This negative evidence seems to bear against the role of cAMP (Zor et al., 1969a), but, as discussed earlier, there are many possible explanations for such negative findings, e.g., the use of an ineffective concentration of theophylline.

There is no good evidence that the stimulation of the pentose phosphate pathway by high concentrations of TSH (>10 mU/ml) is mediated by cAMP. DB-cAMP (up to 1 mM), cAMP and methylxanthines

(1 mM) fail to reproduce this effect in beef thyroid slices (Gilman and Rall, 1968b), or to mimic it quantitatively in dog thyroid slices (Pastan, 1966b; Pastan and Macchia, 1967; Rodesch et al., 1969) (Fig. 14). In the latter system DB-cAMP reproduces the weaker effects of low concentrations of TSH. Similarly DB-cAMP (up to 0.45 mM), and cAMP fail to stimulate, like high concentrations of TSH, glucose C-1 oxidation by sheep (500 mU/ml TSH) (Burke, 1968a) and rat (50 mU/ml TSH) (Pastan and Macchia, 1967) thyroid slices. However, this evidence does not disprove the hypothesis of an involvement of cAMP in this effect as the concentrations of DB-cAMP and cAMP may not be comparable to the concentrations of TSH. The stimulation of glucose C-1 oxidation by large concentrations of TSH is not potentiated by methylxanthines in beef, sheep, or dog thyroid slices (Burke, 1968a; Gilman and Rall, 1968b; Rodesch et al., 1969). Furthermore, above 10 mU/ml, increasing the concentration of TSH further enhances glucose C-1 oxidation but not cAMP accumulation by beef thyroid slices (Gilman and Rall, 1968a,b). However, increasing doses of TSH, while not increasing the measurable tissue level of cAMP after 10 minutes, may sustain this level, thus producing a greater overall effect on glucose C-1 oxidation which was measured at 45 minutes. Although the negative evidence outlined above may not be conclusive, it seems likely that the stimulation of the pentose phosphate pathway in thyroid by high concentrations of TSH, unlike that by low concentrations, is not mediated by cAMP.

3. Synthesis of NADP

TSH in vitro enhances considerably the NADP content of dog thyroid slices incubated in the absence of glucose in the medium (Pastan et al., 1963; Dumont and Eloy, 1966; F. R. Butcher and Serif, 1967). This effect is much decreased but still measurable in the presence of glucose (Pastan et al., 1963). It is not apparent in sheep and beef thyroid slices (Jarrett and Field, 1964; Gilman and Rall, 1968b). In rats, hypophysectomized or not, TSH also increases the NADP content of the thyroid (Maayan and Rosenberg, 1966).

In stimulated dog thyroid slices, the increase in NADP content is accompanied by a decrease in NAD content (Pastan et al., 1963; Dumont and Eloy, 1966) (Table IV). The kinetics of the two processes are parallel (Pastan et al., 1963). These data suggest that the increase in NADP content is caused by a stimulation of NADP synthesis rather than by an inhibition of NADP degradation (Pastan et al., 1963). This hypothesis is supported by the observation of increased transfer of ^{14}C and ^{32}P from NAD$^+$ to NADP$^+$ in stimulated dog thyroid slices incubated in the presence of nicotinic acid-^{14}C or orthophosphate-[32]P (F. R. Butcher and Serif, 1967; Oka and Field, 1967). Increased oxidation of 6-phosphogluconate-^{14}C in ATP- and NAD[+]-enriched homogenate of stimulated thyroid slices may indicate an increased synthesis of NADP (Field et al., 1966), but it may perhaps also result from decreased NADP catabolism or increased NADPH oxidation (Dumont and Eloy, 1966). The stimulation of NADP synthesis in dog thyroid slices, as indicated by nicotinic acid-^{14}C incorporation into NADP, appears after 20 minutes of incubation in the presence of TSH. This effect clearly follows the increase of the NADP[+] content of the slices (Oka and Field, 1967). In the presence of glucose this effect is transient, but the steady rise of NADP[+] levels in dog thyroid slices incubated without glucose (Pastan et al., 1963) suggests that in such conditions it may be a more lasting effect.

The known mechanism of NADP synthesis in mammalian cells is the phosphorylation by ATP of NAD[+] to NADP[+] in the presence of NAD kinase. A stimulation of NADP[+] synthesis could therefore be due to an increase in the supply of ATP or NAD[+] or to increased activity of NAD kinase. Depletion of thyroid ATP by a treatment with ethionine inhibits the enhancement by TSH *in vivo* of the NADP content of rat thyroid (Maayan and Rosenberg, 1968). Similarly, severe inhibition of oxidative phosphorylation by 2,4-dinitrophenol (1 mM) greatly decreases the NADP content in resting and stimulated dog thyroid slices (O'Malley and Field, 1964). Therefore, the effect of TSH requires ATP. However, this effect is not caused by an increased formation of ATP in the stimulated gland: TSH simultaneously increases the NADP content and decreases the ATP content in dog thyroid slices (Ohta and Field, 1966). The NAD[+] supply may limit the synthesis of NADP[+] in thyroid slices. In carzinophilin-treated dog thyroid slices, which are severely depleted of NAD[+], TSH only barely enhances the NADP concentration (Field et al., 1965). However, the effect of TSH is observed in slices in which the NAD[+] content is already markedly reduced. Furthermore, treatment of rats with nicotinic acid and nicotinamide increases the thyroid content of NAD but not of NADP (Maayan and Rosenberg, 1968). Therefore, the increased NADP content of the stimulated thyroid is not a consequence of an increased NAD supply.

Having observed that electron acceptors increased the NADP levels in dog thyroid slices, and that glucose inhibited these effects to some extent, Pastan et al. (1963) suggested that since NADH could inhibit liver NAD kinase, NADH and NADPH may control the synthesis of NADP in thyroid slices. Using the data of Pastan et al., Dumont and Eloy (1966) later demonstrated that whatever the conditions of incubation of dog thyroid slices, there was a very good correlation between the total NADP content of the slices and their NADP[+]/NADPH ratio. This suggested a causal relation between an oxidation–reduction equilibrium in the cell, as reflected by the NADP$^+$/NADPH ratio, and the synthesis of NADP. A control of NAD kinase by reduced pyridine nucleotides was proposed to explain this relation (Dumont and Rocmans, 1965; Dumont and Eloy, 1966). The increased NADP synthesis as well as the enhanced activity of the pentose cycle in stimulated thyroid tissue were considered to be the consequences of the activation of NADPH oxidation. Field *et al.*, on the contrary (Field, 1965; Field *et al.*, 1966), consistently advocated the hypothesis that TSH had a more direct effect on NAD-kinase activity. An argument in favor of this thesis is the demonstration of increased 6-phosphogluconate oxidation in ATP- and NAD$^+$-enriched homogenates of stimulated thyroid slices (Field *et al.*, 1966). However, in these experiments increased 6-phosphogluconate oxidation might result from increased NADPH oxidation or decreased NADP degradation as well as from increased NADP synthesis.

Evidence in favor of the hypothesis that increased NADP synthesis in thyroid slices is secondary to the activation of NADPH and perhaps NADH oxidation has been provided: (1) The increased NADP$^+$ synthesis in stimulated thyroid slices follows the rise of the NADP/NADPH ratio (Oka and Field, 1967). (2) Liver NAD-kinase activity is markedly inhibited by NADH and NADPH; this inhibition is competitive with NAD$^+$ (Apps, 1968; Oka and Field, 1968). (3) As stated previously, all the electron acceptors that activate NADPH oxidation also increase the NADP content of dog thyroid slices (Pastan *et al.*, 1963; Dumont and Eloy, 1966; F. R. Butcher and Serif, 1967). One of these agents, carbamylcholine, has even been shown to enhance NADP synthesis in these slices (F. R. Butcher and Serif, 1967).

This hypothesis would be simpler, since it would not imply any effects of TSH other than an activation of NADPH oxidation. However, it is not yet proved.

Macchia *et al.* (1969) showed that cAMP at low concentrations (0.01–1 μM) enhances the oxidation of glucose C-1 by beef thyroid homogenates reinforced with NAD$^+$ and ATP. This effect is increased in the presence of 1 mM theophylline; it is abolished in the presence of NADP$^+$; it is maximal after a preincubation of 15 minutes. Glucose C-1 oxidation in such systems is exquisitively sensitive to NADP$^+$ concentration (Dumont and Eloy, 1966). Therefore, these data suggest that cAMP acts by eliciting the formation of new NADP$^+$, perhaps by activating NAD$^+$-kinase. Alternatively, such an effect could result from the activation by a phosphorylation of an NADPH-consuming reaction such as the generation of H_2O_2. Activation of NAD-kinase would be well in keeping with the increasing evidence relating cAMP role and its action on various kinases (Robison *et al.*, 1968). It remains doubtful that this action of cAMP can explain the stimulation of the hexose monophosphate pathway by TSH since it depends on observations in beef thyroid homogenates, whereas in intact beef thyroid cells, DB-cAMP and physiological concentrations of TSH inhibit rather than activate this pathway. (Gilman and Rall, 1968b).

Burke (1969b) has reported that DB-cAMP reproduces the action of TSH on glucose C-1 oxidation but, contrary to TSH, also increases the cellular levels in reduced pyridine nucleotides in sheep thyroid slices. However, the concentrations of DB-cAMP (0.075 mM) and TSH (50–500 mU/ml) used in these experiments are not comparable. These results are difficult to explain and were not explained.

In conclusion, two mechanisms could account for the increased NADP levels in stimulated thyroid tissue: a decrease in the inhibition of NAD kinase by reduced pyridine nucleotides, and an activation of this enzyme. Although at present much evidence supports the first hypothesis, the second hypothesis is not ruled out.

4. Relation between the Stimulation of the Pentose Phosphate Pathway and Other Effects of TSH

Once stimulation by TSH of the pentose phosphate pathway in thyroid by TSH had been demonstrated, it was proposed as the primary effect of TSH on this tissue (Field *et al.*, 1960). However, it was soon shown that this action was secondary to an enhanced NADP$^+$ supply in the thyroid cell (Dumont, 1961b; Field *et al.*, 1961). Furthermore, many effects of TSH have been shown to be independent of the activation of the pentose cycle and of the synthesis of NADP. Indeed, increased NADPH oxidation and pentose cycle activity are caused by a great variety of agents which do not mimic the effects of TSH (Dumont, 1965). An example of such agents is acetylcholine, which does not induce secretion in perfused dog thyroids (Rocmans and Dumont, 1969b) even though it activates the pentose cycle in dog thyroid slices (Pastan *et al.*, 1961). Many effects of TSH are observed in the absence of glucose in the medium, which suggests that they are not caused by an activation of glucose metabolism (Freinkel, 1963). The argument that in such cases TSH may still stimulate the metabolism of endogenous glucose 6-phosphate originating from glycogenolysis (Hall and Tubmen, 1965) does not seem valid, since in the absence of exogenous glucose the low glycogen levels of the thyroid would allow, even in the presence of TSH, only a very small pentose cycle activity in comparison to the activity of this pathway in resting slices incubated in the presence of glucose (Dumont, 1965). Some effects of TSH are even observed in the absence of a stimulation of the pentose

cycle: increased lactate formation (Gilman and Rall, 1968b), intracellular colloid droplet formation in slices incubated with EDTA and in
the absence of Ca^{2+} in the medium (Willems and Dumont, 1970). Stimulation of the activity of the pentose cycle is, therefore, not a prerequisite
for TSH action on the thyroid.

E. RESPIRATION

1. *Nature of Thyroid Tissue Respiration*

The stimulation of cell respiration in thyroid slices is a well known
in vitro effect of thyrotropin (Freinkel, 1964; Dumont, 1965). This increase in oxygen consumption is observed in all the species studied, but
its relative magnitude varies: 14 to 19% for sheep thyroid slices (Freinkel,
1957, 1960; Schussler and Ingbar, 1961; Dumont, 1962), 30 to 50% for
dog slices (Dumont, 1964; Dumont and Tondeur-Montenez, 1965), and
40 to 70% for calf slices (Turkington, 1963; Stanbury, 1964). It is an
early effect, being observed at the first manometric reading (10 minutes)
after the addition of TSH to the incubation medium (Freinkel, 1957;
Turkington, 1963); it is observed in the absence of exogenous substrates,
i.e., it does not depend on the uptake or metabolism of substrates in the
medium (Freinkel, 1957); it is observed *in vitro* after the *in vivo* administration of TSH (Rocmans and Dumont, 1964).

The oxygen consumption of thyroid tissue is mainly a measure of
mitochondrial respiration. Indeed, thyroid oxygen uptake is strongly
inhibited by mitochondrial inhibitors, some of which have known specific
effects on mitochondrial function: malonate, fluoroacetate, amytal,
rotenone, antimycin, cyanide, and oligomycin (Freinkel and Ingbar,
1955; Suzuki, 1956; Dumont, 1961b, 1962, 1966; Lamy *et al.*, 1967;
Tyler *et al.*, 1968). Moreover, other agents (electron acceptors, agents
uncoupling oxidative phosphorylation, inhibitors of the tricarboxylic acid
cycle) modify thyroid respiration in the same manner as the oxidation
of pyruvate C-3, i.e., as the activity of the tricarboxylic acid cycle
(Dumont, 1962, 1966). Antimycin in sheep thyroid slices and oligomycin
in sheep and dog slices inhibit tissue respiration as completely in the
presence as in the absence of TSH (Lamy *et al.*, 1967). This shows that
cell respiration in stimulated thyroid tissue also mainly represents mitochondrial respiration and suggests that the increment in oxygen uptake
of the TSH-treated slices is due to mitochondrial activation. The latter
conclusion has not yet been rigorously established. Oligomycin and antimycin may also affect extramitochondrial cellular processes. However, the
enhancement of the activity of the tricarboxylic cycle, indicated by the

increased oxidation of pyruvate and acetate in slices, fully supports the conclusion that TSH activates mitochondrial respiration in thyroid (Dumont, 1962; Dumont and Tondeur-Montenez, 1965).

Among the factors that may also contribute to the increased oxygen uptake of stimulated thyroids is the activation of iodide oxidation and organification, metabolic processes which require oxygen (Degroot, 1965). However, these reactions can account for only a minute part of the TSH effect: it can be calculated that with optimal concentrations of iodide, thyroid slices organify approximately 1 nmole of iodide per milligram dry weight of tissue per hour, whereas the observed oxygen uptake of the slices is of the order of 110 nmoles in the resting, and 150 nmoles in the stimulated, dog thyroid. However, if the action of TSH on iodide organification bears on the H_2O_2 generating system (Section IV,C,4,d), there need not be a stochiometric relation between the H_2O_2 formed and the iodide bound to proteins. Activation of the H_2O_2 generating system could therefore account for a much larger part of the oxygen uptake than the rate of iodide binding would suggest.

2. Mechanism—Role of cAMP

Although the work cited above strongly suggests that the TSH-stimulated oxygen uptake of thyroid slices is due at least in part to mitochondrial activation, there is no evidence that TSH acts directly on the mitochondria. TSH does not modify respiration, oxidative phosphorylation, respiratory control, or ATPase activity in isolated thyroid mitochondria (Lamy et al., 1964, 1967; Degroot et al., 1966). Thyroxine was not found to stimulate the respiration of isolated sheep thyroid mitochondria and activated mitochondrial ATPase only slightly (Lamy et al., 1967). With liver mitochondria such effects are observed, but only with concentrations of thyroxine much higher than those one would expect even in stimulated thyroid. Thus TSH-stimulated thyroxine release from thyroglobulin does not account for the increased mitochondrial respiration of stimulated thyroid.

The respiration of thyroid and other mitochondria is regulated by several factors of which the more important are oxygen and substrate supply, and the concentrations of ADP, phosphate, and calcium. In thyroid slices incubated under conditions in which TSH activates oxygen uptake, dinitrophenol considerably enhances respiration (Dumont, 1966) as it also does in isolated mitochondria incubated with exogenous substrates (Lamy et al., 1967). The dinitrophenol-stimulated respiration in intact cells is mitochondrial as indicated by its complete inhibition in the presence of antimycin (Rodesch and Dumont, 1967). Oxygen and substrate supply therefore are not the limiting factors in mitochondrial respiration in the intact cells, as loosening the respiratory control by itself can stimulate the oxygen uptake.

The TSH effect on cellular respiration does not appear to be a function of calcium concentration. Oligomycin inhibits TSH stimulation of respiration although it does not prevent the stimulation of mitochondrial respiration by calcium. TSH increases the concentration of phosphate in sheep thyroid slices (Freinkel, 1957, 1963). However, this effect is small, and the concentration of phosphate in control slices is already at a level which allows maximal stimulation of isolated mitochondria (Lamy et al., 1967).

The most likely factor regulating mitochondrial respiration is ADP concentration, in thyroid as in other tissues. Therefore, a stimulation of mitochondrial respiration should be caused by increased ADP supply, which in turn would follow the enhancement by TSH of any endergonic process. The fact that TSH stimulates many such processes in the thyroid fits in very well with this interpretation. In a cell with satisfactory respiratory control, increased formation of ADP immediately results in increased mitochondrial respiration and ADP phosphorylation; thus the ratio ADP/ATP may not change significantly. In thyroid cells this ratio may also be stabilized by creatine phosphokinase and presumably phosphocreatine (Graig and Smith, 1967). An increase in the ratio ADP/ATP in stimulated thyroid would strongly support our hypothesis. Phosphorylation of ADP is efficient in incubated sheep thyroid slices, as nucleotide triphosphates always represent more than 85% of the total nucleotides (Lamy et al., 1967; Tyler et al., 1968); a satisfactory respiratory control in the mitochondria of these slices is evidenced by the high ratio of dinitrophenol-stimulated to oligomycin-inhibited respiration (Rodesch and Dumont, 1967; Tyler et al., 1968). In stimulated sheep thyroid slices, we have demonstrated a slight but significant increase in the ratio of nucleotide diphosphates to nucleotide triphosphates (Lamy et al., 1967). The decrease in ATP concentration in stimulated dog thyroid slices observed by Ohta and Field (1969) supports these data. No such decrease was observed in calf thyroid slices (Schneider, 1969).

Therefore, there is strong evidence that TSH-stimulated mitochondrial respiration is secondary to an activation of ATP-consuming processes (Fig. 17). TSH activates several ATP-consuming processes which in turn could enhance mitochondrial respiration: cAMP formation, protein synthesis, endocytosis, etc. A study of the kinetics of ATP hydrolysis in stimulated and resting thyroid slices in which ADP phosphorylation were blocked by oligomycin could test this hypothesis.

However, alternative hypothesis are not excluded, such as activation by phosphate in cells, in which, because of compartmentation effects, the medium around the mitochondria would contain limiting amounts of phosphate. cAMP might also directly activate thyroid mitochondria. We have not observed any modification of the respiration, oxidative phosphorylation or respiratory control of isolated thyroid mitochondria in the presence of various concentrations of cAMP (Mockel and Dumont, 1970). It is not even certain that cAMP mediates the stimulation of mitochondrial respiration. TSH stimulates the oxidation of pyruvate to CO_2 by the thyroid. In beef thyroid slices, a significant effect is obtained only for concentrations of TSH (20 mU/ml) higher than those required for enhancing glycolysis and decreasing glucose C-1 oxidation (2 mU/ml). Therefore, it is not surprising that this effect was not mimicked by DB-cAMP (Gilman and Rall, 1968b) at a concentration (1 mM) corresponding to less than 2 mU/ml TSH. Theophylline (1 mM) mimics and potentiates the effect of TSH on pyruvate oxidation (Gilman and Rall, 1968b). On the other hand, increasing the concentration of TSH above 10 mU/ml further enhances pyruvate oxidation, but it does not further increase the tissue concentration of cAMP after 10 minutes' incubation. Therefore, the evidence for the possible mediation by cAMP of the TSH stimulation of pyruvate oxidation is not conclusive.

Iodide enhances oxygen uptake in sheep (Dumont, 1961c) and beef (Green, 1970) thyroid slices. However, the release of iodide from iodotyrosine in the activated gland cannot account for the stimulation of respiration since the effect of iodide, but not of TSH, is abolished by methimazole (Dumont, 1961c; Green, 1970).

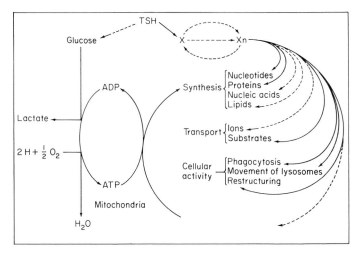

FIG. 17. Regulation of ATP metabolism in the thyroid. Xn = any mediator of thyrotropin (TSH) action, such as cyclic 3',5'-adenosine monophosphate (cAMP).

Even indirect activation of thyroid mitochondrial respiration by TSH cannot account for the other thyroid effects of TSH. Strong inhibition of mitochondrial respiration by fluoroacetate, amobarbital, and antimycin barely decreases the TSH stimulation of glucose C-1 oxidation by sheep thyroid slices (Dumont, 1966). The effects of TSH on iodide organification and secretion in the rat *in vivo* are not inhibited by pretreatment with ethionine, which considerably lowers the ATP content of the thyroid (Maayan and Rosenberg, 1968), or by treatment with 2,4-dinitrophenol (Maayan, 1968). TSH by itself may decrease the ATP (Ohta and Field, 1969) and nucleotide triphosphate (Lamy et al., 1967) levels in stimulated dog thyroid slices.

3. *Energy Metabolism*

Incubations of resting and stimulated dog thyroid slices have provided data which permit the evaluation of ATP formed by the pathways of energy metabolism (Table I).

Lactate accumulation in the medium measures the difference between lactate formation and degradation. In dog thyroid slices, lactate accumulation appears to be a good index of aerobic glycolysis as it accounts for a large part of the glucose taken up (Dumont and Tondeur-Montenez, 1965). It also allows an estimation of ATP formation via aerobic glycolysis as one molecule of ADP is phosphorylated for each molecule of lactate formed.

In isolated thyroid mitochondria, as in other mitochondria (Gonze and Tyler, 1965; Lamy et al., 1964, 1967), oligomycin inhibits the respiration induced by ADP, i.e., the controlled respiration. Thus the fraction of oxygen uptake which is inhibited by oligomycin represents an estimate of the controlled respiration of the thyroid slices. As phosphorylation may still occur in uncontrolled respiration, the measurement of oligomycin-inhibited respiration somewhat underestimates total phosphorylating respiration. However, on the basis of this measurement, assuming a P:O ratio of 3, one can still estimate the oxidative phosphorylation of ADP in the slices. Despite very active aerobic glycolysis, in resting as well as in stimulated dog thyroid slices, the principal energy supply of the cell is mitochondrial oxidative phosphorylation (Dumont, 1965) (Table I).

Investigations by Freinkel and his group (Freinkel, 1963, 1964) have shown that the preferred substrates for oxidation in resting sheep thyroid tissue were the fatty acids. Free fatty acids added to the medium depress the oxidation of exogenous glucose (presumably by a sparing effect), but glucose has no such effect on the oxidation of exogenous free fatty acids. In stimulated tissue, on the contrary, the oxidation of glucose but not the oxidation of free fatty acids is increased. This suggested that TSH stimulation induces a shift of oxidizable substrates from free fatty acids to glucose. Therefore, TSH would not only activate oxidative phosphorylation in thyroid mitochondria, but also make glucose the preferred supply of metabolic substrates for mitochondrial respiration.

VI. Action of TSH on RNA and Ribonucleotide Metabolism

A. RNA Metabolism

1. *In Vivo*

a. Acute Effects. Three to 12 hours after the injection of TSH *in vivo*, the RNA content of chick, guinea pig, and dog thyroid, especially cytoplasmic RNA, begins to increase (Fiala *et al.*, 1957; Creek, 1965; Kerkof and Tata, 1967; Nève and Dumont, 1970). Within a shorter time (less than an hour) TSH enhances the incorporation of precursors ($^{32}P_i$, uridine-^{14}C) into thyroid RNA (Creek, 1965; Kerkof and Tata, 1967). The latter effect is also observed in fetal rat thyroid in culture (Imbenotte *et al.*, 1969). It may be tempting to equate incorporations and RNA synthesis rates. However, total uptake of $^{32}P_i$ and the specific activity of acid-soluble phosphorus are also increased in such activated thyroids (Tala *et al.*, 1955; Creek, 1965; Kerkof and Tata, 1967; Imbenotte *et al.*, 1969). In the chick thyroid, TSH increases in parallel the incorporation of uridine-^{14}C in the acid-soluble and in the RNA fractions of the homogenates (Creek, 1965). Stimulation of the incorporation of precursors into RNA, larger than the stimulation of total uptake of precursors or of acid-soluble radioactivity, have sometimes been interpreted (Kerkof and Tata, 1967; Ochi and Degroot, 1968; Imbenotte, 1969) as sufficient evidence of activation of RNA synthesis. However, in the absence of kinetic data on the radioactivity of the pools of true intracellular precursors of RNA (nucleotide triphosphates), such conclusions may be premature. Therefore, there is no proof of a stimulation of RNA synthesis in the thyroid by TSH *in vivo*. Nevertheless, the combination of increased RNA content and enhanced incorporation of precursors into this RNA is suggestive of such a stimulation.

b. Chronic Effects. In rat thyroids stimulated by feeding the rats a diet deficient in iodine or supplemented with thiouracil (17–21 days), RNA, acid-soluble nucleotides, and incorporation of orotate-^{14}C and uracil-^{14}C into the nucleotides and the RNA increase in parallel (R. H. Lindsay and Cohen, 1965), thus suggesting similar enhancements of nucleotide and RNA synthesis and of nucleotide and RNA pool sizes.

The activities of enzymes involved in ribonucleotide synthesis increase somewhat more. Thus the activated thyroid is characterized by a parallel increase in the size of various pools involved in RNA metabolism (nucleotide, RNA, enzymes), and the turnover rate of these pools, presumably the specific activity of the enzymes remaining unchanged.

2. In Vitro

a. Evidence of an Action on RNA Synthesis or Degradation. In order to study the mechanism of a stimulation of RNA synthesis by TSH, attempts have been made to demonstrate such an effect in vitro. There have been several reports of such a demonstration (Begg and Munro, 1965; H. Shimoda and Yasumasu, 1966; Hall and Tubmen, 1968; Kerkof and Tata, 1969). Begg and Munro (1965) and Shimoda and Yasumasu (1966) observed an enhanced incorporation of adenine-^{14}C, UTP-^{32}P, ^{32}P$_i$, uridine-^{3}H, CTP-^{14}C, into the RNA of isolated sheep and pig thyroid nuclei incubated in the presence of crude TSH. Linear kinetics of incorporation of precursors into RNA were obtained. Both reports conclude that TSH directly stimulates nuclear RNA synthesis. However, calculation of the published data suggests that the radioactivity of the samples was very low and thus may have been much influenced by contamination of the samples and by background radioactivity. Furthermore, we have been unable to obtain, under similar experimental conditions, a significant incorporation of adenine-^{3}H or uridine-^{3}H into the RNA of isolated sheep thyroid nuclei. Increased uptake of formate-^{14}C and adenine into the RNA of TSH-stimulated calf thyroid slices has been taken as evidence of enhanced RNA synthesis (Hall and Tubmen, 1968). However, similar experiments had demonstrated an identical effect of TSH on the incorporation of formate-^{14}C into acid-soluble adenine and RNA-adenine of the slices (Hall, 1963) which rather suggests an effect at the level of nucleotide synthesis. More convincing evidence of an effect of TSH in vitro on RNA synthesis has been provided by Kerkof and Tata (1969). In activated pig thyroid slices ^{32}P$_i$-incorporation into RNA was increased while acid-soluble ^{32}P was slightly decreased. Acid-soluble ^{32}P may not reflect the radioactivity of the immediate precursors of RNA, e.g., the radioactivity of the αP of nucleotide triphosphate. However, in similar slices, the nuclear Mg^{2+}-activated and Mn^{2+}-activated RNA polymerases were stimulated (Adiga et al., 1971), which bears against the hypothesis of an action on precursor pools. TSH also enhances the incorporation of orotate-^{14}C and uridine-^{3}H into the RNA of beef, pig, and sheep thyroid slices (R. H. Lindsay et al., 1969; Lamy et al., 1969). In these cases the radioactivity of the nucleotide precursors was increased to the same extent, thus suggesting a stimulation of nucleotide synthesis but giving no indication concerning RNA synthesis. TSH did not increase the RNA content of the slices in any of these studies. Therefore, there are several indications but no completely satisfactory evidence of a stimulation by TSH *in vitro* of general RNA synthesis in the thyroid.

There is also little evidence on the possibility of stimulation by TSH of the synthesis of specific RNA. TSH enhances the incorporation of uridine-^{3}H into the mRNA of polysomes and increases the proportion of ribosomes bound by mRNA in polysomes in sheep thyroid slices (Lecocq and Dumont, 1967). On the basis of these data we suggested that TSH induces a net synthesis of mRNA in these slices. However, the increased incorporation of uridine into polysomal mRNA was found to reflect an increased radioactivity of the acid-soluble fraction. Moreover, for both the mRNA of the polysomes and the RNA extracted by phenol from the whole tissue, density gradient centrifugation did not demonstrate any qualitative difference between resting and stimulated slices. The data therefore do not allow one to conclude that TSH affects the synthesis of a specific RNA in the thyroid (Dumont *et al.*, 1969a). Progress in this direction could now be made using available techniques of DNA/RNA hybridization, polyacrylamide gel electrophoresis with doubly labeled RNA, etc. The fact that TSH enhances the V_{max} of iodide transport in isolated beef thyroid cells by a process which is inhibited by actinomycin, cycloheximide, and puromycin, suggests the synthesis of a specific mRNA coding for a specific carrier protein (Wilson *et al.*, 1968; Knopp *et al.*, 1970).

Preliminary studies (Lamy and Dumont, 1970) have failed to demonstrate a modification by TSH of RNA degradation rate in sheep thyroid slices. The slices had been labeled with uridine-^{3}H during a preincubation. Incubation in the presence of cold uridine or cold uridine and actinomycin (5 μg/ml) has revealed the existence in the thyroid, as in other tissues (Harris, 1963), of at least 2 pools of RNA: one with a very fast turnover (half-life less than 1 hour), and another with a slower turnover (half-life several hours). No influence of TSH was demonstrated.

b. Role of cAMP. DB-cAMP, but not cAMP or 5'-AMP, qualitatively mimics the stimulation by TSH of ^{32}P$_i$ incorporation into the RNA of pig thyroid slices. The stimulatory effect of DB-cAMP was no longer apparent when the data were corrected for the uptake of ^{32}P$_i$. These data suggested that the action of TSH on RNA biosynthesis was not mediated by cAMP (Kerkof and Tata, 1969). However, this interpretation may not be valid, as it assumes that the size of precursor pools was constant in the different conditions, and that the concentrations of TSH and DB-cAMP used were comparable. Furthermore, recent data

(Adiga *et al.*, 1971) suggest that DB-cAMP mimics the activation by TSH of nuclear RNA polymerase in pig thyroid slices *in vitro*. A possible mechanism for cAMP action on RNA synthesis has been proposed by Langan (1968): cAMP would activate the phosphorylation of histones by a protein kinase and thus unmask DNA. In dog thyroid slices TSH activates the phosphorylation of histones (Lamy and Dumont, 1970). DB-cAMP mimics the stimulation by TSH of iodide transport in isolated beef thyroid cells; this process is inhibited by actinomycin and cycloheximide (Knopp *et al.*, 1970). This suggests that the stimulation by TSH of the synthesis of a mRNA coding for a protein involved in this transport is mediated by cAMP. One is reminded of the cAMP-mediated induction of tyrosine α-ketoglutarate transaminase (Wicks, 1969) and serine dehydratase (Jost *et al.*, 1970) in rat liver. Therefore, the evidence available supports the hypothesis that cAMP mediates TSH effects on the transcription of DNA to RNA.

c. Conclusion. Despite a rather large number of investigations we know relatively little about the action of TSH on RNA metabolism in the thyroid. Progress in this area would require studies on the kinetics of action of a single TSH administration, and on the comparison of resting and chronically stimulated glands, i.e., on the change of one steady state to another and on the nature of the new steady state. Synthesis and degradation rates should be studied not only on the whole RNA but on each major species of RNA (nuclear heterodisperse RNA, cytoplasmic mRNA, ribosomal RNA, and tRNA, etc.). Furthermore, the hormones could act on RNA metabolism by subtler means than mere modification of gross synthesis and degradation rates. For instance, they could alter the selective transport of RNA from the nucleus to the cytoplasm (Shearer and McCarthy, 1970). Consideration of the very useful model of Britten and Davidson (1969) could help in the development of more sophisticated working hypotheses.

B. RIBONUCLEOTIDE SYNTHESIS

1. *Purine Nucleotides*

Hall has shown that TSH *in vitro* stimulates the incorporation of labeled precursors into free and RNA purine nucleotides of calf thyroid slices; glucose and ribose mimicked this effect. He concluded that TSH stimulates de novo purine nucleotide synthesis by activating the pentose phosphate pathway and thus increasing the limiting supply of ribose phosphate (Hall, 1963; Hall and Tubmen, 1965) (Fig. 18).

There is evidence that *in vitro* TSH stimulates the de novo synthesis of purine nucleotides. Objections may be raised to the methodology of

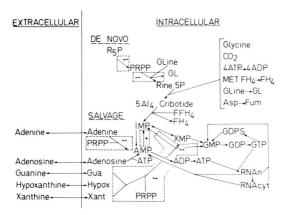

FIG. 18. Metabolism of purines. *5Ai4C:* 5-aminoimidazole-4-carboxamide; *ASP:* aspartate; *fum:* fumarate; *FFH₄:* N^{10}-formylfolate-H₄; *FH₄:* folate-H₄; *GLine:* glutamine; *GDPS:* guanosine diphosphate sugars, e.g., GDP mannose; *Met FH₄:* N^{6-10}-methenyl-folate-H₄; *PRPP:* 5-phosphoribosyl pyrophosphate; *R₅P:* ribose 5-phosphate; *Rine 5P:* ribosamine 5-phosphate; *RNAn:* nuclear RNA; *RNAcyt:* cytoplasmic RNA; areas enclosed by dashed lines: regulated reaction, + positive control (activation), − negative control (inhibition). Adapted from Murray *et al.* (1970).

Hall's experiments (incubation of 1 gm of tissue for 3–6 hours in 4 ml of buffer), but not against the results of Serif (1966), which largely confirm them. De novo synthesis of purine nucleotides is demonstrated by the incorporation of formate-¹⁴C into positions 2 and 8 of RNA adenine (Hall, 1962). Free and RNA purine nucleotide-specific activities are enhanced by TSH. This effect is specific for the tissue (Hall, 1963) and for the hormone (Hall and Tubmen, 1965). The importance of this effect varies much from one thyroid gland to another (141%, 196%, 230%, 263% of the controls) (Table V). The effect was interpreted as a stimulation of de novo purine nucleotide synthesis (Hall, 1963). This interpretation was later supported by the observation that TSH similarly enhances the specific activity of RNA adenine when glycine-¹⁴C is used as a precursor (Hall and Tubmen, 1965). However, effects on the pool sizes of free purine nucleotides, though unlikely (Lamy *et al.*, 1967), have not been excluded (R. H. Lindsay *et al.*, 1967). Whether the stimulation of de novo purine synthesis by TSH is entirely caused by the activation of the pentose phosphate pathway, and consequent increase in ribose phosphate supply, is less clear. Glucose and ribose mimic the effect of TSH on the incorporation of formate-¹⁴C into RNA adenine. In the presence of ribose neither TSH nor glucose further enhances this incorporation (Hall and Tubmen, 1965). Moreover, TSH enhances the

TABLE V

EFFECT OF GLUCOSE, TSH, AIC, AND 5AIC-RIBONUCLEOSIDE ON FORMATE-^{14}C
INCORPORATION INTO RNA ADENINE OF CALF THYROID SLICES[a]

Medium content	Percent of control
Control	100
Glucose	145
TSH	141
Glucose + TSH	171
AIC	842
AIC + glucose	1558
AIC + TSH	1507
AIC + glucose + TSH	1757
AIC ribonucleoside	1429
AIC ribonucleoside + TSH	1883

[a] Glucose, 5 mM; AIC and AIC ribonucleoside, 0.2 mM; TSH 200 mU/ml. AIC = 5-amino-4-imidazole carboxamide. Data from Hall (1963).

incorporation of glucose-^{14}C, but not of ribose-^{14}C, into RNA (Hall and Tubmen, 1965), a finding which suggests that TSH increases the formation of ribose phosphate from glucose, but not the fraction of the ribose phosphate pool used in purine nucleotide synthesis. These data certainly suggest that purine synthesis in calf thyroid slices is limited by ribose phosphate supply and that TSH increases this supply. The latter effect may be accounted for by the increase in the fraction of available glucose phosphate which is metabolized through the pentose phosphate pathway (Dumont and Tondeur-Montenez, 1965) and also, in the absence of exogenous glucose, by the increase in carbohydrate supply through activation of thyroglobulinolysis. A similar mechanism may account for the stimulation of adenine incorporation into RNA and free nucleotide of calf thyroid slices in the presence of TSH and/or glucose (Hall and Tubmen, 1965). However, there is evidence that ribose phosphate supply may not be the only or even the most important limiting factor in de novo purine synthesis in thyroid. Indeed, 5-amino-4-imidazole carboxamide, which already contains one of the two formates incorporated during de novo purine nucleotide synthesis, considerably enhances the incorporation of formate-^{14}C into RNA adenine (Hall, 1963) (Table V). This suggests that enough ribose phosphate is available and that de novo purine nucleotide synthesis may be mainly regulated by end product inhibition at the level of the first reactions of the de novo pathway in the thyroid as in other tissues (Murray et al., 1970). The stimulation by 5-amino-4-imidazole carboxamide would be explained by the bypass of the controlled reactions by this base. Therefore, the effect of TSH may also bear on these very important control mechanisms. TSH also enhances formate incorporation in the presence of 5-amino-4-imidazole carboxamide ribonucleoside (Hall, 1963) at a step where ribose phosphate is no longer necessary for ribosylation. This suggests another point of TSH action at the level of the salvage pathway on nucleoside transport or phosphorylation. In conclusion, there is good evidence that TSH stimulates the de novo pathway of purine nucleotide synthesis in calf thyroid slices. This effect seems to be due, at least in part, to the activation of the pentose phosphate pathway and its consequent ribose phosphate formation. Other, perhaps indirect, effects of TSH on the regulated first steps of the de novo pathway and on the salvage pathway are probable.

2. Pyrimidine Nucleotides

R. H. Lindsay et al. (1967) have shown that TSH stimulates the formation of $^{14}CO_2$ from orotate carboxyl-^{14}C in beef thyroid slices (129%). This decarboxylation measures the synthesis of UMP from OMP (Fig. 19). The validity of the assumption has been demonstrated for this material. Azauridine which as azauridine 5'-monophosphate inhibits intracellular OMP decarboxylase, almost completely inhibits the decarboxylation. Moreover, orotate incorporation into uracil, uridine, uridine nucleotides, and RNA accounts for 98% of the decarboxylated orotate (R. H. Lindsay et al., 1967). The effect of TSH is specific for the hor-

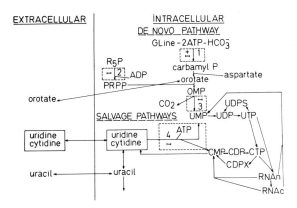

Fig. 19. Metabolism of pyrimidines. X in CDPX: bases, e.g., ethanolamine, diglyceride; GLine: glutamine; PRPP: 5-phosphoribosyl pyrophosphate; RNAn: nuclear RNA; RNAcyt: cytoplasmic RNA; UDPS: uridine diphosphate sugars, e.g., UDP glucose; boxes enclosed by dashed lines: regulated reaction, + positive control (activation), − negative control (inhibition). Adapted from Blakley and Vitols (1968).

mone and for the tissue; it is also observed in dog and pig thyroid slices (R. H. Lindsay et al., 1969).

The action of TSH on orotate incorporation into purine nucleotides appears to be secondary to the activation of the pentose phosphate pathway and its consequent enhancement of ribose phosphate supply. Glucose mimics the action of TSH, but both effects are additive. 2-Deoxyglucose, an inhibitor of glucose metabolism, abolishes the effect. These data suggest that the hormonal effect requires an intact glucose metabolism. Ribose stimulates orotate decarboxylation more than TSH or glucose, and TSH does not further enhance this effect. Inosine and adenosine give similar results (R. H. Lindsay et al., 1970). Therefore, there is good evidence that, in the system used, pyrimidine nucleotide synthesis is limited by the ribose phosphate supply and that TSH increases this supply. The action of TSH on the activity of the pentose phosphate pathway in beef thyroid slices is biphasic: inhibition for low, activation for high TSH concentrations (Merlevede et al., 1963; Gilman and Rall, 1968b). DB-cAMP and theophylline mimic the inhibition; menadione and Synkavit reproduce the activation. In all these conditions, orotate decarboxylation parallels the activity of the pentose phosphate pathway (R. H. Lindsay, 1970). Therefore, there is strong support for the hypothesis that TSH activates orotate incorporation into pyrimidine nucleotides by stimulating the pentose phosphate pathway and thus increasing the supply of ribose phosphate.

The stimulation of orotate decarboxylation by TSH is apparent only at concentrations of orotate higher than 0.67 mM; above this level decarboxylation tends to plateau in control but still increases linearly in TSH-treated slices. In pig and dog thyroid slices, the effect of TSH is apparent only after a preincubation of 1 hour in the presence of high concentrations of cold orotate (2.67 mM) (R. H. Lindsay et al., 1969). This suggests that under normal conditions of operation of the de novo pathway of pyrimidine nucleotide synthesis TSH does not stimulate orotate decarboxylation and that the effect occurs only when ribose phosphate supply becomes artificially limiting due to an increase of orotate concentration and sometimes to depletion of this supply. In beef thyroid slices, activation of orotate decarboxylation as well as activation of the pentose phosphate pathway takes place only for high TSH concentrations (100 mU/ml). Therefore, the physiological significance of these effects is very doubtful.

TSH stimulates the incorporation of uridine-^{3}H into free nucleotides and RNA of sheep thyroid slices (Dumont, 1968; Dumont and co-workers, 1968, unpublished results) (Fig. 20). The extent of this effect is variable

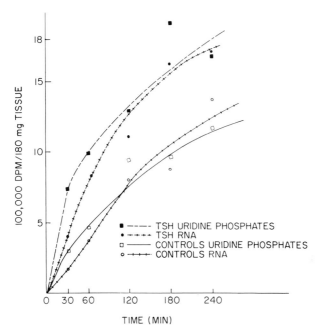

FIG. 20. Effect of thyrotropin (TSH) on the incorporation of uridine-³H into the RNA and the free ribonucleotides of sheep thyroid slices. From Dumont (1968), with the permission of the publisher.

(10–100% increase); it has not been reproduced in beef thyroid slices (R. H. Lindsay, 1970), and is only sporadically observed in dog thyroid slices (Dumont and co-workers, 1968, unpublished results). During a 6-hour incubation of sheep thyroid slices, the concentration of uridine-³H in the medium decreases while the concentration of uracil-³H slowly increases; the rate of incorporation of uridine-³H into uridine phosphates parallels the concentration of uridine-³H. Moreover, the incorporation of uracil-³H into nucleotides or RNA is negligible. Therefore, uridine incorporation into nucleotides probably involves phosphorylation by uridine kinase (Dumont, 1968).

In conclusion, nothing is known about the acute effects of TSH on the de novo pathway of pyrimidine nucleotide synthesis. There is good evidence that TSH stimulates the synthesis of uridine nucleotides from orotate by activating the pentose phosphate pathway and thus increasing the ribose phosphate supply. However, this effect is demonstrated only under conditions in which ribose phosphate supply has been made artificially limiting and with TSH concentrations that are probably too high to be physiologically significant. TSH also stimulates the salvage pathway of pyrimidine nucleotide synthesis from uridine, by activating uridine transport or phosphorylation. However, the significance of this effect is also doubtful as it is not observed in all species.

3. General Remarks

Although one might expect more or less indirect effects of TSH on the first controlling reactions of the de novo pathway of purine and pyrimidine nucleotide synthesis, nothing is known about this subject. The study of the acute effects of TSH on nucleotide synthesis has suggested two mechanisms of action: a stimulation of synthesis secondary to activation of the pentose phosphate pathway and consequent enhancement of ribose phosphate supply and an activation of synthesis from nucleotides by the salvage pathway. The first mechanism would account for the stimulation of de novo purine synthesis, of adenine incorporation into nucleotides by the salvage pathway, and of orotate incorporation into pyrimidine nucleotides. Although this mechanism has been carefully analyzed, its significance is still unknown. It is not certain whether ribose phosphate supply does limit ribonucleotide synthesis under physiological conditions in the thyroid cell. Furthermore, the high concentrations of TSH required to activate the pentose phosphate pathway and nucleotide synthesis in some thyroid tissues cast some doubt on the physiological significance of these effects. Hall (1963) has reported that low concentrations of TSH (0.1 to 1 mU/ml) activate ^{14}C-formate incorporation into purine nucleotides in beef thyroid slices. In general, at such concentrations TSH does not stimulate the activity of the pentose phosphate pathway in the tissue (Gilman and Rall, 1968b). However no concurrent measurement of the two metabolisms was made (Hall, 1963; Hall and Tubmen, 1965). Such measurements would be of great interest. The finding that TSH at low concentrations stimulates de novo purine synthesis while inhibiting the pentose phosphate pathway would indeed suggest an effect of the hormone at the level of the controlling reactions of the de novo pathway and would strongly support the hypothesis that such an effect would have a physiological meaning. The physiological significance of the activation of ribonucleotide synthesis from nucleoside should also be examined. It is not known in which TSH concentration range this effect is obtained; it has not been demonstrated in some species.

Little is known about the possible role of cAMP in ribonucleotide metabolism. Acute effects of TSH on purine and pyrimidine nucleotide synthesis do not seem to require new synthesis of proteins or RNA, as shown by the use of inhibitors of RNA synthesis (actinomycin) and of protein synthesis (puromycin). The stimulation of formate and adenine incorporation into RNA purine nucleotides is not inhibited by puromycin

(Hall and Tubmen, 1968) and the stimulation of orotate decarboxylation resists puromycin and actinomycin (R. H. Lindsay, 1970).

R. H. Lindsay *et al.* (1967) have suggested that "increased formation of RNA would be an expected consequence of an increase in the rate of synthesis of nucleotides." There is little evidence in favor of the hypothesis that RNA synthesis may be regulated by the availability of ribonucleotide triphosphates (Mandel, 1964). However, in cells growing at different rates there may be some parallelism between the size of nucleotide pools and RNA synthesis rate (Canellakis, 1962), although this finding is by no means general (Colby and Eldin, 1970). In chick thyroids *in vivo*, Creek (1965) observed simultaneously an activation of the incorporation of precursors into the TCA-soluble pool and RNA, and an increase in RNA content after TSH stimulation in rat thyroids. Furthermore, under several chronic conditions, R. H. Lindsay and Cohen (1965) found that the acid-soluble phosphate pool and RNA as well as the incorporation of precursors into RNA are similarly modified. Therefore, it is quite possible that some relation exists between nucleotide and RNA syntheses and pool sizes.

VII. Action of TSH on Protein Synthesis and Growth

A. Introduction—*In Vivo*

The thyroid follicular cell synthesizes mainly cellular proteins and thyroglobulin, a protein of molecular weight 660,000 which is secreted into the follicle lumen where it is iodinated and stored. As shown in Section III,B,1, the most striking early effect of TSH on the thyroid is the induction of colloid phagocytosis and its consequences: thyroglobulinolysis, amino acid release, and thyroid hormone secretion into the systemic blood stream. This action of the hormone makes it very difficult to study effects on protein content and protein synthesis in the gland. Even a marked enhancement of protein synthesis would not necessarily compensate for the protein loss by hydrolysis of thyroglobulin. Therefore, thyroid protein content after TSH administration varies much according to experimental conditions: it was increased after 24 hours in the guinea pig (Ekholm and Pantic, 1963) but not in the chick (Creek, 1965); in guinea pigs it was greater 24 hours than 1 hour after TSH injection (Kosanovic *et al.*, 1968). Similarly, measurements of labeled amino acid incorporation into thyroid protein are also certainly influenced by the dilution of cellular pools by amino acids released from thyroglobulin. This may explain why *in vivo* TSH rapidly enhanced this incorporation in mice (Bradley and Wissig, 1966) and rats after more than 2 hours (Cavalieri and Searle, 1967), but not in mice in another laboratory

(Ochi and Degroot, 1969b). Similarly, stimulation of incorporation of labeled amino acids into proteins could not be demonstrated in guinea pig thyroids incubated *in vitro* until 15 hours after TSH had been injected into the animals (Raghupathy *et al.*, 1963). TSH *in vitro* did not modify leucine incorporation into the proteins of sheep thyroid slices (Raghupathy *et al.*, 1964). While there is no doubt about a delayed stimulation of protein synthesis *in vivo*, biochemical evidence of an early effect is not clear. However, hints provided by morphological studies (Section III,B,2), as well as the existence of positive results despite the odds, suggest such an action.

We are not aware of any study on the degradation rates of thyroid proteins and on the effect of TSH on this catabolism.

B. *In Vitro* MECHANISM

1. *Effect in Vitro*

Overflooding of cellular amino acid pools by amino acids released from thyroglobulin is avoided in two experimental systems: isolated beef thyroid cells which are stripped of luminal colloid (Tong, 1967) and dog thyroid slices incubated in the presence of high concentrations of amino acids, i.e., in which the influence of thyroglobulinolysis becomes negligible (Lecocq and Dumont, 1970). TSH stimulates (120–160%) the incorporation of leucine-^{14}C and tyrosine into the proteins of isolated beef thyroid cells. Insulin, but not inactivated TSH or other polypeptide hormones, reproduces this effect. Although most of these experiments were performed with high concentrations of TSH (125 mU/ml), the effect could be reproduced at concentrations (1 mU/ml) which are in the same range as concentrations required to elicit other effects in this system. The action of TSH is already detected in 30 minutes incubations (Tong, 1967). Similar effects of TSH are observed in dog thyroid slices incubated in the presence of high concentrations of amino acids (>2 mM): leucine-^{3}H, tyrosine-^{3}H, lysine-^{3}H. This action is also specific for TSH and is observed in the same range of TSH concentrations as other effects (Fig. 8). The previous failure to demonstrate such an effect in slices (Raghupathy *et al.*, 1964) or in fetal rat thyroid in culture (Nataf, 1968) may have been due to dilution of precursor pools by amino acids released from thyroglobulin. In the dog thyroid slices, TSH increases the formation of TCA-soluble ninhydrin-positive material (mainly amino acids) and, in the absence of carrier leucine, decreases the incorporation of leucine-^{3}H into proteins (Lecocq and Dumont, 1970). In both systems the increased incorporation of amino acids into proteins has been interpreted as a stimulation of total protein synthesis. In dog thyroid slices this interpretation is supported by the fact that the relative stimulation is constant above a concentration of carrier of 2 mM. The effect of TSH is mimicked by DB-cAMP in both systems and by cAMP and caffeine in dog thyroid slices (Wilson et al., 1968; Lecocq and Dumont, 1970). ATP is inactive. This suggests that this effect of TSH is mediated by cAMP.

2. Mechanism—Role of cAMP

Several mechanisms might account for a stimulation of protein synthesis by TSH. New RNA synthesis and increased mRNA or ribosome supply do not explain the rapid action of TSH: the effect occurs early in isolated cells; concentrations of actinomycin which block RNA synthesis do not suppress or markedly inhibit it; no activation of RNA synthesis has been detected (Tong, 1967; Dumont and Lecocq, 1970). There is no evidence that the stimulation of protein synthesis might result from an enhancement of amino acid uptake. TSH at a high concentration (500 mU/ml) does not increase the uptake of natural amino acids in dog or beef thyroid slices (Segal et al., 1966). In isolated beef thyroid cells, TSH and DB-cAMP stimulate the uptake of ^{14}C-AIB (Wilson et al., 1968). However, the kinetics of uptake in the thyroid of this non-metabolizable amino acid and of natural amino acids are very different. Therefore, AIB is not a suitable tracer of amino acid transport in the thyroid (Segal et al., 1966).

In isolated beef thyroid cells, as in dog thyroid slices, labeled amino acid incorporation into protein is increased in the presence of glucose, but the relative effect of TSH is unaffected by glucose (Tong, 1967; Lecocq and Dumont, 1970). Preincubation of isolated cells in the presence of 2-deoxyglucose greatly decreases amino acid incorporation and abolishes its activation by TSH. From these data, Tong (1967) concluded that "the augmentation of protein synthesis following TSH treatment is secondary to a stimulation of glucose metabolism." We would rather interpret the data as showing only that the TSH action requires intact glucose metabolism. Moreover, several facts suggest that the stimulation by TSH of amino acid incorporation into proteins is not secondary to an activation of glucose metabolism. Concentrations of TSH required to stimulate glucose metabolism (pentose phosphate pathway, or glycolysis) in beef thyroid slices (Merlevede et al., 1963; Dumont, 1964; Gilman and Rall, 1968b) seem higher than those which enhance amino acid incorporation into the isolated cells. Furthermore, while the effect of TSH on amino acid incorporation is mimicked by DB-cAMP in isolated cells, DB-cAMP, like low concentrations of TSH, does not stimulate glucose oxidation in beef thyroid slices (Pastan and Macchia, 1967; Gilman and

Rall, 1968b). Parallel studies of the concentration-effect relationship of TSH for the different pathways of glucose metabolism (e.g., pentose phosphate pathway, glycolysis, etc.) and for amino acid incorporation into proteins in isolated cells could help to settle this question.

Another approach might be used in the analysis of the mechanism of TSH and cAMP stimulation of protein synthesis. Its early onset and its resistance to actinomycin suggest that this effect takes place at the level of translation and not of transcription. cAMP may act on translation in several ways. In adrenal homogenates it binds specifically to microsomal proteins, thus suggesting a direct effect on the ribosome (Gill and Garren, 1969). Lissitzky *et al.* (1969) have shown that cAMP enhances phenylalanine-^{14}C incorporation into proteins in thyroid and liver cellfree systems enriched or not with polyU. Trypsin pretreatment also enhances labeled amino acid incorporation into proteins by the polysomes, but the effects of trypsin and cAMP are additive. This might suggest that both trypsin and cAMP would unmask some mRNA. The physiological significance of this finding remains uncertain: the concentrations of cAMP used (0.1 mM) were several orders of magnitude higher than the expected intracellular concentrations (10^{-9} M); an effect was obtained with liver preparations although glucagon and its mediator cAMP do not induce a general stimulation of protein synthesis in liver tissue (Wicks, 1969). Malkin and Lipmann (1969) also reported activation by cAMP of some aminoacyl tRNA synthetases and of phenylalanine polymerization from phenylalanyl tRNA on polyU-charged reticulocyte ribosomes. cAMP also activates the release of proteins from rat liver polysomes *in vitro* (Khairallah and Pitot, 1967). However, in both these cases the action of cAMP is maximal at low concentrations of GTP, and high concentrations of the nucleotide are required (1–10 mM). Therefore, the physiological significance of these findings is very doubtful.

The recent findings that different ribosomal proteins may be phosphorylated in the polyribosomes, in the monosomes, and in the ribosomal subunits (Kabat, 1970), and that physiological concentrations of cAMP may activate the phosphorylation of ribosomal proteins (Loeb and Blat, 1970) suggest the existence of a subtle regulatory control of protein synthesis at the level of translation.

TSH, at the same concentration required to elicit other effects (1 mU/ml) (Fig. 8), including the activation of protein synthesis, brings about a shift in the ribosomes from the monosomes to the polysomes and from the light to the heavy polysomes in dog thyroid slices (Fig. 21) (Dumont *et al.*, 1969a). This effect is mimicked by cAMP and caffeine and by DB-cAMP. Two facts suggest that this effect does not involve the synthesis of new mRNA and takes place at the level of translation:

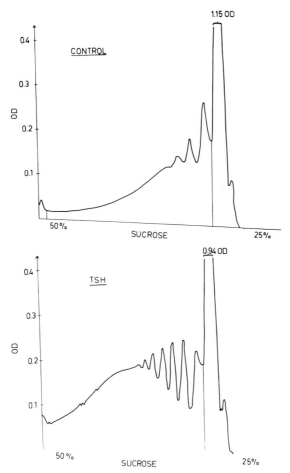

FIG. 21. Effect of thyrotropin (TSH) *in vitro* on the ribosome pattern of dog thyroid slices. Density gradient centrifugation pattern of the deoxycholate-treated 20,000 *g* supernatant (linear gradient 25–50%). TSH 200 mU/ml. OD, optical density. From Dumont *et al.* (1969a), with permission of the publisher.

it is observed 45 minutes after the beginning of the incubation at a time when very little incorporation of uridine-³H has taken place in the polysomes; no stimulation of uridine-³H incorporation into the RNA of the slices is observed. Theoretical study of a model of the ribosome cycle suggests two possible explanations for these findings: an activation of initiation in protein synthesis, and a shift in the population of translated mRNA toward larger mRNA (Vassart and Dumont, 1970).

Heywood (1966) has reported that low concentrations of thyroxine (1 m*M*) inhibited amino acid incorporation in rat thyroid slices and microsomal cellular systems. Such concentrations are unlikely to be encountered *in vivo* but could exist *in vitro*. The possibility that thyroxine inhibits protein synthesis in the thyroid during the first secretory phase of TSH action should be considered.

In conclusion, *in vitro* preparations in which overflooding of the cell amino acid pools by thyroglobulinolysis is avoided allow the demonstration of a rapid stimulation of protein synthesis by TSH. There is some evidence that this effect takes place at the translation level and that it is mediated by cAMP. Present working hypotheses on the nature of the mechanism of this action are activation of protein initiation and unmasking of large mRNA. Evidence that the delayed effects of TSH and cAMP on protein synthesis may involve an action at the level of transcription, i.e., through the synthesis of new RNA, has been presented in Section VI,A,2,a.

C. NATURE OF SYNTHESIZED PROTEINS

Little is known about the action of TSH on the nature of the proteins synthesized in the thyroid, for instance, whether or not TSH selectively enhances the synthesis of thyroglobulin. Acute TSH administration, either *in vitro* (Pavlovic-Hournac *et al.*, 1967) or *in vivo* (Cavalieri and Searle, 1967) does not seem to change the pattern of labeled amino acid incorporation into thyroid soluble proteins, as judged by density gradient centrifugation. However, such studies should be repeated with more sophisticated methods: measurements in all the thyroid subcellular fractions, kinetic analysis, and separation of proteins by techniques giving higher resolution, such as polyacrylamide gel electrophoresis. At 24 hours after the *in vivo* administration of TSH, the pattern of labeled amino acid incorporation in the rat thyroid *in vitro* demonstrates a clear shift in favor of the synthesis of thyroglobulin and its 12 S precursor (Pavlovic-Hournac *et al.*, 1967). Similarly, in chick embryos the onset of TSH secretion is accompanied by the appearance of protein labeling in the colloid. Before the onset of TSH secretion or in decapitated embryos methionine-^{3}H is incorporated only into follicular cells, but not into the colloid (Straznicky and Mess, 1967). These data suggest that a delayed effect of TSH may be to shift the thyroid protein synthesis machinery toward the formation of the specific exportable protein, i.e., thyroglobulin.

D. GROWTH

1. *Protein Synthesis in Chronically Stimulated Thyroid*

Chronic administration of TSH induces growth of thyroid tissue which is characterized mainly by an increase in tissue cell mass (Section

III,C), i.e., a general increase of structural cell components, proteins, phospholipids, and nucleic acids. Thyroid growth requires higher doses of TSH than secretion. In the chicken, enhancement of thyroid weight requires doses of TSH 50 times higher than activation of thyroid iodine depletion (Bates and Condliffe, 1960). Thyroid growth may require other hormones besides TSH: e.g., insulin, growth hormone (Bartke, 1968; Jolin et al., 1968, 1970).

Chronic stimulation of the rat thyroid by iodine deficiency or TSH administration is accompanied by an increased incorporation of labeled amino acids into thyroid proteins (Ochi and Degroot, 1969b; Pisarev et al., 1970), while hypophysectomy decreases this incorporation in in vitro incubated guinea pig thyroid slices (Raghupathy et al., 1963). Thyroglobulinolysis, like secretion, should vary in parallel with the level of thyroid stimulation; therefore intracellular amino acid pools would be expected to be increased in the stimulated gland and decreased in resting tissue. The data on amino acid incorporation therefore suggest that the protein synthesis rate in the thyroid is a function of the tonic level of thyroid stimulation. The population size of cytoplasmic ribosomes seems to vary in the same way (Section III,C,2). In rat thyroids chronically stimulated by thiouracil in the diet, incorporation of phenylalanine-^{14}C by ribosomes in acellular systems is increased while the relative stimulation of this incorporation by polyU is decreased (Greif and Eich, 1969). Under the conditions of these experiments, little initiation would be expected to take place and the Mg^{2+} concentration would allow polyU-directed polyphenylalanine synthesis in the absence of initiation factors. Therefore, these results are compatible with the hypothesis that the proportion of ribosomes actively engaged in protein synthesis, i.e., ribosomes of polysomes, is increased. It is probable therefore that in the chronically stimulated thyroid the number and the activity of the ribosomes is increased.

2. Role of cAMP in the Induction of Thyroid Growth

Kerkof and Tata (1969) have proposed the provocative hypothesis that cAMP may mediate only the rapid effects on cellular permeability and modulation of enzyme activities, but that cAMP does not exert a direct influence on the slower biosynthetic responses to the hormone. The evidence in favor of this concept, i.e., the failure of DB-cAMP to mimic the TSH stimulation of phospholipid and RNA synthesis is certainly not conclusive. Moreover, there are strong indications of cAMP action on protein synthesis at the level of translation (Section VII,B,2) and transcription (Section VI,A,2,b).

Several arguments support the hypothesis that the chronic goitrogenic or growth-promoting action of TSH on the thyroid is mediated by cAMP. Methylxanthines are mildly antithyroid but strongly goitrogenic in the rat. Theophylline causes marked synergistic enhancement of the goitrogenic effect of small doses of PTU. Measurements of plasma TSH levels show that increases in thyroid weight can be obtained without increase in hormonal levels. The order of potency of methylxanthines is like that reported for cAMP phosphodiesterase (Wolff and Varrone, 1969). Chronic administration of cAMP in thyroxine-treated mice *in vivo* mimics the action of TSH on goitrogenesis (thyroid weight and total protein content) and on labeled amino acid incorporation into proteins. AMP or adenosine has no such effect. No increase of plasma TSH was observed at the beginning or at the end (4 days) of the treatment (Pisarev *et al.*, 1970). A stimulation of TSH release by cAMP is not completely ruled out since TSH plasma levels were for the most part below the measurable limit, and measurements were made long enough after cAMP administration (2 hours and 6 hours) for a large discharge of TSH (half-life ±35 minutes; Bakke *et al.*, 1962) to escape detection. However, the possibility that the *in vivo* effect of cAMP is due to a discharge of TSH is unlikely since it is known that T_4 blocks cAMP-induced TSH release from the pituitary (Wilber *et al.*, 1969). Therefore, these data support the hypothesis that the chronic goitrogenic effects of TSH are mediated by cAMP. Similar data supporting the hypothesis of a cAMP mediated action have been presented for the maintenance by ACTH of adrenal weight and function (Ney, 1969).

E. Role of Nucleic Acids and Protein Synthesis in the
    Action of TSH

The stimulation by TSH of RNA synthesis has been proposed several times as the primary action of the hormone (Begg and Munro, 1965; H. Shimada and Yasumasu, 1966; Ochi and Degroot, 1968).

There is now extensive evidence that many early effects of TSH on the thyroid do not depend on a prior stimulation of RNA and/or protein synthesis. Indeed, very marked inhibitions of these processes by inhibitors such as actinomycin D, puromycin, and cycloheximide do not inhibit these early effects.

Actinomycin and puromycin do not relieve the early inhibition by TSH of iodide transport in isolated beef thyroid cells (Wilson *et al.*, 1968), nor do they inhibit the stimulation of iodide binding to proteins or of thyroxine synthesis in fetal rat thyroid in organ culture (Nataf, 1968) or isolated beef thyroid cells (Tong, 1965). Actinomycin, puromycin, and cycloheximide do not inhibit the release of iodine or the secretion of thyroid hormone in TSH-stimulated mouse (McKenzie *et al.*, 1968; Bauduin *et al.*, 1967), rabbit (Taurog and Thio, 1966), or rat (Halmi *et al.*, 1966) thyroids. Actinomycin and puromycin do not inhibit the stimulation by TSH of glucose C-1 and C-6 oxidation in sheep and dog thyroid slices (Field *et al.*, 1963; Dumont and Burelle, 1964; Dumont, 1966; Field *et al.*, 1966). Actinomycin, puromycin, and cycloheximide do not inhibit the early activation by TSH of orotate-^{14}C, adenine-^{14}C and formate-^{14}C incorporation into ribonucleotides of calf or beef thyroid slices (Hall and Tubmen, 1968; R. H. Lindsay *et al.*, 1970).

Only one example so far has been provided of an effect of TSH which might be secondary to a stimulation of some RNA and protein synthesis: the enhancement of iodide trapping in isolated beef thyroid cells (Wilson *et al.*, 1968; Knopp *et al.*, 1970). This effect is delayed (more than 2 hours), and it is inhibited by actinomycin, cycloheximide, and puromycin. Some of the early TSH effects also obviously require the presence in the cell of rapidly metabolized proteins, as suggested in the case of secretion, by the inhibition of TSH secretory action by pretreatment of rats with actinomycin D, puromycin, and cycloheximide (McKenzie, 1968; Halmi *et al.*, 1966; Kriss *et al.*, 1964; Seljelid and Nakken, 1969). It is quite probable that other delayed effects of TSH on the thyroid, such as growth, are also, at least in part, secondary to an activation of RNA and protein synthesis. However, this hypothesis remains unproved; the best argument in favor of it is perhaps the dissociation in ^{131}I-irradiated cockerels of the secretory and the growth-promoting actions of TSH (Skanse, 1948). The difficulty of maintaining for long periods adequate inhibition of RNA and/or protein synthesis *in vivo* or *in vitro*, without provoking phenomena of general toxicity probably explains the lack of evidence on this point. Moreover, growth *in vitro* has not been demonstrated, except in culture systems in which some dedifferentiation is taking place.

VIII. Action of TSH on Phospholipid Metabolism

A. Introduction

Studies in sheep thyroid slices incubated *in vitro* support the validity of current concepts of phospholipid metabolism for this tissue (Fig. 22) (Freinkel, 1958). In particular, the kinetics of phosphate-^{32}P incorporations are compatible with the role of water-soluble phosphorylated bases as precursors and of water-soluble phosphodiesters as catabolic derivatives. These studies have also demonstrated the great heterogeneity of turnover of the various phospholipids. However, the conventional scheme of phospholipid synthesis does not account readily for some find-

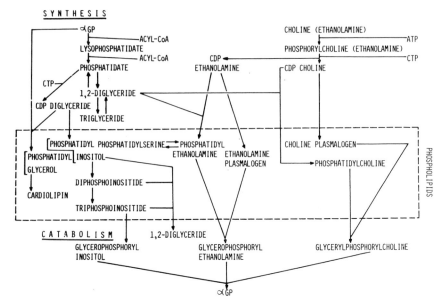

Fig. 22. Phospholipid metabolism. αGP: α-glycerophosphate. Adapted from Dawson (1966).

ings: (1) monophosphatidylinositol P is more heavily labeled than the P in all the other intermediates, including monophosphatidate in dog thyroid slices (Scott *et al.*, 1966b) ; (2) increased labeling in the 1,2-diglyceride fraction of sheep thyroid slices incubated in the presence of palmitate-^{14}C is not followed by increased labeling of phosphatidylcholine or phosphatidylethanolamine (Scott *et al.*, 1968).

B. *In Vivo*

TSH *in vivo* enhances the incorporation of ^{32}P-phosphate into the thyroid phospholipids of sheep (Freinkel, 1957), guinea pigs (Kerkof and Tata, 1967), and mice (Ochi and Degroot, 1968). This effect is accompanied by a relatively smaller increase in the total uptake of ^{32}P$_i$ by the gland (Kerkof and Tata, 1967; Ochi and Degroot, 1968). More specifically, TSH *in vivo* increases the activity of the acid-soluble fraction of the gland (Creek, 1965) and of water-soluble phosphorylated bases (Freinkel, 1957). The fact that phosphate-^{32}P incorporation into the thyroid phospholipids was relatively more increased than total ^{32}P$_i$-uptake of the gland has been taken as evidence of stimulation of phospholipid synthesis (Kerkof and Tata, 1967; Ochi and Degroot, 1968). In the absence of kinetic data on the specific activity of precursors, such findings are merely suggestive. A few hours after TSH injection the phospholipid content of guinea pig thyroid is increased (Kerkof and Tata, 1967).

C. *In Vitro*

1. *Nature of the Effect*

Enhancement of ^{32}P-phosphate incorporation into the phospholipids of stimulated thyroids, and the mechanism of this increase have been extensively studied *in vitro*. TSH stimulates ^{32}P phosphate incorporation into the phospholipids of sheep (230%) (Freinkel, 1957; Jacquemin and Haye, 1970), beef (Morton and Schwartz, 1953; Florsheim *et al.*, 1957; Kögl and Van Deenen, 1961), pig (Kerkof and Tata, 1969; Jacquemin and Haye, 1970, Macchia *et al.*, 1970), and dog (Altman *et al.*, 1966; Pastan and Macchia, 1967; Burke, 1968b) thyroid slices. This effect is hormone and tissue specific (Florsheim *et al.*, 1957; Freinkel, 1957). The enhancement is demonstrated in all cell fractions; the TSH-controlled phospholipids belong to the "bound class" (Kögl and Van Deenen, 1961; Kerkof and Tata, 1969). Extrapolation of isotopic values to zero time has suggested that the TSH action begins within minutes after the beginning of the activation (Freinkel, 1957); it has been demonstrated in 15-minute incubations (Burke, 1968b).

Increased phosphate-^{32}P incorporation into phospholipids does not appear to reflect increased phosphate penetration into the cells: TCA-soluble ^{32}P is not modified (Florsheim *et al.*, 1957; Kerkof and Tata, 1969), and the specific activity of tissue inorganic phosphate or of water-soluble organic phosphorus is not increased (Freinkel, 1957). The TSH stimulation is observed even in beef thyroid slices in which no alteration of the specific activity of the γP of ATP has been detected (Schneider, 1969). TSH also stimulates the incorporation of glucose-^{14}C and ^{14}C-labeled fatty acids into the phospholipids of dog and sheep thyroid slices, respectively (Scott *et al.*, 1968), which also suggests an action on synthesis rather than multiple effects on precursor pool sizes. The kinetics of phospholipid labeling is not so fast as to make it plausible to explain an increased incorporation of ^{32}P into thyroid phospholipids by a slowing down of the catabolic rate (Schwartz and Morton, 1955; Freinkel, 1958; Kerkof and Tata, 1969). Moreover, the effect of TSH does not seem to increase with the time of incubation (Freinkel, 1957). However, these findings do not exclude the former hypothesis. Therefore, there is good evidence that TSH *in vitro* stimulates phospholipid synthesis and that this effect takes place at a step beyond ATP in the anabolic sequence. We do not know whether TSH affects phospholipid degradation, i.e., whether it accelerates the turnover or induces a net synthesis of phospholipids.

2. Classes of Phospholipids

The action of TSH on phosphate-^{32}P incorporation into thyroid phospholipids varies much from one class to another; there is a very great activation for phosphatidylserine (330%) and even more for monophosphatidylinositol (370%), a smaller effect on phosphatidylethanolamine (171%) and phosphatidate (184%), and no consistent effect on phosphatidylcholine (113%) (sheep, Freinkel, 1957); sphingomyelins are not affected (steer, Florsheim et al., 1957). In another study on sheep thyroid slices (Scott et al., 1966a), TSH markedly enhanced ^{32}P$_i$ incorporation into monophosphatidylinositol, phosphatidate, and phosphatidylcholine, but the effect on phosphatidylserine and phosphatidylethanolamine was not constant. In calf thyroid slices TSH markedly enhanced ^{32}P$_i$ uptake in monophosphatidylinositol, had a doubtful effect on phosphatidate, and decreased the uptake in phosphatidylcholine (Vilkki, 1961). In dog thyroid slices the hormonal effect is marked on phosphatidate and monophosphatidylinositol, less important in higher phosphoinositides and phosphatidylcholine, and absent in phosphatidylglycerol, plasmagenic phosphatides, and sphingomyelins (Scott et al., 1966b). Some of the latter observations have been confirmed by Altman et al. (1966).

All these results have been obtained with thyroid slices incubated for several hours in the presence of rather high concentrations of TSH (≥ 100 mU/ml). More specific effects have been obtained by altering this experimental protocol. Acute exposure of dog thyroid slices to TSH for 2–10 minutes (following a 2 hour prelabeling with ^{32}P-phosphate in vitro) enhanced the incorporation of ^{32}P$_i$ into phosphatidate and monophosphatidylinositol; no other phosphatide was consistently affected (Scott et al., 1966b). Similarly, in pig and sheep thyroid slices, with low concentrations of TSH (≤ 1 mU/ml), ^{32}P$_i$ incorporation is specifically increased in monophosphatidylinositol, decreased in phosphatidylcholine, and unchanged in total phospholipids. In the presence of higher TSH concentrations a general enhancement of ^{32}P$_i$-incorporation into phospholipids is observed (Jacquemin and Haye, 1970).

In conclusion, the pattern of the TSH action on individual phospholipids may be summarized as follows. TSH greatly and consistently increases ^{32}P$_i$-incorporation into monophosphatidylinositol and phosphatidate; this effect occurs early after TSH administration and, for monophosphatidylinositol at least, for low TSH concentrations; it corresponds to a realignment in the pattern of phospholipid metabolism. TSH also stimulates ^{32}P$_i$-incorporation into the whole phospholipid fraction; this action reflects both the former effect and an enhanced incorporation into phosphatidylethanilamine, phosphatidylserine, higher phosphoinositides and in some cases phosphatidylcholine. These effects vary from one species to another, and may take place later and for higher, perhaps unphysiological concentrations of TSH. Incorporation of ^{32}P-phosphate into phosphatidylcholine may be increased or decreased by TSH under different conditions. TSH does not seem to affect phosphatidylglycerol, plasmogenic phospholipids, and sphingomyelins.

3. Mechanisms

Increased incorporation of ^{32}P$_i$ into monophosphatidylinositol does not appear to reflect variations in precursor pools sizes, since TSH also increases the incorporation of glucose-^{14}C, glycerol-^{14}C, and ^{14}C-labeled fatty acids in monophosphatidylinositol in both dog and sheep thyroid slices (Scott et al., 1968). For the reasons already developed for the whole phospholipid class, it is probable that increased incorporation of precursors into monophosphatidylinositol reflects increased synthesis, but it is not known whether net synthesis or acceleration of turnover is taking place.

Hormonal stimulation of monophosphatidylinositol metabolism has been observed in many endocrine and nonendocrine tissues when functional activation is induced (Scott et al., 1968). However, the significance of this effect is still unknown. The very early activation in thyroid tissue must be approximately concomitant with the induction of phagocytosis. It has been suggested that increased monophosphatidylinositol synthesis may be related to this rapid membrane activity with the formation of apical pseudopods and the mobilization of lysosomes in the follicular cells (Scott et al., 1966b). The hypothesis is becoming unlikely as more instances of intracellular colloid droplet formation in the absence of evidence of activated phospholipid metabolism are described, e.g., with DB-cAMP in dog and some beef thyroid slices (Pastan and Macchia, 1967), or reportedly (Burke, 1970a) in sheep thyroid slices incubated in the presence of prostaglandins.

TSH consistently and markedly decreases the ratio of radioactive triglycerides to diglycerides in stimulated dog (Freinkel and Scott, 1964) and sheep (Scott et al., 1966a, 1968) thyroid slices incubated with glucose-^{14}C. TSH also increases the proportion of ^{14}C radioactivity from labeled glucose, glycerol, palmitate, and oleate incorporated into 1,2-diglycerides in sheep and dog thyroid slices. Addition of TSH to thyroid slices for 10 minutes, after 2 hours of prelabeling with glycerol-^{14}C, also increased the proportion of radioactivity incorporated into the 1,2-diglyceride fraction (Scott et al., 1968). Since incorporation into total neutral lipids is increased or unchanged, we may assume that these findings reflect an increased formation of 1,2-diglyceride. Increased formation of such precursors of phospholipids would certainly tend to favor phospholipid biosynthesis. It has been suggested that this phenomenon may reflect a new lipogenic equilibrium which selectively favors cytostructural renewal, that is phospholipogenesis (Freinkel and Scott, 1964).

The metabolic steps at which TSH may stimulate the synthesis of phospholipids, especially monophosphatidylinositol and phosphatidate, have not been identified. Incorporation of all precursors of monophosphatidylinositol is activated by TSH. This would be compatible with an effect at the latest step of this synthesis. However, effects of TSH on the 1,2-diglyceride and phosphatidate formation would rather suggest that several steps are involved in this TSH action. In the absence of precise knowledge of all the pathways of phospholipid synthesis, of their rate-limiting steps and of their possible feedback controls' one can do little more than speculate on this subject.

Schneider (1968) has investigated in the guinea pig the possibility that the action of TSH on thyroid phospholipid synthesis could be mediated by an increase in the activity of the enzymes involved in phosphatidate synthesis: acyl-coA synthetase and glycerophosphate acyltransferase. The activity of both enzymes was increased slightly 6 hours and definitely 24 hours after the injection of TSH. No effect was found in calf thyroid slices incubated 1–2 hours with TSH, although ^{32}P-phosphate incorporation into total phospholipids was increased. These data suggest that increases in enzyme levels may account for the late, but not for the early, activation of phospholipid synthesis.

Inclusion of glucose in the incubation medium increases the incorporation of phosphate-^{32}P into all phospholipid species of dog thyroid slices. The action of TSH does not appear to be secondary to increased glucose consumption by the tissue, since it is more specific. In particular the increases of radioactivity of phosphatidylserine and monophosphatidylinositol are much greater with TSH, whereas enhancement of the radioactivity of other phospholipids is much lower (Scott et al., 1966b). Furthermore, the action of TSH on phospholipid metabolism can be observed in the absence of glucose in the medium (Freinkel, 1957). Therefore, the action of TSH does not require a supply of exogenous glucose.

Stimulation of the catabolism of endogenous glucose is unlikely to cause the activation of phospholipid metabolism. The main effect of TSH on glucose metabolism is the activation of the pentose phosphate pathway (Dumont and Tondeur-Montenez, 1965). Activation of this pathway in dog thyroid slices by epinephrine, serotonin, and Synkavit

(Altman *et al.*, 1966) or in sheep thyroid slices by iodotyrosines (Burke, 1968b) or by prostaglandins (Burke, 1970a) is not accompanied by evidence of stimulation of phospholipid metabolism. It has been reported that stimulation of glucose C-1 oxidation in sheep thyroid slices is abolished in physiological saline while the enhancement of $^{32}P_i$ incorporation into phospholipids is further increased (Burke, 1970c). In dog thyroid slices, DB-cAMP has been reported to activate phospholipid metabolism at concentrations which do not influence glucose oxidation (Burke, 1968a). Conversely, in the absence of Na^+ or in the presence of ouabain, the stimulation by TSH of ^{32}P-phosphate incorporation into phospholipids, but not the enhancement of glucose C-1 oxidation, is abolished (Oka and Field, 1966; Burke, 1970c). Prostaglandin E_1 mimics the effect of TSH on glucose oxidation but not on phospholipid metabolism in dog thyroid slices (Zor *et al.*, 1969a). Although these studies included ^{32}P measurements only in the whole phospholipid fraction, this suggests that activation of phospholipid metabolism does not cause the stimulation of the pentose phosphate pathway. Therefore, no relation has been demonstrated between the effect of TSH on phospholipid metabolism and other hormonal effects.

4. *Role of cAMP*

In sheep thyroid slices the stimulation by TSH of $^{32}P_i$ incorporation into phospholipids was mimicked by DB-cAMP, cAMP, and 0.3 mM theophylline. In addition, concentrations of theophylline and of cAMP, AMP, ADP, and ATP, but not of CTP, GTP, or UTP, which were individually ineffective, stimulated phospholipogenesis when added together (Burke, 1968a, 1969a). However, theophylline, at concentrations either stimulatory (0.3 mM) or inactive (30 μM), did not potentiate the effect of TSH or LATS (Burke, 1969a). Perhaps this negative finding may be explained by an action of theophylline on phospholipid metabolism unrelated to the inhibition of phosphodiesterase; in these experiments it is apparent that theophylline inhibited the effects of maximal concentrations of TSH and LATS. For other species, the role of cAMP seems conflicting. In beef thyroid slices, DB-cAMP, 0.15–0.3 mM, increased $^{32}P_i$-incorporation into phospholipids in 6 of 12 experiments, whereas TSH 100 mU/ml was always active. This discrepancy was unexplained (Pastan and Macchia, 1967). However, as discussed previously, the concentrations of DB-cAMP used corresponded to less than 2 mU/ml of TSH and could not therefore be expected to mimic effects of 100 mU/ml TSH. In dog thyroid slices, DB-cAMP but not cAMP reproduced the TSH stimulation of $^{32}P_i$ incorporation into phospholipids (Pastan, 1966b). In a later paper Pastan and Macchia (1967) failed to reproduce the effect of DB-cAMP. No comment was made on this discrepancy with their previous results. DB-cAMP did not mimic the TSH stimulation of inositol-^{3}H incorporation into phospholipids either. However, the concentrations of TSH (100 mU/ml) and DB-cAMP (less than 0.4 mM) used in the latter experiments are not comparable. Burke (1968c) has confirmed the effect of DB-cAMP on ^{32}P incorporation into dog thyroid phospholipids and obtained a similar effect with higher concentrations of cAMP but not with 5'-AMP. Differences in tissue sensitivities may account for the discordant results of the two groups. In pig thyroid slices, DB-cAMP, but not cAMP, stimulated, like TSH, the incorporation of ^{32}P$_i$ into phospholipids (Kerkof and Tata, 1969). Theophylline, 50 μM, did not potentiate the effect of TSH (Zor et $al.$, 1969a); but, as recognized by the authors, it is doubtful whether the concentration used was sufficient to inhibit phosphodiesterase activity significantly.

Burke (1969d) reported that in sheep thyroid slices submaximal concentrations of dl-propanolol and phentolamine (0.1 mM) stimulated phosphate-^{32}P incorporation into phospholipids, and increased the effect of maximal concentrations of TSH and DB-cAMP on these variables. Since phentolamine and propanolol (0.5 mM) prevented the colloid droplet formation elicited by TSH and DB-cAMP, Burke concluded "that phospholipogenesis in thyroid is unrelated to adenyl cyclase activation." In view of the different concentrations of the inhibitors used in the study of the two variables this conclusion is unwarranted. Of more interest is the report that in sheep thyroid slices, TSH at 50 mU/ml stimulated the incorporation of ^{32}P into thyroid phospholipids, while it enhanced glucose-C-1 oxidation, elicited colloid droplet formation in slices and activated adenyl cyclase in particulates, but only at a concentration of 250 mU/ml (Burke, 1970c).

A very strong argument against the hypothesis that cAMP mediates the action of TSH on phospholipid metabolism has been provided by Jacquemin and Haye (1970). These authors showed that in sheep thyroid slices DB-cAMP (25–500 μg/ml) failed to mimic the action of low (<1 mU/ml) (incorporation of ^{32}P$_i$ increased in phosphatidylinositol, decreased in phosphatidylcholine) and of higher concentrations (1 mU/ml to 100 mU/ml) (general increase of ^{32}P$_i$ incorporation in the phospholipids) of TSH. However, no proof of the activity of DB-cAMP on other metabolic variables was given in these experiments. In conclusion, the available evidence makes it very doubtful that cAMP mediates the entire action of TSH on phospholipid metabolism. The stimulation of phospholipid metabolism by TSH may be the result of several mechanisms, and it is still possible that some of these may involve cAMP.

In pig thyroid slices DB-cAMP, like TSH, stimulates the incorporation of $^{32}P_i$ into phospholipids. However, when this incorporation was corrected for the increased uptake of $^{32}P_i$, the increase in phospholipid labeling, although still observable with TSH, was no longer apparent in the DB-cAMP stimulated slices. From these experiments, it has been concluded that if DB-cAMP enhances the incorporation of phosphate into phospholipids in thyroid slices, it does not mimic the stimulation of phospholipid synthesis (Kerkof and Tata, 1969). This interpretation is subject to some reservations. A parallel increase in the radioactivity of the precursor pool and in the radioactivity of the product cannot be taken as evidence of increased synthesis, but it does not exclude it. If the precursor pools were enlarged, such data would indeed demonstrate an increased synthesis. In this regard, cAMP and even its acylated derivatives could dilute the specific activity of the adenine nucleotides and perhaps even of a phosphate pool. Furthermore, the concentrations of TSH (130 mU/ml) and DB-cAMP (0.30 mM) used in these experiments were not truly comparable, and it is quite possible that lower concentrations of TSH would have given results similar to those obtained with DB-cAMP, i.e., parallel increases of radioactivity of precursors and phospholipids. The fact that in these experiments DB-cAMP quantitatively mimicked the stimulation by TSH of iodide organification does not bear against this argument as this TSH effect reaches a plateau for low concentrations of TSH (Rodesch et al., 1969). Therefore, it is not certain that there is a qualitative difference between the action of TSH on phospholipid turnover and on phospholipid synthesis.

IX. Action of TSH on Membranes

A. Electrophysiology of the Follicular Cell

Krüskemper and Reichertz (1960) reported that injection of TSH into guinea pigs induced in 1–2 minutes a monophasic depolarization reaction in the thyroid. More recently, Williams (1970) has shown that 20–40 minutes after TSH addition to the perfusion fluid of a rabbit thyroid, there is a decrease of the resistance and an enhancement of the capacitance of the follicular cell wall. Similarly, in mouse thyroids incubated in vitro TSH rapidly induces a decrease of the membrane potential of acinar cells (Konno and McKenzie, 1970). The most likely explanation of these effects is a fall in specific resistance across the follicular epithelium at the apical or basal membrane. Such a fall is equivalent to an increase in permeability to one or more ions (Williams, 1970). TSH induces a marked increase in the 10 minute-uptake of radiosodium in chick thyroid (Solomon, 1961). Therefore, increased permeability in the stimulated gland may involve primarily Na$^+$. The physiological significance of this effect is unknown.

Chronic stimulation by PTU treatment decreases cellular polarization in the guinea pig (Woodbury and Woodbury, 1963) and in the frog (Gorbman and Ueda, 1963) thyroid. There is an inverse parallelism during the development of the tadpole between thyroid functional level, on the one hand, and cell potential and follicular wall resistance, on the other hand (Gorbman and Ueda, 1963). Similarly PTU treatment in the rabbit (Williams, 1970) and TSH treatment in the frog (Gorbman and Ueda, 1963) decrease follicular wall resistance and increase follicular wall capacitance. These effects have been related to an increase of the membrane area due to folding of cellular basal membranes (Williams, 1970). Whereas the acute effects of TSH on cell polarization would therefore be explained by enhancement of permeability, the chronic effects would merely reflect the hypertrophy of the basal cell membrane.

B. Na$^+$/K$^+$ ACTIVATED ATPASE

Turkington (1962) reported that TSH *in vitro* stimulated the Na$^+$/K$^+$ activated ATPase of thyroid cell membrane. This effect was inhibited by ouabain. It was suggested that the primary effect of TSH on the thyroid cell was the activation of Na$^+$ transport (Turkington, 1962, 1963). Wolff and Halmi (1963) did not observe a stimulation by TSH of Na$^+$/K$^+$ activated ATPase in an acellular system. Stanbury and Hugues (1964) could reproduce this effect with crude, but not with purified, TSH.

If the stimulation of Na$^+$/K$^+$ activated ATPase was the primary effect of TSH, other hormonal effects should disappear when this enzyme is inhibited, i.e., in the presence of ouabain, or in the absence of Na$^+$. It was reported (Turkington, 1963) that the stimulation of calf thyroid slice respiration by TSH was inhibited by ouabain, in the absence of Na$^+$, or in the presence of high concentrations of K$^+$. Under similar conditions, Stanbury (1964) did not observe this effect of ouabain. Another effect of TSH is not inhibited by ouabain or the absence of Na$^+$ in the medium: the activation of the pentose phosphate pathway (Dumont and Burelle, 1964; Stanbury, 1964; O'Malley and Field, 1964; Dumont and Van Sande, 1966; Oka and Field, 1966). Therefore, there is no support for the hypothesis that the stimulation of Na$^+$/K$^+$ activated ATPase may be the primary effect of TSH on the thyroid cell. However, the integrity of the Na$^+$/K$^+$ pump is required for some TSH effects: for instance, the enhancement of ^{32}P incorporation into thyroid phospholipids is inhibited in the absence of Na$^+$ in the medium or in the presence of ouabain (Oka and Field, 1966; Burke, 1969c).

In guinea pig and rat thyroids chronically stimulated by PTU or TSH treatments the activity of Na^+/K^+ stimulated ATPase is increased (Wolff and Halmi, 1963; Brunberg and Halmi, 1966). However, this effect seems to reflect mainly thyroid hypertrophy and hyperplasia.

C. SUBSTRATE TRANSPORT

1. Amino Acids

TSH stimulates the uptake of ^{14}C-α-aminoisobutyrate (AIB) in bovine and dog thyroid slices (Debons and Pittman, 1962). This effect is small (20% increase) and specific for the tissue, but it is not specific for the hormone, as it is mimicked by insulin and growth hormone (Debons and Pittman, 1966). It is not due to a variation in water distribution in the tissue (Debons and Pittman, 1962). A similar action has been demonstrated in isolated bovine thyroid cells (Tong, 1964b). No such effect was observed in sheep thyroid slices (Raghupathy et al., 1964). However, the responsitivity of this system was not checked by demonstrating other TSH effects. Segal et al. (1966) also observed that TSH enhances AIB accumulation by dog and bovine thyroid slices. However, the kinetics of uptake in thyroid slices is very different for AIB and other amino acids: in the case of AIB this uptake increases linearly for 4 hours whereas for other amino acids, including cycloleucine, it reaches a plateau after 30 minutes. Therefore, AIB uptake is not a valid index of the transport of natural amino acids in the thyroid. Whatever its meaning may be, the stimulation by TSH of AIB-uptake in isolated beef thyroid cells is mimicked by DB-cAMP (Wilson et al., 1968).

TSH enhances the uptake of AIB, but not of other amino acids according to Segal et al., 1966. However, only one very high concentration of TSH was used in these experiments. Moreover, interpretation of these experiments presents great difficulties because of the TSH-induced thyroglobulinolysis and the consequent variations of intracellular amino acid pool sizes. In this regard, it is regrettable that only the accumulation of AIB was studied in the isolated cells where thyroglobulinolysis does not cloud the picture. The hypothesis of a stimulation by TSH of amino acid uptake in the thyroid is therefore not excluded, even though as yet unsupported.

After 2 days of TSH administration, the uptake of arginine-^{14}C and tyrosine in the thyroid is increased (Klitgaard et al., 1965). However, in the absence of data on free amino acid pool sizes or on the kinetics of amino acid uptake in the soluble and protein fractions, it is not known if the increased uptake reflects an effect on amino acid transport, on protein synthesis or on both.

2. Sugars, Nucleosides, Phosphate, Iodide

TSH increases the uptake of glucose in thyroid slices of various species (Section V,B,1). It has been reported that the hormone stimulates the uptake of stereospecific nonmetabolizable sugars in bovine thyroid slices (Tarui and Nonaka, 1963; Tarui et al., 1963). Such data suggest that the effect of TSH on sugar uptake may reflect an activation of sugar transport into the cell.

Increased nucleotide formation from nucleosides in TSH-stimulated thyroid cells may also be related to activated nucleoside transport (Section VI,B,3).

TSH increases the inorganic phosphate content of sheep thyroid slices in vitro (Freinkel, 1957). This effect has been reproduced in slices incubated in the absence of phosphate in the medium (Freinkel, 1963); therefore, it does not reflect a stimulation of phosphate transport, although the possibility that such an effect also takes place is not excluded. It has been suggested that the increased inorganic phosphate content of stimulated thyroid slices results from an activation of phosphatases (Freinkel, 1963). It may also reflect the activation of endergonic nucleotide triphosphate-requiring processes, for instance, the activation of adenyl cyclase (Fig. 17). Indeed, TSH slightly decreases the nucleotide triphosphate content of dog thyroid slices (Lamy et al., 1967) (Section V,E,2).

The action of TSH on iodide transport in the thyroid has been discussed before (Section IV,B). The immediate effect of the hormone is an increased efflux of iodide which has been related to increased cell permeability; the delayed action is an enhancement of iodide transport which may be secondary to the synthesis of new transport systems.

3. General

Many acute effects of TSH on the thyroid do not seem to require enhancement of substrate uptake by the cell. Several such effects are observed in the absence of substrates in the medium: increase of Q_{O_2} (Freinkel, 1963), of intracellular inorganic phosphate concentration (Freinkel, 1963), of tissue TPN level (Pastan et al., 1963; Dumont and Eloy, 1966) stimulation of phosphorus turnover in phospholipids (Morton and Schwartz, 1953; Florsheim et al., 1957; Freinkel, 1957), of glucose oxidation (Dumont and Eloy, 1966), and of thyroid secretion (Willems et al., 1970). Therefore, effects on substrate uptake by the thyroid do not seem to be required for the early phase of TSH action. However, as discussed previously (Freinkel, 1964), such effects "may represent mechanisms for facilitating and sustaining the full response to TSH through exogenous contributions to net energy balance" and pools of precursors for biosynthetic pathways.

Although the effects of TSH on membrane transport may not be required for the expression of hormonal action, there is much evidence that the integrity of the plasma membrane is a necessary condition of this action. Treatment of sheep (Dumont and Burelle, 1964) or beef (Larsen and Wolff, 1967) thyroid slices with crude phospholipase C or of dog thyroid slices with a purified enzyme (Macchia and Pastan, 1967) abolishes the stimulation by TSH of glucose C-1 oxidation (sheep, dog) and $^{32}P_i$ incorporation into phospholipids (beef, dog). As the DB-cAMP effects were also suppressed (Pastan and Macchia, 1967), it was concluded that the inhibition bore on a step beyond cAMP formation. When pig thyroid slices were treated with a more purified enzyme, specific for lecithin, the effects of TSH but not those of DB-cAMP were suppressed (Macchia et al., 1970). These latter data suggest that lecithinase C acts on cAMP formation at the level of adenyl cyclase and/or the TSH receptor.

D. Conclusion

In conclusion, in the early phase of its action, TSH seems to increase thyroid cell permeability, which would explain the decrease in cell polarization and in follicular wall resistance, the increase of the iodide efflux and of the rate of Na^+ penetration into the thyroid. There is some support for the hypothesis that TSH may stimulate the uptake of stereo-specific sugars, including glucose, but it is not known whether it affects amino acid transport. There is no support for the hypothesis that TSH stimulates Na^+/K^+ activated ATPase. Effects on membrane permeability or transport do not seem to cause the other early hormonal effects. The action of TSH may be abolished by specific membrane alterations involving the TSH receptor adenyl cyclase system. Less specific alterations of the membrane may also prevent the expression of the action of cAMP on its target systems.

X. Action on the Thyroid of Agents Which Enhance or Decrease cAMP Accumulation

A. Agents That Increase cAMP Accumulation

If an effect of TSH is mediated by cAMP, any agent which increases the intracellular concentration of this nucleotide in the thyroid should reproduce the hormonal effect, unless the agent independently inhibits a more distal step in the cause-effect sequence.

1. Epinephrine

Epinephrine has been reported to enhance cAMP accumulation in beef thyroid slices. This effect was inhibited by a β-receptor inhibitor (dichloroisoproterenol), but not by an α-inhibitor (phenoxybenzamine) (Gilman and Rall, 1968a). However, Pastan and Katzen (1967) did not observe any stimulation of adenyl cyclase activity by epinephrine in beef thyroid homogenate. Epinephrine reproduces several effects of TSH; it enhances glucose carbon-1 oxidation by thyroid slices (Pastan et al., 1962; Hupka and Dumont, 1963); in isolated calf thyroid cells, it activates iodide binding to protein and iodothyronine formation, it stimulates the incorporation of ^{14}C-labeled mixed amino acids into proteins (Maayan and Ingbar, 1970). Epinephrine does not modify the incorporation of ^{32}P$_i$ into the phospholipids of isolated calf thyroid cells. Phentolamine (α inhibitor), but no propanolol (a β inhibitor), inhibits the action of epinephrine on glucose oxidation and iodine metabolism in isolated cells (Maayan and Ingbar, 1968, 1970). These effects of epinephrine are complex. The activation of glucose oxidation is, at least in part, secondary to an increased oxidation of NADPH by the adrenochrome derived from epinephrine (Pastan et al., 1962; Hupka and Dumont, 1963). The stimulation of iodide metabolism might also reflect a direct oxidizing action of epinephrine or adrenochrome (e.g., on H_2O_2 generation). However, epinephrine activates adenyl cyclase activity in isolated cells prepared in a hypotonic medium. This action might also account for the activation of iodide oxidative metabolism and for the stimulation of amino acid incorporation into proteins. It is more doubtful that it may account for the increase of glucose oxidation, as this effect in beef slices may not be mediated by cAMP (Section V,D,2). It is not surprising that epinephrine does not reproduce TSH action on phospholipid metabolism as it is becoming unlikely that this TSH effect is mediated by cAMP (Section VIII,C,4).

2. Prostaglandins

Prostaglandin E_1 (PGE$_1$) inhibits the activation of adenyl cyclase by several hormones in fat cells, but enhances the accumulation of cAMP in numerous tissues, e.g., lung, spleen, diaphragm, testis (R. W. Butcher and Baird, 1968). Various prostaglandins, including PGE$_1$, activate sheep, beef, and dog thyroid adenyl cyclase (Ahn and Rosenberg, 1970a; Burke, 1970a; Wolff and Jones, 1970). PGE$_2$ increases the cAMP content (Zor et al., 1969b) and PGE$_1$ enhances the formation of ^{14}C-cAMP from adenine (Ahn and Rosenberg, 1970a) and the cAMP content (Dekker and Field, 1970) in dog thyroid slices. If PGE$_1$ increases cAMP accumulation in thyroid tissue, it should mimic the cAMP-mediated TSH effects. Indeed PGE$_1$ activates iodide organification (Rodesch et al., 1969; Ahn and Rosenberg, 1970a) and iodothyronine synthesis (Ahn and Rosenberg, 1970a), glucose carbon-1 oxidation (Rodesch et al., 1969; Zor et al.,

1969a; Onaya and Solomon, 1970) and, contrary to a previous report, (Rodesch *et al.*, 1969) intracellular colloid droplet formation in dog thyroid slices (Onaya and Solomon, 1970; Willems *et al.*, 1970). The latter results have been confirmed by electron microscopy, which showed in addition that PGE_1, like TSH, induces the formation of numerous pseudopods at the apex of the follicular cells (Nève and Dumont, 1970b). PGE_1 and other prostaglandins also enhance the release of ^{131}I from prelabeled mouse thyroid *in vivo* (Burke, 1970a; Onaya and Solomon, 1970). This effect may take place at the level of the pituitary. However, PGE_1 also enhances thyroid secretion from dog thyroid slices *in vitro* (Ahn and Rosenberg, 1970b; Willems *et al.*, 1970). The latter effect is not constant and the range of effective PGE_1 concentrations may vary.

PGE_1 failed to mimic the TSH-stimulation of $^{32}P_i$ incorporation into the phospholipids of dog thyroid slices (Zor *et al.*, 1969a). However, the concentration of PGE_1 used stimulated glucose carbon-1 oxidation to the same extent as TSH (0.5 mU/ml), and the results suggest that such a concentration of TSH would also have little effect on phospholipid turnover. Similarly, Burke (1970a) reported that while various prostaglandins mimicked the effects of TSH on adenyl cyclase, glucose oxidation, and droplet formation in sheep thyroid particulates and slices, they did not reproduce the stimulation of $^{32}P_i$-incorporation into phospholipids. Unfortunately, the authors did not check whether the prostaglandins by themselves had any inhibitory action on the latter TSH effect. Furthermore, while in the adenyl cylcase experiment prostaglandins only approached the efficiency of TSH at 10–20 mU/ml, concentrations of TSH of 250–500 mU/ml were used in the slice experiment. Therefore, these experiments are not conclusive.

The available evidence suggests that PGE_1 enhances cAMP accumulation in dog thyroid slices and by this mechanism mimics the effects of TSH on glucose C-1 oxidation, iodide organification, and colloid phagocytosis. The failure of prostaglandins to mimic the TSH stimulation of phospholipid metabolism, although not completely established, supports the conclusion that at least part of this TSH effect is not mediated by cAMP.

3. *Fluoride*

Fluoride is the most potent activator of adenyl cyclase in homogenates of thyroid (Pastan and Katzen, 1967) and of other tissues. It is reported not to act in intact cells presumably because of its poor penetration (Robison *et al.*, 1968). However, in relatively high concentrations (10 mM) fluoride inhibits glycolysis in sheep thyroid slices the same as in other tissues (Dumont, 1966), which demonstrates its penetration into the cells. At high enough concentrations, fluoride should therefore mimic the cAMP-mediated TSH effects that it does not inhibit by different mechanisms. Indeed, fluoride activates glucose carbon-1 oxidation in sheep (Dumont and Burelle, 1964), beef (Pastan et al., 1968), and dog (O'Malley and Field, 1964; Rodesch et al., 1969) thyroid slices, glucose C-6 oxidation in sheep and beef thyroid slices (Dumont, 1966; Pastan et al., 1968), iodide organification (Rodesch et al., 1969; Ahn and Rosenberg, 1970a) and iodothyronine synthesis (Ahn and Rosenberg, 1970a) in dog thyroid slices and ^{32}P-phosphate incorporation into phospholipids in beef (Pastan and Macchia, 1967) and sheep (Burke, 1970f) thyroid slices. Burke (1970f) reported that when Krebs-Ringer bicarbonate medium was replaced by physiological saline the stimulation of phospholipid metabolism by TSH and NaF was enhanced while the effects of both agents on glucose C-1 oxidation were nearly abolished. Whatever its mechanism, the mimicry by fluoride of TSH action is striking. However, there are discrepancies.

Fluoride is not a specific agent. Besides its action on adenyl cyclase, it inhibits many enzymes, e.g., enolase, tributyrinase, mitochondrial ATPase, etc. Therefore, it is not surprising that the actions of TSH and NaF on the thyroid *in vitro* differ in several respects. At high concentrations, NaF (>9 mM) enhances more glucose C-6 than glucose C-1 oxidation (Dumont, 1966; Pastan et al., 1968). This has been interpreted as evidence that at such concentrations fluoride does not affect enolase (Pastan et al., 1968). This argument is not valid, because glucose C-6 oxidation is not a good index of glycolysis, but measures the amount of glucose which is completely oxidized through the Embden-Meyerhof pathway and the Krebs cycle, i.e., only a small proportion of the glucose metabolized through the Embden-Meyerhof pathway (Dumont and Tonteur-Montenez, 1965). In fact, NaF, 50 mM, greatly inhibits the Embden-Meyerhof pathway and mitochondrial activity (as shown by reductions in lactate formation of 78%, glucose uptake of 33%, and oxygen uptake of 27%), but still increases glucose carbon-6 oxidation by 101%, presumably by increasing considerably the proportion of pyruvate that is completely oxidized (Dumont, 1966). Therefore, the action of NaF on glucose oxidation seems to reflect two effects: the activation of the pentose phosphate pathway and the inhibition of glycolysis. The latter effect becomes more prevalent at high concentrations.

Another difference between the actions of TSH and NaF on the thyroid is the failure of NaF to induce the formation of colloid droplets in the follicular cells of dog thyroid slices (Pastan et al., 1968; Rodesch et al., 1969). This discrepancy would weigh against the hypothesis that NaF activates thyroid adenyl cyclase, if, as reported by Pastan et al. (1968),

NaF by itself did not inhibit the formation of intracellular colloid droplets induced by TSH. However, in our preparations, with concentrations of NaF (5 mM) giving reproducible stimulation of glucose C-1 oxidation, and concentrations of TSH equal to or lower than the concentrations giving a maximal effect on colloid droplet formation (1 mU/ml), NaF completely inhibits the effect of TSH on colloid droplet formation (Willems and Dumont, 1969). As NaF *per se* appears to inhibit colloid droplet formation, it is not surprising that it fails to elicit this response. In the experiments of Pastan *et al.* (1968), the inhibitory effect of NaF may have been masked because a supramaximal concentration of TSH was used (50 mU/ml).

Three arguments are presented by Burke (1970f) against the hypothesis that fluoride and TSH might act at the same site in thyroid slices: (1) There was no synergism between the effects of these compounds on glucose oxidation or phosphate-^{32}P incorporation into phospholipids in sheep thyroid slices; in fact the effects were additive. (2) Ineffective concentrations of TSH were not potentiated by NaF. (3) Stimulation of glucose oxidation or phospholipid metabolism by maximally effective concentrations of NaF was enhanced by the addition of TSH (Zor *et al.*, 1969a; Burke, 1970f). In fact, since NaF action is clearly biphasic, maximally effective concentrations of NaF may well have both stimulatory and inhibitory actions.

We believe that these arguments do not bear very heavily against the validity of the hypothesis. However, it is probable that NaF and TSH act on different sites of the thyroid adenyl cyclase system just as NaF and hormones do in other tissues. Burke (1970b) has reported that phentolamine and propanolol greatly inhibit the action of TSH but not of NaF on the particulate enzyme system.

A very much more relevant argument against the hypothesis that NaF mimics the TSH effects on the intact follicle cell by activating adenyl cyclase is the failure of NaF, 10 mM, to increase the cAMP content of dog thyroid slices (Kaneko *et al.*, 1969; Zor *et al.*, 1969b; Ahn and Rosenberg, 1970a). Even this argument is not completely convincing in the absence of data on the kinetics and concentration–action relationship of NaF action.

In conclusion, the available evidence tends to be against the hypothesis that NaF affects the metabolism of intact thyroid cells by activating adenyl cyclase but does not rule it out. If this hypothesis is rejected, other explanations will have to be found for the striking similarities in the action of TSH, cAMP, and NaF. A worthwhile working hypothesis might be that NaF mimics some effects of cAMP by activating the kinases or inhibiting the phosphatases which are involved in the phosphorylation caused by cAMP (Fig. 23). For instance, fluoride inhibits liver glycogen phosphorylase phosphatase (Stalmans *et al.*, 1970) and glycogen synthetase phosphatase activating enzyme (De Wulf *et al.*, 1970). If such were the case, the reproduction of TSH effects by NaF would hint at effects secondary to cAMP-mediated phosphorylations.

4. *Iodide*

Iodide activates the pentose phosphate pathway in sheep thyroid slices; this effect is inhibited by methimazole (Dumont, 1961a; Green and Ingbar, 1963); it is specific for sheep tissue (Jarrett and Field, 1964). Iodide has been reported to activate adenyl cyclase and to inhibit the activation of this enzyme by TSH and PGE$_1$ in a sheep thyroid mitochondrial microsomal fraction. These effects would be inhibited by methimazole (Burke, 1970a). Iodide increases glucose C-1 oxidation in the sheep thyroid slices and would inhibit the action of TSH and PGE$_1$, but also of DB-cAMP on this variable; it would not elicit, as do TSH, PGE$_1$, and DB-cAMP, the formation of intracellular colloid droplets, nor inhibit this action (Burke, 1970d). Unfortunately, no study was performed on the thyroids of another species, the TSH concentrations used with slices and with particulates were very different (500 mU/ml *vs.* 10 mU/ml, respectively), no attempt was made to check whether methimazole relieved the inhibition by iodide in slices, etc. Therefore, it is difficult to reach a firm conclusion at the present time. Nevertheless, the apparent specific action of iodide on sheep thyroids could provide a very useful experimental tool in the study of the role of cAMP in thyroid activation.

B. Agents That Decrease cAMP Accumulation

If effects of TSH are mediated by cAMP, inhibition of TSH action at the level of adenyl cyclase, or inhibition of cAMP accumulation should depress these effects.

1. *α- and β-Adrenergic Inhibitors*

Phentolamine and *dl*-propanolol, α- and β-adrenergic inhibitors, respectively, inhibit the activation by TSH of adenyl cyclase in dog and in beef thyroid homogenates (Levey *et al.*, 1969). These compounds have also been reported to inhibit TSH and prostaglandin activation of adenyl cyclase in sheep thyroid particulates *in vitro* (Burke, 1970a). The observation that the effect of *dl*-propanolol was reproduced by *d*-propanolol and phentolamine suggested that a specific β-adrenergic blockade was not responsible for the inhibition. These compounds did not act on cAMP phosphodiesterase (Levey *et al.*, 1969). In intact cells, inhibitors acting at the adenyl cyclase level should inhibit cAMP-mediated TSH effects but not the action of DB-cAMP or of cAMP. Phentolamine suppresses the stimulation by TSH of glucose C-1 oxidation in dog thyroid slices, at concentrations lower (0.3 mM) than those which have been shown to abolish nearly completely the TSH stimulation of adenyl cyclase activity (0.75 mM) (Levey et al., 1969). However, the published data suggest that phentolamine also decreased the basal level of glucose oxidation and inhibited its activation by DB-cAMP. dl-Propanolol (0.15–0.3 mM) largely reduced the stimulation by TSH of glucose C-1 oxidation in dog thyroid slices (Levey et al., 1969; Zor et al., 1969a). While Levey et al. (1969) observed only a slight decrease and often no inhibition of the DB-cAMP effect, Zor et al., (1969a) observed equal inhibition of the TSH, DB-cAMP, and carbamylcholine effects. Onaya and Solomon (1969) observed that dl-propanolol equally inhibits the actions of TSH and DB-cAMP on glucose oxidation and colloid droplet formation in dog thyroid slices. Similarly, Burke (1969d) reported that dl-propanolol and phentolamine inhibit to the same extent the stimulation by TSH and by DB-cAMP of glucose oxidation and colloid droplet formation by sheep thyroid slices. Therefore, it is doubtful that these effects of dl-propanolol are specific and bear only on adenyl cyclase. When slices were incubated with dl-propanolol and then washed, in a subsequent incubation, glucose C-1 oxidation could still be activated by DB-cAMP but not by TSH (Levey et al., 1969). Under such conditions, dl-propanolol seems to act at the level of adenyl cyclase. Therefore, these data further suggest that the TSH stimulation of glucose C-1 oxidation in dog thyroid slices is mediated by cAMP. On the other hand, concentrations of propanolol which inhibited beef thyroid adenyl cyclase failed to modify the enhancement of glucose C-1 oxidation in beef thyroid slices incubated in the presence of high concentrations of TSH (Levey et al., 1969). These data cast some further doubt on the hypothesis that cAMP may mediate the latter effect of TSH.

2. Other Inhibitors of Adenyl Cyclase: Chlorpromazine, Polyene Antibiotics, Li^+ Ion

Chlorpromazine (0.03 mM), thymol (1.5 mM), and Na dodecyl sulfate (0.25 mM) completely block the activation of beef thyroid adenyl cyclase by TSH. These compounds (chlorpromazine > 0.3 mM) enhance the action of NaF. It has been hypothesized that these effects might result from membrane expansion (Wolff and Jones, 1970). Chlorpromazine (0.2 mM) abolishes the formation of intracellular colloid droplets and inhibits the activation of glucose oxidation in stimulated dog thyroid slices (Onaya et al., 1969). These effects were attributed to "lysosomal stabilization" (Onaya et al., 1969), but Wolff and Jones (1970) explained them by an inhibition of adenyl cyclase. Since chlorpromazine at high concentrations (1 mM) greatly decreases colloid droplet formation in DB-cAMP treated dog thyroid slices (Onaya et al., 1969), it is apparent that such compounds may act at a level beyond adenyl cyclase also. Selective inhibition of adenyl cyclase may require the use of chlorpromazine in a narrow range of concentrations.

Polyene antibiotics (nystatin and filipin) inhibit basal and TSH-stimulated adenyl cyclase activity in dog thyroid particulates (9000 g) preparations; they also depress cAMP levels in stimulated thyroid slices (F. R. Butcher and Serif, 1969). As these antibiotics also inhibit the stimulation by TSH of glucose C-1 oxidation, the authors presented their data as a further argument in favor of the hypothesis that the activation by TSH of glucose oxidation in the thyroid is mediated by cAMP. However, this argument appears irrelevant: in the same study it was shown that the polyene antibiotics equally inhibit the stimulation of glucose oxidation by DB-cAMP and by carbamylcholine.

Li^+ ion (10 mM) inhibits the TSH activation of beef thyroid membrane adenyl cyclase in an acellular system (Wolff et al., 1970). This action may account for some of the acute effects of Li^+ in vivo, e.g., the slowing down of radioiodine release from the thyroid (Berens et al., 1970). It would be of great interest to use this effect for studies on slices.

3. Activators of cAMP Phosphodiesterase

If an effect of TSH is mediated through cAMP, enhancement of cAMP hydrolysis should inhibit this effect of TSH. Little information is available on this topic. Nicotinic acid, which activates phosphodiesterase in other tissues (Robison et al., 1968), was reported not to inhibit the stimulation by TSH of glucose C-1 oxidation in dog thyroid slices (Field et al., 1963). In our dog thyroid slice preparations, imidazole, 5 mM, which is also reported to activate phosphodiesterase (Robison et al., 1968) did not inhibit the stimulation by TSH of glucose C-1 oxidation or iodide organification (Willems and Dumont, 1969). In the absence of any evidence that these compounds actually activated cAMP hydrolysis in the intact cells, interpretation of such data is impossible.

XI. CONCLUSION

Thyrotropin activates thyroid adenyl cyclase and thereby causes the accumulation of cyclic 3′,5′-AMP in the thyroid. There is strong evidence that the TSH stimulation of iodide trapping, iodide organification, iodothyronine synthesis, colloid endocytosis, thyroid hormone secretion, glycolysis, glucose oxidation by the pentose phosphate pathway in dog thyroid slices, and amino acid incorporation into proteins and the TSH inhibition of glucose oxidation by the pentose phosphate pathway in beef and human thyroid slices are mediated by intracellular cAMP. Thus there is strong support for the hypothesis that TSH exerts these effects by the stimulation of thyroidal adenyl cyclase. Nevertheless, even for these effects, all criteria proposed to assess the validity of a mechanism of hormonal action have not yet been fulfilled. In particular, correlations between TSH concentration-effect relationships for cAMP accumulation in acellular systems or in intact thyroid cells and for the various effects which seem to be mediated by cAMP are lacking. There is some support for the hypothesis that cAMP also mediates the TSH stimulation of glucose uptake, NADP synthesis, RNA synthesis and growth, and, therefore, that these effects are also secondary to the activation of adenyl cyclase by TSH. For two TSH effects, the stimulation of phospholipid metabolism and the activation of the pentose phosphate pathway by high concentrations of hormone, there are good indications that cAMP may not be involved. While the latter effect is of doubtful physiological significance, the former seems to be of great, if still unknown, importance in the action of TSH.

The problem of the mechanism of action of cAMP in the thyroid follicle cell is part of the more general problem of the action of the nucleotide in differentiated cells. The specificity of this action in a cell is determined by the differentiated state of this cell. From the numerous recent studies on the action of cAMP in different types of cells, a general working hypothesis is emerging (Fig. 23). cAMP would activate protein kinase(s) which by phosphorylating different proteins would in its/their turn activate these proteins. The action of cAMP would correspond to the activation of reactions catalyzed by the phosphorylated proteins (Corbin and Krebs, 1969; Kuo and Greengaard, 1969). cAMP would activate protein kinase by binding to a regulatory subunit of the enzyme, thus detaching this inhibitory subunit and activating the catalytic subunit (Gill and Garren, 1970; Tao et al., 1970). Bovine thyroid contains cAMP-activated protein kinase(s) (Kuo et al., 1970). The proteins phosphorylated by protein kinase(s) could also be protein kinases. Such a mechanism would add further steps in the cascade (Bowness, 1966; Larner, 1966) of cAMP action. Effects of cAMP secondary to protein phosphorylation may involve effects at the level of the enzyme system (e.g., in the activation of lipase or lipase activating system) (Corbin et al., 1970; Huttunen et al., 1970) and effects at the level of enzyme synthesis [e.g., in the stimulation of the synthesis of hepatic enzymes by

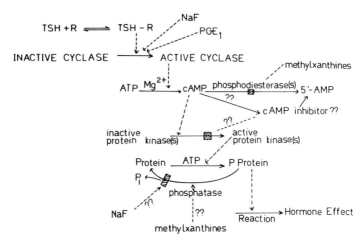

FIG. 23. Hypothetical scheme of cascade effects and feedback loop in the mechanism of action of thyrotropin (TSH) by the cyclic 3′,5′-adenosine monophosphate (cAMP) system. *P Protein:* phosphorylated protein; *R*: TSH receptor; - - - - - ->: activation; - - - - - - ▨ : inhibition.

glucagon, perhaps secondary to histone phosphorylation (Wicks, 1969; Langan, 1969)]. In fact, until now no effect of cAMP in nucleated cells has been proved not to be due to the activation of the phosphorylation of an enzyme. The only case in which there is some indication of such a process is the activation of phosphofructokinase (Mansour, 1966; Hoskins and Stephens, 1970). However, in this case the concentration of cAMP required is high. The cascade concept of hormone and cAMP action which emerges would explain many facets of hormone action: the great amplification from stimulus to action, the wide range of time response relationships, the great possibilities of regulation.

Although the scheme outlined represents a very useful conceptual framework, many questions should still be asked about TSH action within and beyond this framework. Are there other adenyl cyclases in subcellular organelles other than the plasma membrane? How does TSH interact with its "receptor" and the receptor with adenyl cyclase? Is the level of adenyl cyclase regulated, for instance, does it increase in chronically stimulated tissue? With regard to cAMP action, the problem of storage and redistribution of cAMP in the cell should be investigated. Indeed, the release of large amounts of cAMP in the incubation medium of stimulated fat cells (Moskowitz and Fain, 1970) suggests that permeability barriers to cAMP could play an important role in hormone action. In this regard it would be of the utmost importance to compare TSH concentration-effect relationships for cAMP accumulation and other TSH effects. To facilitate such comparisons despite the variability of tissue sensitivity and hormone, perhaps the study of this relationship for one type of effect should always include a reference curve for another well defined TSH effect. The stimulation of iodide organification, which is an easy, sensitive, and reproducible effect of TSH, could be such a reference (Rodesch et al., 1969). The number and characteristics of thyroid phosphodiesterase(s), protein kinase(s), and phosphatases, the substrate specificities of the latter enzymes, as well as the possible role of the cAMP inhibitor derived from cAMP (Murad et al., 1969) and the mechanism of cAMP action on protein synthesis and tissue growth are questions of great interest. The action of NaF and methylxanthines on the phosphatases or phosphatase activating enzyme(s) could explain the striking mimicry of TSH action by fluoride, and the divergent results obtained on the action of methylxanthines on intact cells.

Besides this cascade model, other hypotheses should be investigated. One of these is the possible existence of cellular secondary messengers in the organ, i.e., the possibility that in response to TSH some thyroid cells would release secondary messengers (e.g., prostaglandins) which would then activate the follicle cells. The comparison of the response to TSH in systems with intact structural spatial relationship such as the slice, to disorganized systems, such as the isolated cell, in which secondary messengers would be diluted in the large volume of incubation medium, could provide clues about the existence of such messengers. The mechanisms of non-cAMP-mediated TSH effects and the possibility that these effects could be secondary to the accumulation of other intracellular messengers than cAMP (e.g., cGMP) should be considered. The role of Ca^{2+} in TSH action should be clarified. It is already known that in Ca^{2+}-depleted cells some TSH effects are abolished or inhibited, such as the activation of the pentose phosphate pathway (Dumont and Van Sande, 1965; Zor et al., 1968), or of iodide organification (Willems and Dumont, 1970), whereas other effects are not affected, such as the stimulation of cAMP accumulation (Dekker and Field, 1970), of phospholipid metabolism (Zor et al., 1968), of colloid endocytosis, and of secretion (Willems and Dumont, 1970).

ACKNOWLEDGMENTS

The work from this laboratory which is reported in this review was mainly carried out under Contract Euratom–University of Brussels–University of Pisa (No. 026-63-4 BIAC) (contribution No. 649 of the Biology Department, Euratom), and was helped through grants No. 022 of the Fonds de la Recherche Fondamentale Collective and No. 1011 of the Fonds de la Recherche Scientifique Médicale.

The author thanks Miss C. Borrey and Miss J. Hennaux, who prepared the manuscript and drew the figures.

REFERENCES

Abraham, S., Kopelovich, L., Kerkof, P. R., and Chaikoff, I. L. (1965). *Endocrinology* **76**, 178.

Adiga, P. R., Murthy, P. V. N., and McKenzie, J. M. (1971). *Biochemistry* **10**, 702.

Ahn, C. S., and Rosenberg, I. N. (1967). *Endocrinology* **81**, 1319.

Ahn, C. S., and Rosenberg, I. N. (1968). *Proc. Nat. Acad. Sci. U. S.* **60**, 830.

Ahn, C. S., and Rosenberg, I. N. (1970a). *Endocrinology* **86**, 396.

Ahn, C. S., and Rosenberg, I. N. (1970b). *Endocrinology* **86**, 870.

Ahn, C. S., and Rosenberg, I. N. (1970c). *Abstr. Int. Thyroid Conf., 6th, 1970*, p. 109.

Ahn, C. S., Athans, J. C., and Rosenberg, I. N. (1969). *Endocrinology* **85**, 224.

Al-Hindawi, A. Y., and Wilson, G. M. (1965). *Clin. Sci.* **28**, 555.

Altman, M., Oka, H., and Field, J. B. (1966). *Biochim. Biophys. Acta* **116**, 586.

Ansell, G. B., and Hawthorne, J. N. (1964) "Phospholipids," p. 273. Elsevier, Amsterdam.

Apps, D. K. (1968). *Eur. J. Biochem.* **5**, 444.

Bakke, J. L., Lawrence, N., and Roy, S. (1962). *Endocrinology* **22**, 352.

Balasubramaniam, K., and Deiss, W. P. (1965). *Biochim. Biophys. Acat* **110**, 564.

Balasubramaniam, K., Deiss, W. P., Tan, W. C., and Powell, R. C. (1965). *Endocrinology* **77**, 54.

Bartke, A. (1968). *Gen. Comp. Endocrinol.* **11**, 246.

Bastomsky, C. H., and McKenzie, J. M. (1967). *Amer. J. Physiol.* **213**, 753.

Bastomsky, C. H., and McKenzie, J. M. (1968). *Endocrinology* **83**, 309.

Bastomsky, C. H., and Rosenberg, I. N. (1966). *Endocrinology* **79**, 505.

Bates, R. W., and Condliffe, P. G. (1960). *Recent Progr. Horm. Res.* **16**, 309.

Bates, R. W., and Warren, L. (1963). *Endocrinology* **73**, 1.

Bauduin, H., Reuse, J., and Dumont, J. E. (1967). *Life Sci.* **6**, 1723.

Bauer, W. C., and Meyer, J. S. (1965). *Lab. Invest.* **14**, 1795.

Begg, D. J., and Munro, H. N. (1965). *Nature (London)* **207**, 483.

Belotti, R., and Ravera, M. (1954). *Arch. "E. Maragliano" Patol. Clin.* **9**, 1077.

Bénard, J., and Brault, J. (1970). *Abstr. Int. Thyroid Conf., 6th, 1970* p. 101.

Bénard, B., and Degroot, L. J. (1969). *Biochim. Biophys. Acta* **184**, 48.

Bengmark, S., Heiman, P., and Tengroth, B. (1963). *Acta Morphol. Neer.-Scand.* **5**, 361.

Berens, S. C., Bernstein, R. S., Robbins, J., and Wolff, J. (1970). *J. Clin. Invest.* **49**, 1357.

Blakley, R. L., and Vitols, E. (1968). *Annu. Rev. Biochem.* **37**, 201.

Blecher, M., Ro'Ane, J. T., and Flynn, P. D. (1970). *J. Biol. Chem.* **245**, 1867.

Borell, V. (1945). *Acta Med. Scand., Suppl.* **161**.

Botkin, A. L., Eskelson, C. D., Firsheim, H. E., and Jensen, H. (1954). *J. Clin. Endocrinol. Metab.* **14**, 1219.

Bowness, J. M. (1966). *Science* **152**, 1370.

Bradley, A. S., and Wissig, S. L. (1966). *J. Cell Biol.* **30**, 433.

Britten, R. J., and Davidson, E. H. (1969). *Science* **165**, 349.

Brown, J., and Munro, D. S. (1967). *J. Endocrinol.* **38**, 439.

Brown, J. R. (1959). *Acta Endocrinol. (Copenhagen)* **32**, 289.

Brown-Grant, K. (1969). *J. Basic Eng.* **12**, 313.

Brown-Grant, K., von Euler, C., Harris, G. W., and Reichlin, S. (1954). *J. Physiol. (London)* **126**, 1.

Brunberg, J. A., and Halmi, N. S. (1966). *Endocrinology* 79, 801.
Burke, G. (1968a). *J. Clin. Endocrinol. Metab.* 28, 1816.
Burke, G. (1968b). *Endocrinology* 83, 495.
Burke, G. (1968c). *Endocrinology* 83, 1210.
Burke, G. (1969a). *Endocrinology* 84, 1055.
Burke, G. (1969b). *Metab., Clin. Exp.* 18, 132.
Burke, G. (1969c). *Metab., Clin. Exp.* 18, 720.
Burke, G. (1969d). *Metab., Clin. Exp.* 18, 961.
Burke, G. (1970a). *Amer. J. Physiol.* 218, 1445.
Burke, G. (1970b). *Endocrinology* 86, 346.
Burke, G. (1970c). *Endocrinology* 86, 353.
Burke, G. (1970d). *J. Clin. Endocrinol. Metab.* 30, 76.
Burke, G. (1970e). *Life Sci.* 9, 789.
Burke, G. (1970f). *Metab., Clin. Exp.* 19, 35.
Butcher, F. R., and Serif, G. S. (1967). *Biochim. Biophys. Acta* 141, 8.
Butcher, F. R., and Serif, G. S. (1968). *Biochim. Biophys. Acta* 156, 59.
Butcher, F. R., and Serif, G. S. (1969). *Biochim. Biophys. Acta* 192, 409.
Butcher, R. W., and Baird, C. E. (1968). *J. Biol. Chem.* 243, 1713.
Canellakis, E. S. (1962). *Annu. Rev. Biochem.* 31, 271.
Cavalieri, R. R., and Searle, G. L. (1967). *Proc. Soc. Exp. Biol. Med.* 126, 459.
Chow, S. Y., and Woodbury, D. M. (1965). *Endocrinology* 77, 825.
Clayton, J. A., and Szego, C. M. (1967). *Endocrinology* 80, 689.
Colby, C., and Edlin, G. (1970). *Biochemistry* 9, 917.
Corbin, J. D., and Krebs, E. G. (1969). *Biochem. Biophys. Res. Commun.* 36, 328.
Corbin, J. D., Reimann, E. M., Walsh, D. A., and Krebs, E. G. (1970). *J. Biol. Chem.* 245, 4849.
Creek, R. O. (1965). *Endocrinology* 76, 1124.
Daniel, P. M., Plaskett, L. G., and Pratt, O. E. (1967a). *J. Physiol. (London)* 188, 25.
Daniel, P. M., Pratt, O. E., Roitt, I. M., and Torrigiani, G. (1967b). *Immunology* 12, 489.
Dawson, R. M. C. (1966). *Essays Biochem.* 2, 69.
Debons, A. F., and Pittman, J. A. (1962). *Endocrinology* 70, 937.
Debons, A. F., and Pittman, J. A. (1966). *Amer. J. Physiol.* 210, 395.
de Duve, C., and Wattiaux, R. (1966). *Annu. Rev. Physiol.* 28, 435.
Degroot, L. J. (1965). *N. Engl. J. Med.* 272, 243.
Degroot, L. J., and Dunn, A. D. (1968). *Endocrinology* 78, 1032.
Degrott, L. J., Dunn, A. D., and Jaksina, S. (1966). *Endocrinology* 79, 28.
Dekker, A., and Field, J. B. (1970). *Metab., Clin. Exp.* 19, 453.
Delcroix, C., and Dumont, J. E. (1969). Unpublished data.
Dempsey, E. W., and Peterson, R. R. (1955). *Endocrinology* 56, 46.
De Robertis, E. (1941). *Anat. Rec.* 80, 219.
Desbarats-Schönbaum, M. L., Sellers, E. A., Laansoo, M., Koues, E., and Schönbaum, E. (1970). *Acta Endocrinol. (Copenhagen)* 64, 133.
De Wulf, H., Stalmans, W., and Mers, H. G. (1970). *Eur. J. Biochem.* 15, 1.
Dickson, J. A. (1966). *Endocrinology* 79, 721.
Douglas, W. W. (1968). *Brit. J. Pharmacol.* 34, 451.
Dumont, J. E. (1961a). *Biochim. Biophys. Acta* 46, 195.
Dumont, J. E. (1961b). *Biochim. Biophys. Acta* 50, 506.
Dumont, J. E. (1961c). *C. R. Soc. Biol.* 155, 2225.

Dumont, J. E. (1962). *Biochim. Biophys. Acta* **56**, 382.

Dumont, J. E. (1964). *Bull. Soc. Chim. Biol.* **46**, 1131.

Dumont, J. E. (1965). *Ann. Soc. Roy. Sci. Med. Natur. Bruxelles* **18**, 111.

Dumont, J. E. (1966). *Bull. Soc. Chim. Biol.* **48**, 419.

Dumont, J. E. (1968). *Bull. Soc. Chim. Biol.* **50**, 2401.

Dumont, J. E., and Burelle, R. (1964). *C. R. Soc. Biol.* **158**, 2500.

Dumont, J. E., and Eloy, J. (1966). *Bull. Soc. Chim. Biol.* **48**, 155.

Dumont, J. E., and Lecocq, R. E. (1970). Unpublished results.

Dumont, J. E., and Rocmans, P. (1964). *J. Physiol. (London)* **174**, 26.

Dumont, J. E., and Rocmans, P. (1965). *Proc. Int. Congr. Endocrinol., 2nd, 1964* p. 81.

Dumont, J. E., and Tondeur-Montenez, T. (1965). *Biochim. Biophys. Acta* **111**, 258

Dumont, J. E., and Van Sande, J. (1965). *Bull. Soc. Chim. Biol.* **47**, 321.

Dumont, J. E., Lecocq, R., and Lamy, F. (1969a). *Proc. Int. Congr. Endocrinol., 3rd, 1968* p. 659.

Dumont, J. E., Nève, P., and Otten, J. (1969b). *In* "Endemic Goiter" (J. B. Stanbury, ed.), p. 14. World Health Organ., Washington, D. C.

Ekholm, R., and Elmqvist, L. G. (1967). *Exp. Cell Res.* **48**, 640.

Ekholm, R., and Pantic, V. (1963). *Nature (London)* **199**, 1203.

Ekholm, R., and Smeds, S. (1966). *J. Ultrastruct. Res.* **16**, 71.

Ekholm, R., Smeds, S., and Stranberg, U. (1966). *Exp. Cell Res.* **43**, 506.

Ensor, J. M., and Munro, D. S. (1969). *J. Endocrinol.* **43**, 477.

Farnararo, M., Sgaragli, G., Bigazzi, M., and Melani, F. (1968). *Life Sci.* **7**, 667.

Fiala, S., Sproul, E. E., and Fiala, A. E. (1957). *Proc. Soc. Exp. Biol. Med.* **94**, 517.

Field, J. B. (1965). *Curr. Top. Thyroid Res., Proc. Int. Thyroid Conf., 5th, 1965* p. 581.

Field, J. B. (1968). *Metab., Clin. Exp.* **17**, 226.

Field, J. B., Pastan, I., Johnson, P., and Herring, B. (1960). *J. Biol. Chem.* **235**, 1863.

Field, J. B., Pastan, I., Herring, B., and Johnson, P. (1961). *Biochim. Biophys. Acta* **50**, 513.

Field, J. B., Johnson, P., Kendig, E., and Pastan, I. (1963). *J. Biol. Chem.* **238**, 1189.

Field, J. B., Remer, A. K., and Epstein, S. M. (1965). *J. Biol. Chem.* **240**, 883.

Field, J. B., Epstein, S. M., Remer, A. K., and Boyle, C. (1966). *Biochim. Biophys. Acta* **121**, 241.

Florsheim, W. H., Moskowitz, N., Schwartz, J. R., anid Morton, M. E. (1957). *Endocrinology* **60**, 683.

Freinkel, N. (1957). *Endocrinology* **61**, 448.

Freinkel, N. (1958). *Biochem. J.* **68**, 327.

Freinkel, N. (1960). *Endocrinology* **66**, 851.

Freinkel, N. (1961). *J. Clin. Invest.* **40**, 476.

Freinkel, N. (1963). *Nature (London)* **198**, 889.

Freinkel, N. (1964). *In* "The Thyroid Gland" (R. Pitt-Rivers and W. R. Trotter, eds.), p. 131. Butterworth, London.

Freinkel, N. (1965). *In* "Metabolism and Physiological Significance of Lipids" (R. M. C. Dawson and D. N. Rhodes, eds.), p. 455. Wiley, New York.

Freinkel, N., and Ingbar, S. H. (1955). *J. Clin. Endocrinol. Metab.* **15**, 598.

Freinkel, N., and Scott, T. W. (1964). *Nature (London)* **204**, 1313.

Futterman, S., and Kinoshita, J. H. (1959). *J. Biol. Chem.* **234**, 3174.

Gedda, O. P. (1960). *Acta Endocrinol. (Copenhagen), Suppl.* **56**, 1, 93.

Gersh, I., and Casperson, T. (1940). *Anat. Rec.* **78**, 303.

Gholson, R. K. (1966). *Nature (London)* **212**, 933.

Gibadulin, R. A. (1962). *Bull. Exp. Biol. Med. (USSR)* **54**, 84.

Gill, G. N., and Garren, L. D. (1969). *Proc. Nat. Acad. Sci. U. S.* **63**, 512.

Gill, G. N.. and Garren. L. D. (1970). *Biochem. Biophys. Res. Commun.* **39**, 335.

Gilman, A. G., and Rall, T. W. (1968a). *J. Biol. Chem.* **243**, 5867.

Gilman, A. G., and Rall, T. W. (1968b). *J. Biol. Chem.* **243**, 5872.

Gonze, J., and Tyler, D. D. (1965). *Biochim. Biophys. Res. Commun.* **19**, 67.

Goodman, D. P., Rasmussen, H., Dibella, F., and Guthrow, C. E. (1970). *Proc. Nat. Acad. Sci. U. S.* **67**, 652.

Gorbman, A., and Ueda, K. (1968). *Gen. Comp. Endocrinol.* **3**, 308.

Goss, R. J. (1967). *In* "Control of the Cellular Growth in the Adult Organisms" (H. Teir and I. Rytömaa, eds.), p. 3. Academic Press, New York.

Graig, F. A. (1967). *Endocrinology* **81**, 708.

Graig, F. A., and Smith, J. C. (1967). *Science* **156**, 254.

Green, W. L. (1970). *Endocrinology* **86**, 706.

Green, W. L., and Ingbar, S. H. (1963). *J. Clin. Invest.* **42**, 1802.

Greer, M. A. (1959). *Endocrinology* **64**, 724.

Greif, R. L., and Eich, E. F. (1969). *Endocrinology* **85**, 855.

Greig, W. R., Smith, J. F. B., Duguid, W. P., Foster, C. J., and Orr, J. S. (1969). *Int. J. Radiat. Biol.* **16**, 211.

Gross, J., and Gafni, M. (1968). *Abstr. Int. Congr. Endocrinol., 3rd, 1968* p. 15.

Gulyassi, P. F. (1968). *J. Clin. Invest.* **47**, 2548.

Gyllensten, L., Jalling, B., and Tiden, U. (1959). *Acta Physiol. Scand.* **47**, 328.

Hajos, F., Straznicky, K., and Mess, B. (1964). *Acta Biol. Acad. Sci. Hung.* **15**, 237.

Hall, R. (1962). *Biochim. Biophys. Acta* **61**, 530.

Hall, R. (1963). *J. Biol. Chem.* **238**, 306.

Hall, R., and Tubmen, J. (1965). *J. Biol. Chem.* **240**, 3132.

Hall, R., and Tubmen, J. (1968). *J. Biol. Chem.* **243**, 1598.

Halmi, N. S. (1961). *Vitam. Horm. (New York)* **19**, 133.

Halmi, N. S., Granner, D. K., Doughman, D. J., Peters, B. H., and Muller, G. (1960). *Endocrinology* **67**, 70.

Halmi, N. S., Westra, J. P., and Polly, R. E. (1966). *Endocrinology* **79**, 424.

Harris, H. (1963). *Progr. Nucl. Acid Res.* **2**, 19.

Hershman, J. M. (1967). *Metab., Clin. Exp.* **16**, 279.

Hess, M. E., Hottenstein, D., Shanfeld, J., and Haugaard, N. (1963). *J. Pharmacol. Exp. Therap.* **141**, 274.

Heywood, S. M. (1966). *Biochim. Biophys. Acta* **123**, 188.

Hilz, H., and Tarnowski, W. (1970). *Biochem. Biophys. Res. Commun.* **40**, 973.

Hoskins, D. D., and Stephens, D. T. (1970). *Biochim. Biophys. Acta* **191**, 292.

Hupka, S., and Dumont, J. E. (1963). *Biochem. Pharmacol.* **12**, 1023.

Huttunen, J. K., Steinberg, D., and Mayer, S. E. (1970). *Proc. Nat. Acad. Sci. U. S.* **67**, 290.

Imbenotte, J., Nataf, B., and Harel, J. (1969). *Bull. Soc. Chim. Biol.* **51**, 428.

Ingbar, S. H., and Galton, V. A. (1963). *Annu. Rev. Physiol.* **25**, 361.

Inoue, K., Grimm, Y., and Greer, M. A. (1967). *Endocrinology* **81**, 946.

Irie, M., and Slingerland, D. W. (1963). *Endocrinology* **73**, 265.

Isaacs, G. H., and Rosenberg, I. N. (1967). *Endocrinology* **81**, 981.

Isaacs, G. H., Athans, J. L., and Rosenberg, I. N. (1966). *J. Clin. Invest.* **45**, 758.

Jacquemin, C., and Haye, B. (1970). *Bull. Soc. Chim. Biol.* **52**, 153.

Jarrett, R. J., and Field, J. B. (1964). *Endocrinology* **75**, 711.

406   J. E. DUMONT

Jolin, T., Morreale de Escobar, G., and Esocbar del Rey, F. (1968). *Endocrinology* **83**, 620.
Jolin, T., Morreale de Escobar, G., and Escobar del Rey, F. (1970). *Endocrinology* **87**, 99.
Jost, J. P., Hsie, A., Hugues, S. D., and Ryan, L. (1970). *J. Biol. Chem.* **245**, 351.
Junqueira, L. C. (1947). *Endocrinology* **40**, 286.
Kabat, D. (1970). *Biochemistry*, **9**, 4160.
Kaellis, E., and Goldsmith, E. D. (1965). *Acta Endocrinol. (Copenhagen)* **48**, Suppl. 95, 1.
Kakiuchi, S., Rall, T. W., and McIlwain, M. (1969). *J. Neurochem.* **16**, 485.
Kaneko, T., Zor, U., and Field, J. B. (1969). *Science* **163**, 1062.
Kaneko, T., Zor, U., and Field, J. B. (1970). *Metab., Clin. Exp.* **19**, 430.
Kapitola, J., Schullerova, M., and Schreiberova, O. (1970). *Acta Endocrinol. (Copenhagen)* **65**, 435.
Karnoŭsky, M. L. (1962). *Physiol. Rev.* **42**, 143.
Katakai, S., Yamada, T., and Schichijo, K. (1966). *Metab., Clin. Exp.* **15**, 271.
Katz, J., and Wood, H. G. (1963). *J. Biol. Chem.* **238**, 517.
Kendall-Taylor, and Munro, D. S. (1970). *J. Endocrinol.* **47**, 333.
Kerkof, P. R., and Tata, J. R. (1967). *Biochem. Biophys. Res. Commun.* **28**, 111.
Kerkof, P. R., and Tata, J. R. (1969). *Biochem. J.* **112**, 729.
Kerkof, P. R., Raghupathy, E., and Chaikoff, I. L. (1964). *Endocrinology* **75**, 537.
Khairallah, E. A., and Pitot, H. C. (1967). *Biochem. Biophys. Res. Commun.* **29**, 269.
Kirkham, K. E. (1966). *Vitam. Horm. (New York)* **24**, 173.
Klainer, L. M., Chi, Y. M., Freidberg, S. L., Rall, T. W., and Sutherland, E. W. (1962). *J. Biol. Chem.* **237**, 1239.
Klitgaard, H. M., Meade, R. C., Trocke, D. K., Palay, H. J., and Lorscheider, F. L. (1965). *Proc. Soc. Exp. Biol. Med.* **119**, 334.
Knopp, J., Stolc, V., and Tong, W. (1970). *J. Biol. Chem.* **245**, 4403.
Kögl, F., and Van Deenen, L. L. M. (1961). *Acta Endocrinol. (Copenhagen)* **36**, 9.
Kondo, Y. (1961a). *J. Biochem. (Tokyo)* **50**, 135.
Kondo, Y. (1961b). *J. Biochem. (Tokyo)* **50**, 145.
Kondo, Y. (1961c). *J. Biochem. (Tokyo)* **50**, 210.
Konno, N., and McKenzie, J. M. (1970). *Metab., Clin. Exp.* **19**, 724.
Kosanovic, M., Ekholm, R., Strandberg, U., and Smeds, S. (1968). *Exp. Cell Res.* **52**, 147.
Kotani, M., Seiki, K., Higashida, M., Imanishi, Y., Yamashita, A., Miyamoto, M., and Horii, I. (1968). *Endocrinology* **82**, 1047.
Kriss, J. P., Pleshakov, V., and Chien, J. R. (1964). *J. Clin. Endocrinol. Metab.* **24**, 1005.
Krüskemper, H. L., and Reichertz, P. (1960). *Acta Endocrinol. (Copenhagen)* **34**, 390.
Kuo, J. F., and Greengaard, P. (1969). *Proc. Nat. Acad. Sci. U. S.* **64**, 1349.
Kuo, J. F., Krueger, B. K., Sanes, J. S., and Greengaard, P. (1970). *Biochim. Biophys. Acta* **212**, 79.
Kytomaki, O., and Rinne, U. K. (1963). *Experientia* **19**, 543.
Lamberg, B. A., and Olin-Lamberg, C. (1955). *Acta Endocrinol. (Copenhagen)* **19**, 249.
Lamy, F., and Dumont, J. E. (1970). Unpublished results.

Lamy, F., Rodesch, F., and Dumont, J. E. (1964). *C. R. Soc. Biol.* **158**, 2504.

Lamy, F. M., Rodesch, F. R., and Dumont, J. E. (1967). *Exp. Cell Res.* **46**, 518.

Lamy, F. M., Willems, C., and Dumont, J. E. (1969). Unpublished results.

Langan, T. A. (1968). *Science* **162**, 579.

Langan, T. A. (1969). *Proc. Nat. Acad. Sci. U. S.* **64**, 1276.

Larner, J. (1966). *Trans. N. Y. Acad. Sci.* [2] **29**, 192.

Larsen, P. R., and Wolff, J. (1967). *Science* **155**, 335.

Lecocq, R. E., and Dumont, J. E. (1967). *Biochem. J.* **104**, 13C.

Lecocq, R. E., and Dumont, J. E. (1970). Unpublished results.

Levey, G. S., Roth, J., and Pastan, I. (1969). *Endocrinology* **84**, 1009.

Lindsay, R. H., and Cohen, P. P. (1965). *Endocrinology* **76**, 737.

Lindsay, R. H. (1970). Personal communication.

Lindsay, R. H., Cash, A. G., and Hill, J. B. (1967). *Biochem. Biophys. Res. Commun.* **29**, 850.

Lindsay, R. H., Cash, A. G., and Hill, J. B. (1969). *Endocrinology* **84**, 534.

Lindsay, R. H., Cash, A. G., and Hill, J. B. (1970). *Abstr. Int. Thyroid Conf., 6th, 1970* p. 99.

Lindsay, S. (1963). *Arch. Pathol.* **76**, 257.

Lindsay, S., and Jenks, P. R. (1961). *Advan. Thyroid Res., Trans. Int. Goitre Conf., 4th, 1960* p. 215.

Lissitzky, S., Mante, S., Attali, J. C., and Cartouzou, G. (1969). *Biochem. Biophys. Res. Commun.* **35**, 437.

Loeb, J. E., and Blat, C. (1970). *FEBS Lett.* **10**, 105.

Lupulescu, A., and Petrovici, A. (1968). *In* "Ultrastructure of the Thyroid Gland," p. 150. Heinemann, London.

Maayan, M. L. (1964). *Endocrinology* **75**, 747.

Maayan, M. L. (1968). *Endocrinology* **83**, 938.

Maayan, M. L., and Ingbar, S. H. (1968). *Science* **162**, 124.

Maayan, M. L., and Ingbar, S. H. (1970). *Endocrinology* **87**, 588.

Maayan, M. L., and Rosenberg, I. N. (1963). *Endocrinology* **73**, 38.

Maayan, M. L., and Rosenberg, I. N. (1966). *Endocrinology* **78**, 1049.

Maayan, M. L., and Rosenberg, I. N. (1968). *Endocrinology* **82**, 1223.

Macchia, V., and Pastan, I. (1967). *J. Biol. Chem.* **242**, 1864.

Macchia, V., and Pastan, I. (1968). *Biochim. Biophys. Acta* **152**, 704.

Macchia, V., Meldolesi, M. F., and Maselli, P. (1969). *Endocrinology* **85**, 895.

Macchia, V., Tamburrini, O., and Pastan, I. (1970). *Endocrinology* **86**, 787.

McKenzie, J. M. (1960). *Physiol. Rev.* **40**, 398.

McKenzie, J. M. (1967). *Recent. Progr. Horm. Res.* **23**, 1.

McKenzie, J. M. (1968). *Physiol. Rev.* **48**, 252.

McKenzie, J. M., Adiga, P. R., and Murthy, P. V. N. (1968). *Endocrinology* **83**, 1132.

Malkin, M., and Lipmann, F. (1969). *Proc. Nat. Acad. Sci. U. S.* **64**, 973.

Maloof, F., and Soodak, M. (1963). *Pharmacol. Rev.* **15**, 43.

Mandel, P. (1964). *Progr. Nucl. Acid Res. Mol. Biol.* **3**, 299.

Mansour, T. E. (1966). *Pharmacol. Rev.* **18**, 173.

Matovinovic, J., and Vickery, A. L. (1959). *Endocrinology* **64**, 149.

Matsuda, K., and Greer, M. A. (1965). *Endocrinology* **76**, 1012.

Matsuda, K., Shimoda, S. I., and Greer, M. A. (1964). *Life Sci.* **3**, 251.

Merlevede, W., Weaver, G., and Landau, B. R. (1963). *J. Clin. Invest.* **42**, 1160.

Mockel, J., and Dumont, J. E. (1970). Unpublished data.

Morton, M. E., and Schwartz, J. R. (1953). *Science* **117**, 103.

Moskowitz, J., and Fain, J. N. (1970). *J. Biol. Chem.* **245**, 1101.

Mulvey, P. F., Kelleher, J. J., and Slingerland, D. U. (1962). *Endocrinology* **70**, 481.

Murad, F., Rall, T. W., and Vaughan, M. (1969). *Biochim. Biophys. Acta* **192**, 430.

Murray, A. W., Elliott, D. C., and Atkinson, M. R. (1970). *Progr. Nucl. Acid Res. Mol. Biol.* **10**, 87.

Nadler, N. J., Sarkar, S. K., and Leblond, C. P. (1962). *Endocrinology* **71**, 120.

Nagataki, S., Shizume, K., and Okinaka, S. (1961). *Endocrinology* **69**, 199.

Nataf, B. M. (1968). *Gen. Comp. Endocrinol.* **10**, 159.

Nataf, B. M., and Chaikoff, I. L. (1964). *Endocrinology* **75**, 547.

Nataf, B. M., Rivera, E. M., and Chaikoff, I. C. (1965). *Endocrinology* **76**, 35.

Nève, P., and Dumont, J. E. (1970a). *Z. Zellforsch. Mikrosk. Anat.* **103**, 61.

Nève, P., and Dumont, J. E. (1970b). *Exp. Cell. Res.* **63**, 285.

Nève, P., Rodesch, F., and Dumont, J. E. (1968). *Exp. Cell Res.* **51**, 68.

Nève, P., Willems, C., and Dumont, J. E. (1970). *Exp. Cell Res.* **63**, 457.

Nève, P., Balasse, C., Willems, C., and Dumont, J. E. (1971). Unpublished data.

Ney, R. L. (1969). *Endocrinology* **84**, 168.

Ochi, Y., and Degroot, L. J. (1968). *Biochim. Biophys. Acta* **170**, 201.

Ochi, Y., and Degroot, L. J. (1969a). *Metab., Clin. Exp.* **18**, 331.

Ochi, Y., and Degroot, L. J. (1969). *Endocrinology* **85**, 344.

Ohta, M., and Field, J. B. (1969). *Endocrinology* **79**, 732.

Oka, H., and Field, J. B. (1966). *Amer. J. Physiol.* **211**, 1357.

Oka, H., and Field, J. B. (1967). *Endocrinology* **81**, 1291.

Oka, H., and Field, J. B. (1968). *J. Biol. Chem.* **243**, 815.

Olin-Lamberg, C., and Lamberg, B. A. (1953). *Acta Endocrinol.* **14**, 83.

O'Malley, B. W., and Field, J. B. (1964). *Biochim. Biophys. Acta* **90**, 349.

Onaya, T., and Solomon, D. H. (1969). *Endocrinology* **85**, 1010.

Onaya, T., and Solomon, D. H. (1970). *Endocrinology* **86**, 423.

Onaya, T., Solomon, D. H., and Davidson, W. D. (1969). *Endocrinology* **85**, 150.

Otten, J., and Dumont, J. E. (1970). Unpublished results.

Panda, J. N., and Turner, C. W. (1966). *Proc. Soc. Exp. Biol. Med.* **123**, 553.

Pantic, V. (1967). *Z. Zellforsch. Mikrosk. Anat.* **81**, 487.

Pastan, I. (1961). *Endocrinology* **68**, 924.

Pastan, I. (1966a). *Annu. Rev. Biochem.* **35**, 369.

Pastan, I. (1966b). *Biochem. Biophys. Res. Commun.* **25**, 14.

Pastan, I., and Almqvist, S. (1965). *Biochem. Biophys. Res. Commun.* **18**, 332.

Pastan, I., and Almqvist, S. (1966). *Endocrinology* **78**, 361.

Pastan, I., and Field, J. B. (1962). *Endocrinology* **70**, 656.

Pastan, I., and Katzen, R. (1967). *Biochem. Biophys. Res. Commun.* **29**, 792.

Pastan, I., and Macchia, V. (1967). *J. Biol. Chem.* **242**, 5757.

Pastan, I., and Wollman, S. H. (1967). *J. Cell Biol.* **35**, 266.

Pastan, I., Herring, B., Johnson, P., and Field, J. B. (1961). *J. Biol. Chem.* **236**, 340.

Pastan, I., Herring, B., Johnson, P., and Field, J. B. (1962). *J. Biol. Chem.* **237**, 287.

Pastan, I., Johnson, P., Kendig, E., and Field, J. B. (1963). *J. Biol. Chem.* **238**, 3366.

Pastan, I., Macchia, V., and Katzen, R. (1968). *Endocrinology* **83**, 157.

Pavlovic-Hournac, M., Rappaport, L., and Nunez, J. (1967). *Bull. Soc. Chim. Biol.* **49**, 1309.

Peake, R. L., Balasubramaniam, K., and Deiss, W. P. (1967). *Biochim. Biophys. Acta* **148,** 689.

Philp, J. R., Crooks, J., MacGregor, A. G., and McIntosh, J. A. R. (1969). *Brit. J. Cancer* **23,** 515.

Pisarev, M. A., Degroot, L. J., and Wilber, J. F. (1970). *Endocrinology* **87,** 339.

Pitt-Rivers, R., and Trotter, W. R., eds. (1964). "The Thyroid Gland." Butterworth, London.

Poffenbarger, P. L., Powell, R. C., and Deiss, W. P. (1963). *J. Clin. Invest.* **42,** 239.

Posternak, T., Sutherland, E. W., and Henion, W. F. (1962). *Biochim. Biophys. Acta* **65,** 558.

Powell, R. C., Rahman, M. A., and Deiss, W. P. (1964). *Endocrinology* **74,** 395.

Raghupathy, E., Tong, W., and Chaikoff, I. L. (1963). *Endocrinology* **72,** 620.

Raghupathy, E., Abraham, S., Kerkof, P. R., and Chaikoff, I. L. (1964). *Endocrinology* **74,** 468.

Raghupathy, E., Kerkof, P. R., and Chaikoff, I. L. (1965). *Biochim. Biophy. Acta* **97,** 118.

Rawson, R. W. (1949). *Ann. N. Y. Acad. Sci.* **50,** 491.

Robison, G. A., Butcher, R. W., and Sutherland, E. W. (1968). *Annu. Rev. Biochem.* **37,** 149.

Rocmans, P. A., and Dumont, J. E. (1964). Unpublished results.

Rocmans, P. A., and Dumont, J. E. (1968). Unpublished data.

Rocmans, P. A., and Dumont, J. E. (1969a). *Biochim. Biophys. Acta* **192,** 350.

Rocmans, P. A., and Dumont, J. E. (1969b). Unpublished data.

Rodbell, M., Jones, A. B., Chiappe de Cingolani, G. E., and Birnbauer, L. (1968). *Recent Progr. Horm. Res.* **24,** 215.

Rodesch, F., and Dumont, J. E. (1967). *Exp. Cell Res.* **47,** 386.

Rodesch, F., and Fontaine, Y. A. (1968). *Gen. Comp. Endocrinol.* **11,** 64.

Rodesch, F., Jortay, A., and Dumont, J. E. (1968). *Experientia* **24,** 268.

Rodesch, F., Nève, P., Willems, C., and Dumont, J. E. (1969). *Eur. J. Biochem.* **8,** 26.

Rodesch, F., Nève, P, and Dumont, J. E. (1970). *Exp. Cell Res.* **60,** 354.

Rosenberg, I. N., and Bastomsky, C. H. (1965). *Annu. Rev. Physiol.* **27,** 71.

Rosenberg, I. N., Athans, J. C., and Behar, A. (1960). *Endocrinology* **66,** 185.

Rosenberg, I. N., Athans, J. C., Ahn, C. S., and Behar, A. (1961). *Endocrinology* **69,** 438.

Rosenberg, I. N., Athans, J. C., and Isaacs, G. H. (1965). *Recent Progr. Horm. Res.* **21,** 33.

Rosenfeld, P. S., and Rosenberg, I. N. (1966). *Endocrinology* **78,** 621.

Sage, M., and Robins, P. C. (1970). *Gen. Comp. Endocrinol.* **14,** 601.

Sasson, C. Y., and Rosenberg, I. N. (1963). *Endocrinology* **73,** 155.

Schell-Frederick, E., and Dumont, J. E. (1970). In "Biochemical Actions of Hormones" (G. Litwack, ed.), p. 415. Academic Press, New York.

Schneider, P. B. (1968). *Endocrinology* **82,** 969.

Schneider, P. B. (1969). *J. Biol. Chem.* **244,** 4490.

Schussler, G. L., and Ingbar, S. H. (1961). *J. Clin. Invest.* **40,** 1394.

Schwartz, J. R., and Morton, M. E. (1955). *Proc. Soc. Exp. Biol. Med.* **88,** 50.

Scott, T. W., Jay, S. M., and Freinkel, N. (1966a). *Endocrinology* **79,** 591.

Scott, T. W., Good, B. F., and Ferguson, K. A. (1966b). *Endocrinology* **79,** 949.

Scott, T. W., Mills, S. C., and Freinkel, N. (1968). *Biochem. J.* **109,** 325.

Scrutton, M. C., and Utter, M. F. (1968). *Annu. Rev. Biochem.* **37,** 249.

Seed, R. W., and Goldberg, I. H. (1965). *Science* **149**, 1380.

Segal, S., Roth, H., Blair, A., and Bertoli, D. (1966). *Endocrinology* **79**, 675.

Seljelid, R. (1967a). *J. Ultrastruct. Res.* **17**, 195.

Seljelid, R. (1967b). *J. Ultrastruct. Res.* **17**, 401.

Seljelid, R. (1967c). *J. Ultrastruct. Res.* **18**, 1.

Seljelid, R. (1967d). *J. Ultrastruct. Res.* **18**, 237.

Seljelid, R. (1967e). *J. Ultrastruct. Res.* **18**, 479.

Seljelid, R., and Nakken, K. F. (1969). *Scand. J. Clin. Lab. Invest., Suppl. 106*, p. 125.

Serafimov, N., and Sestakov, G. (1967). *Experientia* **23**, 809.

Serif, G. S. (1966). *Biochim. Biophys. Acta* **119**, 229.

Shearer, R. W., and McCarthy, B. J. (1970). *J. Cell. Physiol.* **75**, 97.

Sheldon, H., McKenzie, J. M., and Van Nimwegan, D. (1964). *J. Cell Biol.* **23**, 200

Sheline, G. E. (1969). *Cell Tissue Kinet.* **2**, 123.

Shimoda, H., and Yasumasu, I. (1966). *Gumma Sympo. Endocrinol.* [*Proc.*] **3**, 47

Shimoda, S. I., Kendall, J. W., and Greer, M. A. (1966). *Endocrinology* **79**, 921

Shishiba, Y., Solomon, D. H., and Davidson, W. D. (1970). *Endocrinology* **86**, 183.

Skanse, B. N. (1948). *J. Clin. Endocrinol.* **8**, 707.

Sobel, H. J. (1962). *Anat. Rec.* **143**, 389.

Sobel, H. J., and Geller, J. (1965). *Amer. J. Physiol.* **46**, 149.

Söderberg, U. (1959). *Physiol. Rev.* **39**, 777.

Söderberg, U. (1958). *Acta Physiol. Scand.* **42**, Suppl., 147.

Solomon, D. H. (1961). *Endocrinology* **69**, 939.

Solomon, D. H., Prujan, R. L., and Triplett, H. W. (1963). *Amer. J. Physiol.* **205**, 549.

Solomon, S. S., Brush, J. S., and Kitabchi, A. E. (1970). *Science* **169**, 387.

Sonenberg, M. (1958). *Vitam. Horm. (New York)* **16**, 205.

Speight, J. W., Baba, W. I., and Wilson, G. M. (1968). *J. Endocrinol.* **41**, 577.

Stalmans, W., De Wulf, H., Lederer, B., and Hers, H. G. (1970). *Eur. J. Biochem.* **15**, 9.

Stanbury, J. B. (1960). *Ann. N. Y. Acad. Sci.* **82**, 417.

Stanbury, J. B. (1964). *Naunyn-Schmiedebergs Arch. Exp. Pathol. Pharmakol.* **248**, 279.

Stanbury, J. B., and Hugues, V. (1964). *Medicine (Baltimore)* **43**, 407.

Stein, O., and Gross, J. (1964). *Endocrinology* **75**, 787.

Steiner, A. L., Peake, G. T., Utiger, R. D., Karl, I. E., and Kipnis, D. M. (1970). *Endocrinology* **86**, 1354.

Straznicky, K., and Mess, B. (1967). *Acta Biol. Acad. Sci. Hung.* **18**, 221.

Sutherland, E. W., and Robison, G. A. (1966). *Pharmacol. Rev.* **18**, 145.

Sutherland, E. W., and Robison, G. A. (1969). *Diabetes* **18**, 797.

Sutherland, E. W., Oye, I., and Butcher, R. W. (1965). *Recent Progr. Horm. Res.* **21**, 623.

Suzuki, M. (1956). *Endocrinol. Jap.* **3**, 291.

Tala, P., Lamberg, B. A., and Uotila, V. (1955). *Acta Endocrinol. (Copenhagen)* **19**, 255.

Tao, M., Salas, M. L., and Lipmann, F. (1970). *Proc. Nat. Acad. Sci. U. S.* **67**, 408.

Tarui, S., and Nonaka, K. (1963). *Endocrinol. Jap.* **10**, 260.

Tarui, S., Nonaka, K., Ikura, Y., and Shima, K. (1963). *Biochem. Biophys. Res. Commun.* **13**, 329.

Taurog, A., and Thio, D. T. (1966). *Endocrinology* **78**, 103.

Taurog, A., Tong, W., and Chaikoff, I. L. (1958a). *Endocrinology* **62**, 646.

Taurog, A., Tong, W., and Chaikoff, I. L. (1958b). *Endocrinology* **62,** 664.
Taurog, A., Potter, G. D., and Chaikoff, I. L. (1959). *Endocrinology* **64,** 1038.
Taurog, A., Porter, J. C., and Thio, D. T. (1964). *Endocrinology* **74,** 902.
Tellkä, A., and Kuusisto, A. N. (1955). *Ann. Med. Intern. Fenn.* **44,** 89.
Tong, W. (1964a). *Endocrinology* **74,** 304.
Tong, W. (1964b). *Endocrinology* **75,** 527.
Tong, W. (1964c). *Endocrinology* **75,** 968.
Tong, W. (1965). *Endocrinology* **76,** 163.
Tong, W. (1967). *Endocrinology* **80,** 1101.
Tonoue, T., Tong, W., and Stolc, V. (1970). *Endocrinology* **86,** 271.
Turkington, R. W. (1962). *Biochim. Biophys. Acta* **65,** 386.
Turkington, R. W. (1963). *J. Biol. Chem.* **238,** 3463.
Tyler, D., Gonze, J., Lamy, F., and Dumont, J. E. (1968). *Biochem. J.* **106,** 123.
Vanderlaan, W. P., and Greer, M. A. (1950). *Endocrinology* **47,** 36.
Van Sande, J., and Dumont, J. E. (1970). Unpublished results.
Vassart, G., and Dumont, J. E. (1970). Unpublished results.
Vilkki, P. (1961). *Advan. Thyroid Res., Trans. Int. Goitre Conf., 4th, 1960* p. 231.
Wahlberg, P. (1955). *Acta Endocrinol. (Copenhagen)* **20,** 240.
Wenner, C. E. (1959). *J. Biol. Chem.* **234,** 2472.
Werner, S. C., and Nauman, J. A. (1968). *Annu. Rev. Physiol.* **30,** 213.
Wetzel, B. K., Spicer, S. S., and Wollman, S. H. (1965). *J. Cell Biol.* **25,** 593.
Wicks, W. D. (1969). *J. Biol. Chem.* **244,** 3941.
Wilber, J. F., Peake, G. T., and Utiger, R. D. (1969). *Endocrinology* **84,** 758.
Willems, C., and Dumont, J. E. (1968). Unpublished results.
Willems, C., and Dumont, J. E. (1969). Unpublished results.
Willems, C., and Dumont, J. E. (1970). Unpublished results.
Willems, C., and Dumont, J. E. (1971). *FEBS Lett.* **19,** 323.
Willems, C., Rocmans, P. A., and Dumont, J. E. (1970). *Biochim. Biophys. Acta* **223,** 474.
Williams, J. A. (1970). *Endocrinology* **86,** 1154.
Wilson, B., Raghupathy, E., Tonoue, T., and Tong, W. (1968). *Endocrinology* **83,** 877.
Wissig, S. L. (1963). *J. Cell Biol.* **16,** 93.
Wissig, S. L. (1964). *In* "The Thyroid Gland" (R. Pitt-Rivers and W. R. Trotter, eds.), p. 32. Butterworth, London.
Wolff, J. (1964). *Physiol. Rev.* **44,** 45.
Wolff, J., and Halmi, N. S. (1963). *J. Biol. Chem.* **238,** 847.
Wolff, J., and Jones, A. B. (1970). *Proc. Nat. Acad. Sci. U. S.* **65,** 454.
Wolff, J., and Varrone, S. (1969). *Endocrinology* **85,** 410.
Wolff, J., Bernes, S. C., and Jones, A. B. (1970). *Biochem. Biophys. Res. Commun.* **39,** 77.
Wollman, S. H. (1969). *In* "Lysosomes in Biology and Pathology" (J. T. Dingle and H. B. Fell, eds.), p. 483. North-Holland Publ., Amsterdam.
Wollman, S. H., and Breitman, T. R. (1970). *Endocrinology* **86,** 322.
Wollman, S. H., and Reed, F. E. (1959). *Amer. J. Physiol.* **196,** 113.
Wollman, S. H., and Warren, L. (1961). *Biochim. Biophys. Acta* **47,** 251.
Wollman, S. H., Spicer, S. S., and Burstone, M. S. (1964). *J. Cell Biol.* **21,** 191.
Wollman, S. H., Andros, G., Cannon, G. B., and Eagleton, G. B. (1969). *In* "Thyroid Neoplasia" (Podoba, ed.), p. 201.
Woodbury, D. M., and Woodbury, J. W. (1963). *J. Physiol. (London)* **169,** 553.

Yamashita, K., and Field, J. B. (1970). *Biochem. Biophys. Res. Commun.* **40**, 171.
Zakarija, M., Bastomsky, C. H., and McKenzie, J. M. (1969). *Endocrinology* **84**, 1310.
Zimmerman, A. E., and Yip, C. C. (1968). *Can. J. Physiol. Pharmacol.* **46**, 449.
Zor, U., Lowe, I. P., Bloom, G., and Field, J. B. (1968). *Biochem. Biophys. Res. Commun.* **33**, 649.
Zor, U., Bloom, G., Lowe, I. P., and Field, J. B. (1969a). *Endocrinology* **84**, 1082.
Zor, U., Kaneko, T., Lowe, I. P., Bloom, G., and Field, J. B. (1969b). *J. Biol. Chem.* **244**, 5189.

Author Index

Numbers in italics refer to the pages on which the complete references are listed.

A

Aach, R. D., 259, *279*
Abdel-Aziz, M. T., 211, *279*
Abou-El-Makarem, M. M., 271, 272, *279*
Aboul-Khair, S. A., 130, *141*
Abraham, G., 99, *147*
Abraham, S., 336, 372, 389, *402, 409*
Abrams, C. L., 123, *145*
Abrams, R. L., 124, *141*
Adam, P. A. J., 132, *142*
Adesman, J., 217, *282*
Adiga, P. R., 262, 364, 378, 379, *402, 407*
Adlercreutz, H., 202, 218, 219, 223, 232, 243, 244, 261, 262, 265, 268, *279, 280, 283*
Adrias, I. M., 256, *284*
Ahlquist, R. P., 133, *151*
Ahn, C. S., 293, 294, 299, 314, 315, 316, 318, 319, 321, 322, 323, 326, 327, 329, 332, 350, 392, 393, 394, 395, *402, 409*
Akasu, F., 128, *142*
Albepart, T., 209, 248, *283*
Albert, A., 100, 101, 103, 104, 112, *142, 147*
Aldred, J. P., 60, *89*
Aldrich, T. B., 8, *37*
Alessandri, H., 258, *282*
Al-Hindawi, A. Y., 312, 313, *402*
Allan, J. S., 259, *280*
Allen, C. F., 155, *196*
Allen, C. M., 172, *196*
Allen, J. G., 212, 214, *280*
Allen, W. M., 109, *147*
Almqvist, S., 327, *408*
Alonso, C., 102, *142*
Altman, M., 381, 382, 385, *402*
Alworth, W., 172, *196*
Amelotti, J., 155, *198*
Amos, J., 34, *37*
Amoss, M., 11, 13, 18, 21, 28, 33, *35, 38, 39*
Anberg, A., 265, 268, *280*
Andros, G., 312, 313, *411*
Ansell, G. B., 307, *402*
Aono, T., 103, 104, *144*

A

Apps, D. K., *402*
Arai, T., 184, *197*
Archer, S. E. H., 209, *280*
Arias, I. M., 259, *280, 282*
Arimura, A., 2, 6, 7, 9, 10, 11, *38*
Arison, B. H., 157, *197*
Arnaud, C., 57, *93*
Arnaud, C. D., 55, 87, *88*
Arnold, D., 177, *196*
Arntzen, C. J., 178, *196*
Arquilla, E. R., 100, *145*
Asami, M., 6, 8, *39*
Aschner, B., 97, *142*
Ask-Upmark, M. E., 108, *142*
Assali, N. S., 130, *142*
Astor, M. A., 100, *145*
Astwood, E. B., 48, *88*
Athans, J., 314, 315, 316, 318, 319, 323, 324, 325, *402, 405, 409*
Atkins, W., 118, *145*
Atkinson, M. R., 365, 366, *408*
Attali, J. C., 374, *407*
Atwood, B. L., 115, 117, *146*
Aubert, M. L., 126, *144*
Audley, B. G., 178, 185, 186, 187, 188, 189, *198, 200*
Aurbach, G. D., 48, 49, 50, 51, 52, 53, 55, 56, 67, 69, 74, 75, 80, 83, 87, 88, *88, 89, 90, 91, 92*
Averill, R. L. W., 23, *35*
Azerad, R. G., 158, 159, 161, 164, 165, 166, 167, 168, 169, 173, 174, 175, *196, 197, 198*

B

Baba, W. I., 312, 313, *410*
Back, N., 210, 211, 217, *283*
Badinand, A., 131, *142*
Baechler, C., 104, *142*
Baggenstoss, A. H., 260, 261, *280*
Baghdiantz, A., 57, *89*
Bagshawe, K. D., 103, 106, 107, 114, *142, 148, 151*
Bahl, O. P., 99, *142*

413

Subject Index